2nd International Adalat® Symposium

W0105904

2nd International Adalat® Symposium

New Therapy of Ischemic Heart Disease

Edited by

Wilhelm Lochner · Wolfgang Braasch
Günther Kroneberg

With 206 Figures

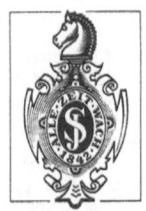

Springer-Verlag Berlin Heidelberg GmbH 1975

President: Professor Dr. WILHELM LOCHNER

2nd International Adalat Symposium

Date: October 4 to 5, 1974
Place: Amsterdam, Okura-Hotel

ISBN 978-3-662-38770-2   ISBN 978-3-662-39666-7 (eBook)
DOI 10.1007/978-3-662-39666-7

Adalat is the registered trade mark of Bayer AG, Leverkusen (Germany). Nifedipine is the generic-name, the research code number was BAY a 1040.

Library of Congress Cataloging in Publication Data. International Adalat Symposium. 2nd. Amsterdam. 1974. New therapy of ischemic heart disease. Bibliography: p. Includes index. 1. Adalat®-Congresses. 2. Coronary heart disease-Congresses. I. Lochner, Wilhelm, 1922. II. Braasch, Wolfgang, 1931. III. Kroneberg, Günther, 1919. IV. Title. [DNLM: 1. Pyridines Therapeutic use Congresses. 3. Coronary Disease Drug therapy Congresses. W3 IN789 1974n/WG 300 161 1974n]. RM666.N53157.1974. 616.1'2. 75–28123.

This work is subject to copyright. All rights are reserved, whether the whole or part of the material is concerned, specifically those of translation, reprinting, re-use of illustrations, broadcasting, reproduction by photocopying machine or similar means, and storage in data banks. Under § 54 of the German Copyright Law, where copies are made for other than private use, a fee is payable to the publisher, the amount of the fee to be determined by agreement with the publisher.
© by Springer-Verlag Berlin Heidelberg 1975
Originally published by Springer-Verlag Berlin Heidelberg New York in 1975.

The use of registered names, trademarks, etc. in this publication does not imply, even in the absence of a specific statement, that such names are exempt from the relevant protective laws and regulations and therefore free for general use.

Preface

The First Adalat Symposium held in Tokyo in 1973, presented important experimental and clinical results which had been collected in Europe and Japan with the new coronary therapeutic agent. The European scientists had an opportunity to discuss the problems and results personally with their Japanese colleagues.

The Second Adalat Symposium was held in Amsterdam within a year with the purpose of bringing together mainly scientists within Europe. The results discussed in Tokyo have been extended and supplemented through additional experiences. Contributions in basic science are presented, but most important are those clinical studies, which support and extend proof of the drug's efficacy in humans.

The editors wish to express their appreciation to all those responsible for contributing to this report and, in particular, to Dr. M. SPENGLER, Dr. F. EBNER and Dr. K. BRANDAU for their editorial help, and to Dr. W. BÖTTGER for the preparation of the Subject Index. We hope that this publication will be a valuable contribution toward conveying information to physicians and scientists.

Düsseldorf/Wuppertal, Autumn 1975

W. LOCHNER · W. BRAASCH · G. KRONEBERG

Contents

Session III. Clinical Pharmacology

(Chairmen: K. HASHIMOTO and R. J. ESPER)

Session IV. Clinical Pharmacological Efficacy

(Chairmen: W. KAUFMANN and B. TABATZNIK)

Session V. Clinical Aspects: Hemodynamics, Onset and Duration

(Chairmen: H. LYDTIN and P. F. ANGELINO)

List of Participants

Prof. Dr. P. F. ANGELINO
   Ospedale Civile S. Croce, Div. Cardiologia, 12100 Cuneo/Italy

Dr. W. ANGEHRN
   Dept. f. Innere Medizin, Med. Universitäts-Klinik, Kardiologie, Kantonsspital, Zurich/Switzerland

Dr. B. ARLT
   4690 Herne/Fed. Rep. Germany, Hölkeskampring 40

Dr. E. ARLT
   4690 Herne/Fed. Rep. Germany, Hölkeskampring 40

Dr. G. AROLD
   5000 Köln/Fed. Rep. Germany, Belfortstr. 9

Dr. M. ARTAZA ANDRADE
   Servicio de Cardiologia Clinica, Puerta de Hierro, CI San Martin de Porres, 4, Madrid (35)/Spain

Prof. Dr. BARTORELLI
   Chief University, Clinic of General Medicine and Medical Therapy II, Milano/Italy

Dr. H.-J. BECKER
   Abt. f. Kardiologie, Zentrum Innere Medizin des Klinikums der Universität, 6000 Frankfurt/M. 70/Fed. Rep. Germany, Theodor-Stern-Kai 7

Dr. J. BELLINGHAUSEN
   5400 Koblenz/Fed. Rep. Germany, Markenbildchenplatz 36

Prof. Dr. A. BERKI
   Universitätsklinik Cebeci, Kardiyoloji Klinigi, Medical School, Cebeci, Ankara/Turkey

Dr. L. BJÖRK
   Roentgenabt., Akademiska Sjukhuset, Fack, 750 14 Uppsala 14/Sweden

Dr. Th. J. J. M. BLOEM
   Kennedylaan 44, Goirle/Netherlands

Dr. G. BLÜMCHEN
   Landesversicherungsanstalt Rheinprov., Klinik Roderbirken, 5672 Leichlingen/Fed. Rep. Germany

Dr. F. BOSSERT
   Bayer AG, Chem. Wiss. Lab., Pharma Forschungszentrum, 5600 Wuppertal 1/Fed. Rep. Germany, Postfach 130105

Dr. H. G. D. BOUMA
   Windelaan 7, Almelo/Netherlands

Dr. M. V. D. BRAND
   Faculteit der Geneeskunde, Erasmus Universiteit, Thoraxcentrum (Cardiologie), Postbus 1738, Rotterdam/Netherlands

Dr. A. O. BRUBAKK
   Section of Cardiology, Regional Hospital and Div. of Engineering Cybernetics, Technical University of Norway, Trondheim/Norway

Dr. R. BUCHWALSKY
   Schüchtermann-Klinik, 4502 Bad Rothenfelde/Fed. Rep. Germany, Ulmenallee 1

Prof. Dr. F. Camerini
Ospedali Riuniti, Div. Cardiologia, 34129 Trieste/Italy

Dr. R. Carsburg
Kreiskrankenhaus, 3410 Northeim/ Fed. Rep. Germany

Dr. R. Casares-Potau
Servicio de Cardiologia, Hospital Sagrado Corazon, CI Paris, 83, Barcelona (15)/Spain

Dr. W. Daniel
MHH – Kardiologie, 3000 Hannover 61/Fed. Rep. Germany, Karl-Wiechert-Allee 9

Dr. L. A. G. Davidson
82 Cathedral Road, Cardiff/Great Britain

Prof. Dr. H. Denolin
Groupment Scientifique pour le Diagnostic et le Traitement des Cardiopathies, Hôpital Universitaire St. Pierre, 1000 Bruxelles/Belgium

Dr. M. Diewitz
Medizinische Klinik, Städt. Krankenanstalten, 5650 Solingen/Fed. Rep. Germany

Prof. Dr. D. Durrer
Rubenstraat 73, Amsterdam/Netherlands

Dr. F. Ebner
Bayer AG, Ressort Medizin, Pharma Forschungszentrum, 5600 Wuppertal 1/Fed. Rep. Germany, Postfach 130105

Dr. L.-G. Ekelund
Dept. of Clinical Physiology, Karolinska Sjukhuset, 10401 Stockholm 60/Sweden

Prof. Dr. R. J. Esper
Arcos 2400 P. B., Buenos Aires (Suc. 28)/Argentina

Prof. Dr. A. Fleckenstein
Physiologisches Institut der Universität, 7800 Freiburg/Fed. Rep. Germany, Hermann-Herder-Str. 7

Dr. G. Fleckenstein-Grün
Physiologisches Institut der Universität, 7800 Freiburg/Fed. Rep. Germany, Hermann-Herder-Str. 7

Dr. A. Franco
Tr. de s. Vicente, 14, 1 esg, Lisboa/ Portugal

Miss D. Galke
8033 Planegg/Fed. Rep. Germany, Pasinger Str. 8

Dr. W. Gattenlöhner
Med. Univ.-Klinik, 8700 Würzburg/ Fed. Rep. Germany, Luitpold-Krankenhaus

Dr. J. Grégoire
Recherche thérapeutique, R. P. Specia, 28, Cours Albert, 75 – Paris VIII/France

Dr. R. Gross
1. Physiologisches Institut der Universität, 6900 Heidelberg/Fed. Rep. Germany, Akademiestr. 3

Dr. M. Hagman
Med. Klinik I, Sahlgrenska Sjukhuset, 41345 Gothenburg/Sweden

Dr. K. Hagemann
Abt. Inn. Medizin I der RWTH Aachen, 5100 Aachen/Fed. Rep. Germany, Goethestr. 27/29

Dr. F. Hagemeijer
Faculteit der Geneeskunde, Erasmus Universiteit, Thoraxcentrum (Cardiologie), Postbus 1738, Rotterdam/ Netherlands

Dr. M. Hascher
Lab. Roger Bellon, 159, Av. du Roule, 92201 Neuilly/s. S./France

Prof. Dr. K. HASHIMOTO (sen.)
Pharmacology, Tohoku University, School of Medicine, 2–1 Seiryocho, Sendai/Japan

Dr. T. HASHIMOTO (jun.)
Universitätsklinik, 5300 Bonn/Fed. Rep. Germany

Dr. H. HEEGER
II. Med. Abt. d. Hanusch-Krankenhauses, Heinrich-Collin-Str. 30, 1140 Wien/Austria

Prof. Dr. R. HEINECKER
Med. Klinik II, Stadtkrankenhaus Kassel, 3500 Kassel/Fed. Rep. Germany

Dr. U. HENKELS
Landesversicherungsanstalt Rheinprov., Klinik Roderbirken, 5672 Leichlingen/Fed. Rep. Germany

Prof. Dr. H. H. HILGER
Med. Univ.-Klinik u. Poliklinik Köln, Abt. Kardiologie, 5000 Köln 41/Fed. Rep. Germany, Joseph-Stelzmann-Str. 9

Prof. Dr. H. HOCHREIN
Rudolf-Virchow-Krankenhaus, III. Inn. Abt., 1000 Berlin/Fed. Rep. Germany, Augustenburger Platz 1

Prof. Dr. W. HOLLMANN
Inst. f. Kreislaufforschung und Sportmedizin, Deutsche Sporthochschule, 5000 Köln 41/Fed. Rep. Germany, Carl-Diem-Weg

Prof. Dr. F. A. HORSTER
II. Med. Klinik der Universität, 4000 Düsseldorf/Fed. Rep. Germany, Moorenstr. 5

Dr. I. IDRIS
8033 Planegg/Fed. Rep. Germany, Pasinger Str. 8

Dr. F. S. JACKSON
Cardiology Department, Newcastle General Hospital, Newcastle-upon-Tyne/Great Britain

Prof. Dr. H. JAHRMÄRKER
Med. Fakultät der Ludwig-Maximilian-Univ. München, 8000 München 40/Fed. Rep. Germany, Geschwister-Scholl-Platz 1

Dr. C. L. JOINER
Guys Hospital, London, SEL/Great Britain

Prof. Dr. W. KAUFMANN
II. Med. Univ.- u. Poliklinik, 5000 Köln 91/Fed. Rep. Germany, Ostmerheimer Str.

Prof. Dr. R. KERN
I. Physiolog. Institut der Universität, 6900 Heidelberg 1/Fed. Rep. Germany, Im Neuenheimer Feld 326

Prof. Dr. H. KIRCHHEIM
I. Physiolog. Institut der Universität, 6900 Heidelberg 1/ Fed. Rep. Germany, Im Neuenheimer Feld 326

Dr. J. KITZING
2000 Hamburg 67/Fed. Rep. Germany, Lottbeker Feld 46

Dr. A. KLIEGIS
2300 Kiel/Fed. Rep. Germany, Lorentzendamm 45

Dr. I. KLIEGIS
2300 Kiel/Fed. Rep. Germany, Lorentzendamm 45

Prof. Dr. K. KLÜTSCH
Stadtkrankenhaus, Med. Abteilung, 6330 Wetzlar/Fed. Rep. Germany

Dr. G. KOBER
Kardiolog. Abteilung, Zentrum der Inneren Medizin, Klinikum der Universität, 6000 Frankfurt/M. 70/Fed. Rep. Germany

Dr. K. KODAMA
Sakurabashi Watanabe Hospital,
Dept. of Internal Medicine, 19
Umeda-machi, Kita-ku, Osaka/
Japan

Prof. Dr. J. A. KÖHLER
Städt. Krankenhaus Landshut, Med.
Abteilung, 8300 Landshut/Fed. Rep.
Germany, Robert-Koch-Str. 1

Prof. Dr. O. KRAUPP
Pharmakologisches Institut, 1090
Wien/Austria, Währingerstr. 13a

Prof. Dr. G. KRONEBERG
Bayer AG, Pharma Research De-
velopment, 5600 Wuppertal 1/ Fed.
Rep. Germany, Postfach 130105

Dr. A. KURITA
Cedars-Sinai Medical Center, Cedars
of Lebanon Hospital Div., Box 54265,
Los Angeles, CA 90054/USA

Dr. U. LAASER
Städt. Krankenanstalten, Med. Klinik, 5000 Köln 91/Fed. Rep. Germany, Ostmerheimer Str. 200

Dr. K. LANDMARK
Rikshospitalet, Modisinsk Avdeling
B, Universitetsklinikk, Pilestredet 32,
Oslo/Norway

Dr. A. H. LEMMERZ
Intern. Fachklinik f. Herz- u. Kreis-
lauferkrankungen, Grand Hotel,
6350 Bad Nauheim/Fed. Rep. Germany, Ernst-Ludwig-Ring 2

Prof. Dr. P. LICHTLEN
Dept. f. Inn. Medizin, Med. Hoch-
schule Hannover, 3000 Hannover-
Kleefeld/Fed. Rep. Germany, Karl-
Wiechert-Allee 9

Prof. Dr. A. LINDNER
Institut für Allgemeine u. Experimen-
telle Pathologie, 1090 Wien/Austria,
Währingerstr. 13

Prof. Dr. H. LINKE
Kurklinik Pitzer KG, 6208 Bad
Schwalbach/Fed. Rep. Germany,
Genthstraße 7–9

Prof. Dr. W. LOCHNER
Physiolog. Institut der Universität,
4000 Düsseldorf/Fed. Rep. Germany,
Moorenstr. 5

Dr. N. LOUVROS
Messologiu Str. 4, Athine/Greece

Prof. Dr. D. W. LÜBBERS
Max-Planck-Institut für Arbeitsphy-
siologie, 4600 Dortmund/Fed. Rep.
Germany, Rheinlanddamm 201

Prof. Dr. H. LYDTIN
Med. Poliklinik der Universität, 8000
München 2/Fed. Rep. Germany,
Pettenkoferstr. 8a

Prof. Dr. G. C. MAGGI
Primario Cardiologo Ospedale Bas-
sini, Via Panfilo Castaldi, 8, 20124
Milano/Italy

Dr. H. MAHR
Sanatorium Grödel, 6350 Bad Nau-
heim/Fed. Rep. Germany, Terrassen-
straße 2–4

Dr. V. MANNINEN
I. Sisätautiklinikka, Meilahden Sai-
raala, Haartmaninkatu 4, 00290 Hel-
sinki 29/Finnland

Dr. J. D. MCARTHUR
University Department of Medical
Cardiology, Royal Infirmary, Glas-
gow/Great Britain

Dr. G. MCILWRAITH
23, Kenilworth Road, Penge, London
SE 20/Great Britain

Dr. J. MENNA
Sección Ergometria y Rehabilitación,
Cardio-vascular, Hospital Italiano,
Sociedad Italiana de Beneficencia en
Buenos Aires, Gascon 450, Buenos
Aires/Argentina

Dr. MESSIN-DEMARET
Hôpital St. Pierre, 1000 Bruxelles/
Belgium

Dr. H. MÖRL
Med. Univ. Klinik, 6900 Heidelberg/
Fed. Rep. Germany, Bergheimer
Straße 58

Dr. F. NAGER
Med. Klinik, Kantonsspital, 6000
Luzern/Switzerland

Dr. G. H. A. C. NORRO
St. Philipsland 131, Amstelveen/
Netherlands

Dr. P. OPHERK
Med. Fakultät der Univ. Heidelberg,
Kardiologie, 6900 Heidelberg/Fed.
Rep. Germany, Grabengasse

Dr. L. ORÖ
Karolinska Sjukhuset, Med. IV,
10401 Stockholm 60/Sweden

Dr. K. PATZSCHKE
Bayer AG, Isotopen-Institut, 5600
Wuppertal 1/Fed. Rep. Germany,
Postfach 130105

Dr. L. PESCHL
Kaiserin-Elisabeth-Spital, Huglgasse
1–3, 1152 Wien/Austria

Dr. W. PFEIFFER
8035 Gauting/Fed. Rep. Germany,
Buchendorfer Str. 15

Dr. K. O. RAWLINGS
Dept. of Medicine, Farnborough
Hospital, Farnborough Common,
Orpington, Kent/Great Britain

Dr. H. REFSUM
Rikshospitalet, Medisinsk Avdeling
B, Universitetsklinikk, Pilestredet 32,
Oslo/Norway

Dr. W. J. REMME
Kastanjestraat 32, Spijkenisse/
Netherlands

Dr. E. REUS
Stadtkrankenhaus, Med. Klinik II,
3500 Kassel/Fed. Rep. Germany,
Mönchbergstr. 41/43

Dr. R. ROKSETH
Regionsykehuset, Trondheim/
Norway

Dr. R. ROST
Deutsche Sporthochschule, 5000
Köln 41/Fed. Rep. Germany, Carl-
Diem-Weg

Prof. Dr. F. ROVELLI
Diagnose-Abt. f. Herzkrankheiten,
Ospedale Maggiore, Milano/Italy

Prof. Dr. W. RUDOLPH
Deutsches Herzzentrum, 8000 München 19/Fed. Rep. Germany, Loth-
straße 11

Prof. Dr. W. RUTISHAUSER
Kantonsspital Zürich, Dept. f. Innere
Medizin der Universität, Med. Poli-
klinik, Rämistr. 100, 8006 Zürich/
Switzerland

Prof. Dr. A. SAKUMA
Dept. of Clinical Pharmacology,
Medical Research Institute, Tokyo
Medical and Dental University, no.
5–45, 1-Chome, Yushima, Bunkyo-
ku, Tokyo 113/Japan

Dr. S. SCARDI
Ospedali Riuniti, Div. Cardiologia,
34129 Trieste/Italy

Dr. G. SCHÄCKE
Inst. f. Arbeits- u. Sozial-Medizin u.
Poliklinik f. Berufskrankheiten der
Universität, 8520 Erlangen/Fed. Rep.
Germany, Schillerstr. 25/29

Prof. Dr. J. SCHAEFER
I. Med. Klinik der Universität Kiel,
Abt. für Spezielle Kardiologie, 2300
Kiel/Fed. Rep. Germany, Schitten-
helmstr. 12

Dr. K. SCHLOSSMANN
Bayer AG, Institut für Pharmakologie, 5600 Wuppertal 1/Fed. Rep. Germany, Postfach 130105

Prof. Dr. J. SCHMIER
Abt. für experimentelle Chirurgie, Chir. Univ.-Klinik, 6900 Heidelberg/ Fed. Rep. Germany, Bergheimstr. 147, Haus „Landfried"

Dr. D. SCHNELL
5220 Waldbröl/Fed. Rep. Germany, Kaiserstr. 62

Mr. W. SCHWERDTFEGER
5000 Köln 1/Fed. Rep. Germany, Belfortstr. 9/XII

Dr. F. J. SLOOFF
Stichting St. Antonius Ziekenhuis, J. van Scorelstraat 2, Utrecht/Netherlands

Prof. Dr. H. A. SNELLEN
Afdeling Cardiologie, Academisch Ziekenhuis, Leiden/Netherlands

Dr. T. STAVNAR
Sandefjord/Norway

Dr. G. STEIN
Curschmann Klinik, 2408 Timmendorfer Strand/Fed. Rep. Germany

Dr. G. STOCKMANN
6900 Heidelberg/Fed. Rep. Germany, Friedrichstr. 10a

Dr. B. STRAUER
Klinikum Gross-Hadern, 8000 München 70/Fed. Rep. Germany

Dr. B. TABATZNIK
Dept. of Cardiology, North Charles General Hospital, 2724 North Charles Street, Baltimore, MD 21218/USA

Prof. Dr. N. TAIRA
Tohoku University, School of Medicine, Dept. of Pharmacology, Sendai 980/Japan

Dr. P. TORTORE
Ospedale Civile S. Croce, Div. Cardiologia, 12100 Cuneo/Italy

Dr. D. VALLÉE
Lungenklinik Heidehaus, 3000 Hannover/Fed. Rep. Germany, Stöckenerstr. 320

Dr. W. VATER
BAYER AG, Inst. f. Pharmakologie, 5600 Wuppertal 1/Fed. Rep. Germany, Postfach 130105

Dr. J. VUORI
Kansaneläkelattoksen, Kontoutustutkimuskeskus, Peltolantie 3, 20720 Turku/Finland

Dr. B. A. G. J. WITTEVEEN
Splinterlaan 153, Leiderdorp/Netherlands

Mr. G. WITZSTROCK
7570 Baden-Baden/Fed. Rep. Germany, Postfach 509

Dr. S. YASUI
1st. Dept. of Internal Medicine, Nagoya University, School of Medicine, Tsurumai-cho, Showa-ku, Nagoya/Japan

Dr. P. VAN ZELLER
Quinta de forbes, Praia da granja/ Portugal

Prof. Dr. P. A. VAN ZWIETEN
Lab. voor Biofarmacie, Plantage Muidergracht 24, Amsterdam/Netherlands

Introduction

W. LOCHNER

Ladies and Gentlemen,

As the president of this symposium, I have the pleasure and the honour to welcome all of you and to declare the congress opened. The aim of our meeting is to present and to discuss thoroughly all the results of the pharmacological investigations and the clinical studies on Adalat, a new antianginal drug.

As we all know, the problem of therapy of ischemic heart disease, despite great efforts, has not been solved sufficiently. A new drug like Adalat, being not only a new therapeutic agent, but also a new tool for understanding, offers new opportunities for investigating the mechanism of action of antianginal drugs and creates new hopes for more successful therapy.

Therefore, if we are going to discuss and to evaluate in this meeting the pharmacological and clinical properties of the new drug Adalat, we should at the same time discuss the concepts underlying the therapy of ischemic heart disease in general.

These theoretical concepts form the background of our discussion and serve as the network in which to place the new insights on Adalat. Our present theoretical concepts are the scale with which we evaluate the new facts, until perhaps one day, we can enlarge this network or even change it, as new knowledge allows new theories.

But let me add and accentuate one point: theoretical concepts and experimental studies are necessary, are indispensible for the development and evaluation of a new antianginal drug. Nevertheless the final answer on the usefulness of such a drug at the present state of knowledge can only come from controlled clinical investigations.

At the end of our two days here, I hope that we shall arrive at the following two main results:

1. I hope that we shall have learned about ischemic heart disease and the theoretical concepts of its therapy;

2. I hope that we shall have gained an overall view of the present state of knowledge on the pharmacological and clinical properties of Adalat.

All of you, I believe, will agree when I express our gratefulness to the organizer and sponsor of the symposium, the Bayer AG, represented here by Prof. KRONEBERG and others. There can be no doubt that it will prove extremely worthwhile to have discussed here extensively and with all the necessary critics, the available results with Adalat. I am sure that we all shall derive benefit from the discussions, and I wish the symposium to be a successful and fruitful one. Thank you very much.

Present Basis of Coronary Therapy

W. LOCHNER

Physiologisches Institut der Universität Düsseldorf, Fed. Rep. Germany

The question concerning the basis of coronary therapy today means, what is the basis of antianginal therapy, the therapy of ischemic heart disease. In this symposium we shall not deal with the treatment or prevention of arteriosclerosis as the main cause of ischemic heart disease. We shall discuss rather the improvement of the relationship between oxygen supply and oxygen consumption of the heart, both in the acute state of angina and as long-term treatment.

Oxygen consumption of the heart depends on several factors that are interrelated in a rather complicated manner (Fig. 1). The main factors are: heart rate, arterial pressure, diastolic and systolic intraventricular pressure, size of the heart and the contractility, measured as the rate of intraventricular pressure rise, dp/dt_{max}. I shall not give an analysis of the complicated relationships between these parameters and oxygen consumption because I believe that it is unnecessary for the discussion of our problem today and tomorrow. But knowledge of the directional change of oxygen consumption if one of the named parameters changes is indispensable.

The higher the heart rate, the arterial pressure, the intraventricular pressure and the contractility, the higher the oxygen consumption will be. Any therapy that influences one of the parameters mentioned, whether directly or indirectly, changes oxygen consumption.

The oxygen delivery to the heart equals coronary flow times oxygen concentration of the arterial blood (Fig. 2). I shall not discuss the oxygen concentration in detail. There is no doubt that in the diseased heart, angina can be brought about by too low a concentration of oxygen, which therefore should be as normal as possible. A lowering of the oxygen concentration can be caused by a diminution of hemoglobin concentration or by a decrease in the oxygen saturation of the hemoglobin. The latter is usually connected with respiratory failure.

Coronary flow is determined by the arteriovenous pressure difference and resistance to flow. It is clear from the equation that an increase in arterial pressure and/or a decrease in venous pressure in the right auricle can be a beneficial therapeutic measure, because it increases oxygen delivery to the heart. But we must remember, as explained above, that the higher the arterial pressure, the higher is the oxygen consumption of the heart.

The question arises of whether the enhancement of flow by increased pressure is sufficient to meet the higher oxygen need. We lack enough reliable experimental data on this problem to give a more precise statement than the following: in a

Oxygen consumption of the heart
depends on

heart rate
arterial pressure
intraventricular pressure
heart size
dp/dt_{max}

Fig. 1

oxygen delivery =
coronary flow × oxygen concentration

$$\text{coronary flow} = \frac{P_A - P_V}{R}$$

Fig. 2

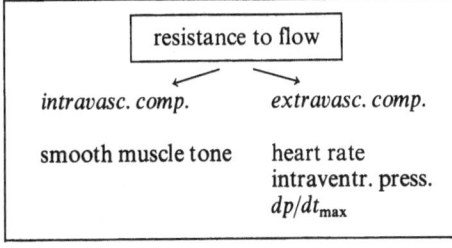

resistance to flow

intravasc. comp.   extravasc. comp.

smooth muscle tone   heart rate
intraventr. press.
dp/dt_{max}

Fig. 3

Fig. 1. dp/dt_{max} = maximal rate of intra-ventricular pressure rise

Fig. 2. P_A = arterial pressure; P_V = venous pressure; R = resistance to flow

Fig. 3. Factors which influence resistance to flow

mean range of pressure, the increased flow meets the higher oxygen demand when pressure increases. This pressure ranges approximately between 70 and 150 mm Hg.

Resistance to flow is more important in the flow equation than the pressure difference, because it can vary much more than the pressure difference. It may decrease to almost 1/5 of the normal value, in a normal heart with a normal vascular system, of course. Pressure can vary too, but never in this range, and it is never used to adapt coronary flow to the oxygen consumption of the heart. The heart performs this adaptation by the regulation of resistance.

The overall resistance to flow must be divided into two components: 1. the intravascular component of coronary resistance and 2. the extravascular component (Fig. 3). No one doubts that there are drugs, more or less specific, which dilate coronary vessels, thus decreasing resistance and improving coronary flow, provided that the vessels can be dilated at all and are not stiff. It is also clear that these drugs can have different mechanisms of action.

The dilating effect of these drugs can be demonstrated easily in animal experiments and also in humans. The question is, does the drug also dilate in the pathologic states of anoxia, ischemia, or infarction. This question is unfortunately hard to answer.

One group of investigators believes that in anoxia or ischemia the vessels are always in a state of maximal dilation and that therefore application of a coronary dilator is necessarily useless and eventually makes the situation worse because it lowers arterial pressure and produces the so-called "steal effect".

Others reject this apodictic statement. Among other things they quote animal experiments which demonstrate that an experimentally produced infarct can be rendered smaller by treatment with pharmacological dilation.

In this connection, one can mention the "walk through phenomenon". Some of the patients who show a working angina can walk through the angina, when they continue walking, the pain and also the typical changes of ECG can disappear. It is not possible to explain completely the mechanism of this phenomenon, nevertheless we must say that in these patients the optimal adaption of coronary flow to the oxygen need of the heart takes several minutes. One of the underlying causes could be a prolonged onset of the mechanism of coronary dilation, i.e. the intravascular component. It is also possible that the extravascular component plays the more important or even decisive role. If the intravascular component were involved, a prophylactic pharmacological dilation could help.

My conclusion from these reflections is that at the present time we should not reject the therapeutic principle of pharmacologic dilation. A final answer regarding its value cannot be given yet.

Now, the pharmacologic dilation of collateral vessels as a possible therapeutic effect has to be discussed. We all agree that well-developed and dilated collaterals can have a protective effect on an infarcted area. Concerning the pharmacologic influence on collaterals, we must distinguish 1. the influence on number and size during the course of a long-term application of a drug and 2. the dilation in acute ischemia.

There are animal experiments which show that longer treatment with pharmacologic dilators can provoke the development of collaterals; this will certainly have a protective effect, the same effect that can be brought about by muscular training. Although the experts do not agree on the effectiveness of such therapy in humans, it is nevertheless a plausible therapeutic principle that we must continue to investigate.

The other question is, can a drug dilate collaterals more than the other vessels, does it have a specific effect on collaterals? This theory has been proposed for nitroglycerin. The problem is related to the so-called steal phenomenon, which effects the opposite of a specific dilation of collaterals: it reduces flow through collaterals. If one measures in dog experiments under controlled conditions collateral flow in terms of back flow into an infarcted area, and then effects a general pharmacologic dilation of the coronary vascular bed with an overall increase of flow, back flow, i.e. collateral flow, can be reduced. We have observed this steal effect in our own studies.

Some investigators believe that the specific effect on the collaterals can differ, depending on the dilator used. Recent experiments in our laboratory do not support the theory that dilating drugs can have different effects, for example specific effects on collaterals or on the "steal phenomenon".

The suggestion that an antianginal drug should have a coronary dilating effect always refers to a primary dilating effect, not a secondary dilating effect. A primary dilating effect leads to an increase of flow in combination with an increase of coronary venous oxygen pressure, or oxygen saturation. The primary dilating effect of adrenaline is shown in Fig. 4. On an anesthetized dog, coronary sinus outflow was continuously recorded with an electromagnetic flowmeter, and coronary venous oxygen saturation with an oximeter. Intracoronary infusion of adrenaline increases sinus outflow as well as oxygen saturation.

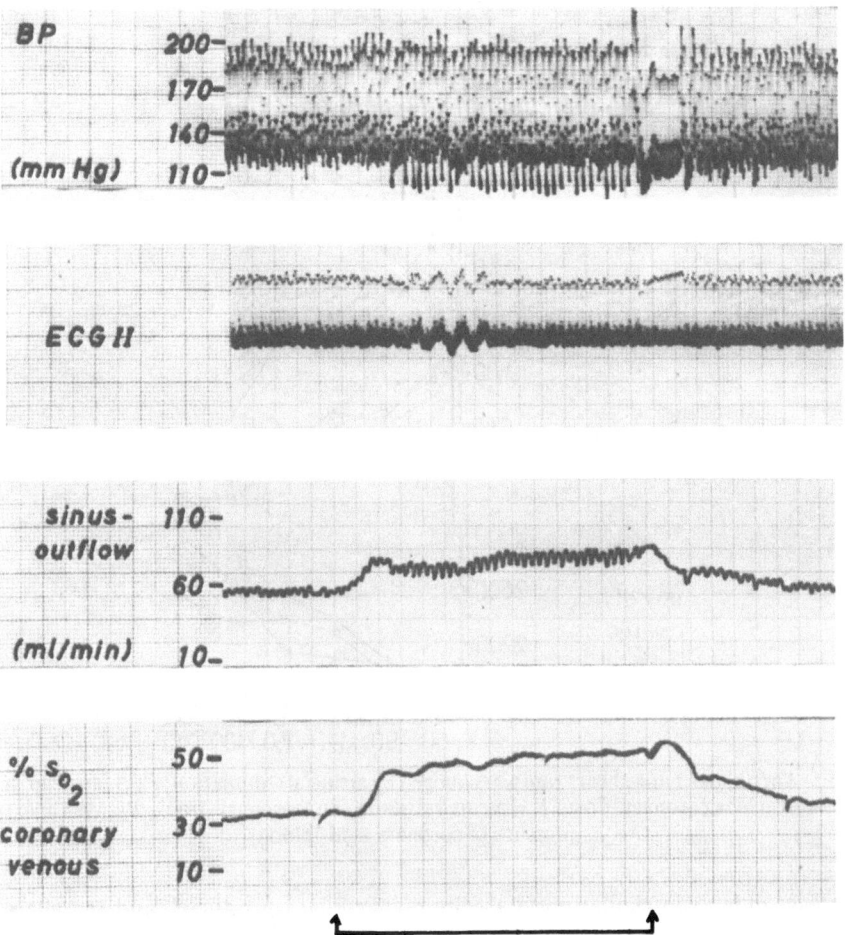

Fig. 4. Anesthetized dog, intracoronary infusion of adrenaline. Coronary sinus outflow was measured with an electromagnetic flowmeter, the chest being closed. BP = arterial pressure; S_{O_2} = oxygen saturation of coronary sinus blood, measured continuously by an oximeter

An example of a secondary dilation is shown in Fig. 5. In dog experiments, heart rate was increased by artificial stimulation; coronary flow increased, certainly because of the increased oxygen demand, but oxygen pressure of coronary venous blood decreased.

The problems so far discussed were connected with the intravascular component of coronary resistance, with the smooth muscle tonus of resistance vessels including collaterals. The following is an elaboration on the extravascular component of coronary resistance, frequently also called extravascular support. The main factors are heart rate, intraventricular pressure and the maximal rate of intraventricular pressure rise, dp/dt_{max}.

In experiments on anesthetized dogs we changed the heart rate from 60 to 220 beats/min. All experiments showed an increase in resistance to coronary flow calculated for the whole cycle, as can be seen in Fig. 6. In other experiments, an

W. LOCHNER

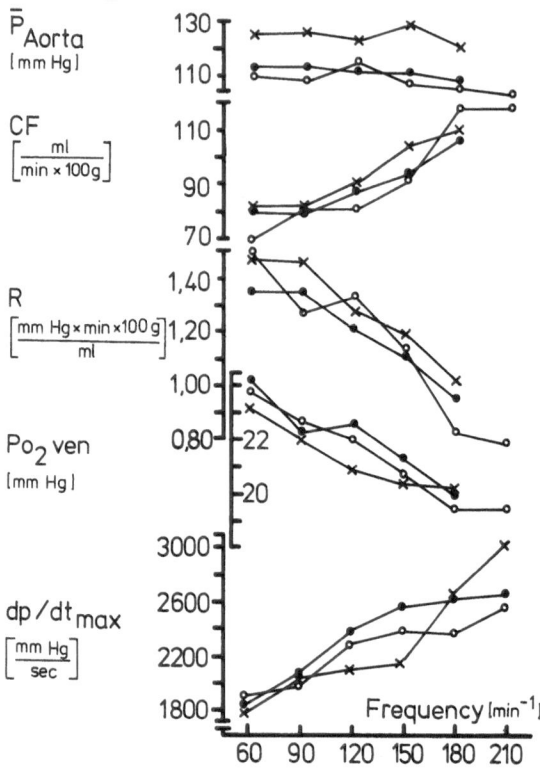

Fig. 5. Anesthetized dog; heart rate was changed by artificial stimulation; $\bar{P}_{Aorta}$ = mean aortic pressure; CF = coronary flow; R = mean resistance to coronary flow; P_{O_2} ven = oxygen pressure of coronary sinus blood

increase of left ventricular enddiastolic pressure was produced, and the effect on the flow, i.e. resistance to flow, measured.

In all cases the result was an increase in the resistance to coronary inflow (Fig. 7). Finally, by intracoronary infusion of isoproterenol, an increase of the maximal rate of rise of intraventricular pressure was produced. This likewise always led to an increase of extravascular support (Fig. 8).

Quantitative evaluation of the change in extravascular support due to alterations in heart rate, enddiastolic intraventricular pressure and dp/dt_{max} leads us to conclude that the factors are of minor importance, if one compares the effects with the maximal dilating capacity of the normal vascular bed. An increase of 100 beats/min in heart rate increases the resistance by only 14%. A change in dp/dt_{max} of ± 1000 mm Hg/sec leads to a 7.5% increase in resistance and finally, an increase of 10 mm Hg in enddiastolic pressure enhances the resistance by only 11%. A normal coronary vascular tree easily compensates for an increase in resistance in this range. However in the case of a sclerotic vascular tree, a 10% increase in resistance might have deleterious effects. Therefore we must consider with great care the extravascular component of coronary resistance.

It is important to know that changes in the significant parameters can be effected through the direct action of a drug on the heart but also by an effect on

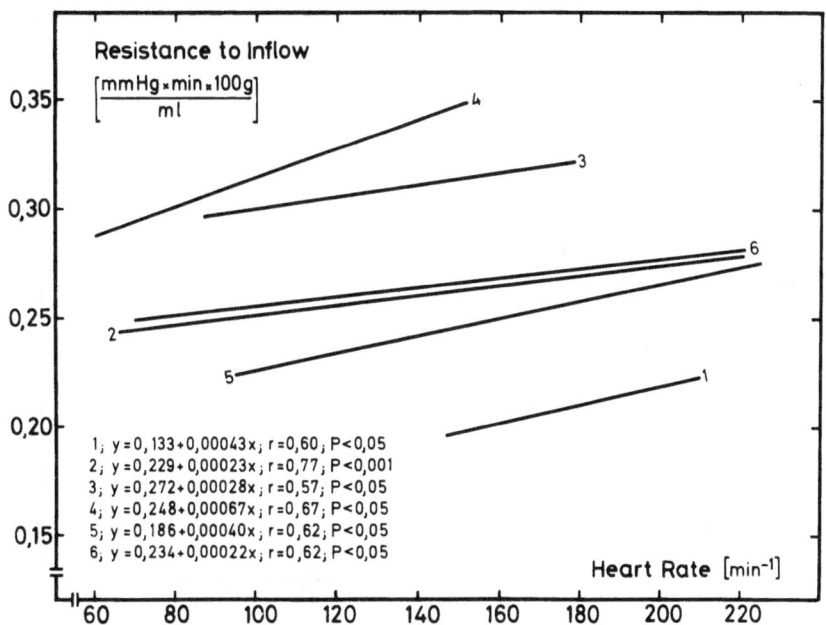

Fig. 6. Anesthetized dogs, heart rate was changed by artificial stimulation (from RAFF, KOSCHE and LOCHNER, Amer. J. Cardiol. **29**, 598 (1972))

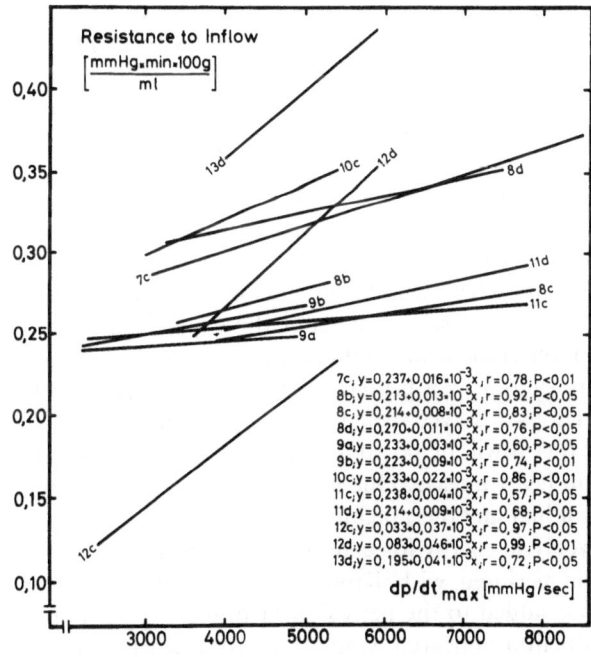

Fig. 7. Anesthetized dogs, left ventricular enddiastolic pressure (LVEDP) was changed by blood transfusion (see Fig. 6)

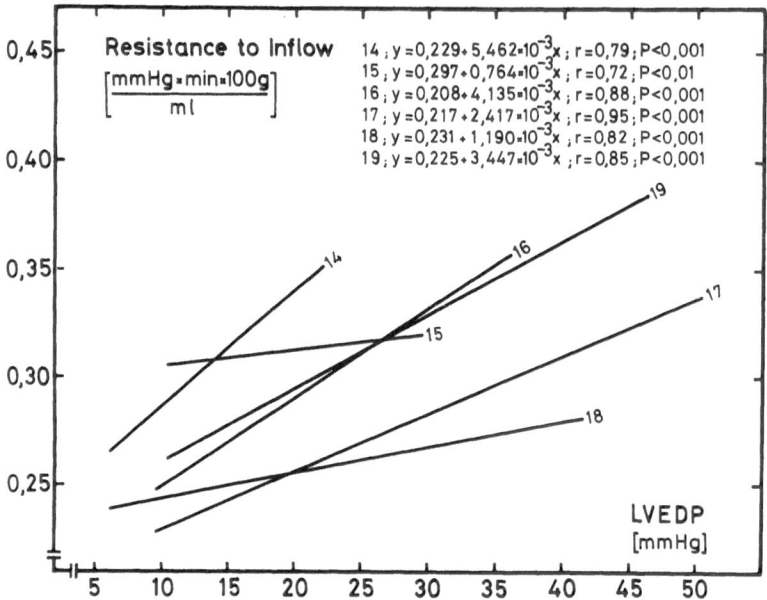

Fig. 8. Anesthetized dogs, rate of intraventricular pressure rise (dp/dt_{max}) was changed by intracoronary infusion of isoproterenol (see Fig. 6)

the peripheral circulation, which relative to the heart is an indirect action. Heart rate can be changed by a direct chronotropic effect on the heart but also by reflexes due to changes in arterial pressure. Enddiastolic filling pressure of the heart can be changed not only by positive or negative inotropic effects on the heart, but also by a decrease or increase in venous return. Venous return again depends on cardiac output, peripheral resistance to flow and to a great degree on the tonus of the capacity vessels.

The maximal rate of intraventricular pressure rise dp/dt_{max} is influenced by a negative or positive stimulus on the heart, but also by the filling pressure, the heart rate and the aortic pressure.

Lastly, I shall make a few remarks on the possible direct influence of a drug on heart metabolism. As I have shown in detail, there are many indirect influences on oxygen consumption of the heart; indirect means that all the changes in metabolism observed are caused by a primary change in the mechanical activity of the heart. All drug actions observed seem to be indirect ones.

It is unlikely that it will be possible to change or to influence the efficiency of energy delivery in heart muscle. One idea is worthwhile mentioning, despite the fact that it has not had any therapeutic consequences so far. We have studied the utilization of glycolytic energy for external heart work in an isolated guinea pig heart preparation perfused with Krebs solution and capable of stroke work. When cyanide was added to the perfusion medium, oxygen uptake was reduced and lactate production appeared, while the stroke work of the heart was kept constant. A steady state of this situation was observed for about 15 min. We concluded that the energy source required for steady-state performance of stroke

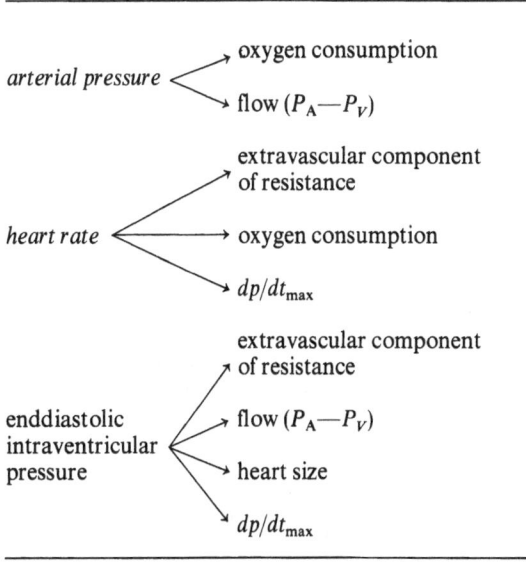

arterial pressure
→ oxygen consumption
→ flow $(P_A - P_V)$

heart rate
↗ extravascular component of resistance
→ oxygen consumption
↘ dp/dt_{max}

enddiastolic intraventricular pressure
↗ extravascular component of resistance
→ flow $(P_A - P_V)$
→ heart size
↘ dp/dt_{max}

Fig. 9. Factors that can influence coronary flow and oxygen consumption of the heart

work can shift at least partly from oxidative to anaerobic metabolism. Energy liberated from carbohydrate breakdown to lactate can be converted to stroke work under steady-state conditions.

Under the conditions of the experiments 12% of the total energy requirement was covered by glycolytic energy. Other investigators have observed a lactate production by the human heart in the state of angina.

I begin my summary with the statement that I made at the onset: our therapeutic goal must be the improvement of the relationship between oxygen supply and oxygen need of the heart. Therefore, in evaluating a drug or any other therapeutic measure, we have to take into consideration all the effects on the factors that can influence coronary flow and oxygen consumption. The effects on the heart can be either direct or indirect. I repeat the significant parameters (Fig. 9): Heart rate influences the extravascular component of resistance, oxygen consumption and dp/dt_{max}. Arterial pressure influences heart work and thus oxygen consumption. The change in oxygen consumption, again in an indirect way, changes resistance to flow. Arterial pressure also influences flow directly by changing the pressure difference. Enddiastolic intraventricular pressure influences the extravascular component of resistance and the pressure difference—it changes heart size and effects dp/dt_{max}.

The effects on the diseased heart can, as pointed out previously, be direct or indirect. Of the indirect effects the most important parameters are the arterial pressure and the tonus of the capacity vessels, i.e. the venous return. This area has been neglected for a long time but is, in my judgement, an important part of the action of nitroglycerin. A decrease in venous return will decrease ventricular filling pressure. This in turn causes a decrease in stroke volume, a decrease in oxygen consumption, a diminution of heart volume, and a decrease in the extra-

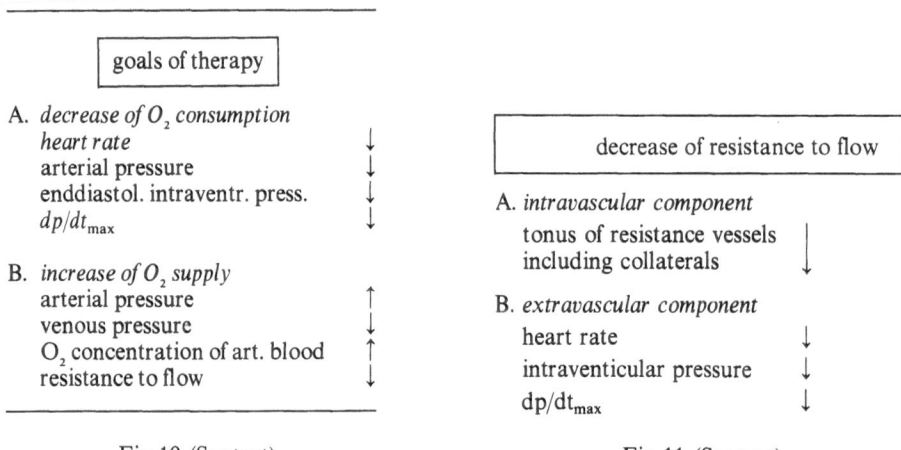

goals of therapy	
A. *decrease of O_2 consumption*	
heart rate	↓
arterial pressure	↓
enddiastol. intraventr. press.	↓
dp/dt_{max}	↓
B. *increase of O_2 supply*	
arterial pressure	↑
venous pressure	↓
O_2 concentration of art. blood	↑
resistance to flow	↓

decrease of resistance to flow	
A. *intravascular component*	
tonus of resistance vessels including collaterals	↓
B. *extravascular component*	
heart rate	↓
intraventicular pressure	↓
dp/dt_{max}	↓

Fig. 10. (See text)   Fig. 11. (See text)

vascular support, all of which will improve the relationship between oxygen need and oxygen supply.

In Fig. 10, our therapeutic goals are summarized. The decrease in oxygen consumption can be effected by decreasing heart rate, arterial pressure, diastolic intraventricular pressure and contractility, here expressed in terms of dp/dt_{max}.

An enhancement of oxygen supply to the heart can be effected by an increase in arterial pressure and oxygen concentration of arterial blood and by a decrease in venous pressure and resistance to flow.

Figure 11 concerns the resistance to flow. A decrease can be brought about by affecting the tonus of resistance vessels including collaterals. In order to decrease the extravascular component, one has to decrease heart rate, intraventricular pressure and contractility.

Ladies and Gentlemen! I hope my survey will prove useful in the analysis and evaluation of the action of Adalat, the drug which we shall be dealing with for the next two days.

Session I

Chemistry and Experimental Pharmacology

Chairmen: A.Fleckenstein (Freiburg), K.Landmark (Oslo)

Pharmacology of Nifedipine

G. KRONEBERG

Pharma Research Center, Bayer AG, Wuppertal, Fed. Rep. Germany

This paper is a brief synopsis of the main pharmacological properties of nifedipine in connection with a concept of its hemodynamic action.

This concept takes into account that the single pharmacological action on a tissue or a special organ of the cardiovascular apparatus is integrated in the intact organism into a systemic hemodynamic action by regulatory mechanisms. Thus it makes the different pharmacological results less inconsistent and the clinical effects more understandable.

First, I would like to present the main subject of our Symposium: BAY a 1040 or nifedipine, trade name Adalat, was found some years ago in the Bayer-laboratories by BOSSERT and VATER [1] and investigated pharmacologically mainly in Germany and Japan (Fig. 1).

Nifedipine is a 1,4-dihydropyridine with a NO_2 group in orthoposition that remains unchanged during the metabolic transformation in the body.

As pointed out by Prof. FLECKENSTEIN [2] and his group in Freiburg, nifedipine inhibits the penetration of extracellular calcium through the cell membrane and the inflow of Ca^{++}-ions from the binding sites at the sarcoplasmatic reticulum into the cell plasma where the ATPase of the myofibrils is located (Fig. 2). This enzyme needs Ca^{++}-ions to be activated and to split ATP for the energy delivering process of muscle contraction. The consequence of the inhibitory action of nifedipine is the relaxation of the muscle fibre—for the heart muscle this means a negative inotropic effect, and for the blood vessel, vasodilation.

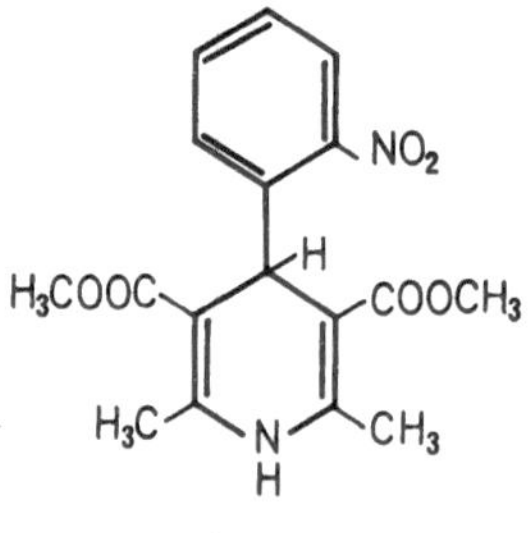

BAY a 1040, Adalat®, (Nifedipine)

Fig. 1

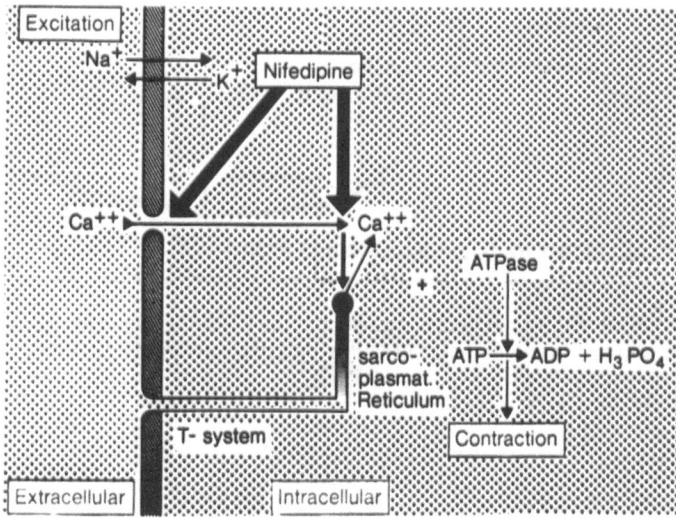

Fig. 2. Site of nifedipine action on the excitation-contraction coupling (scheme)

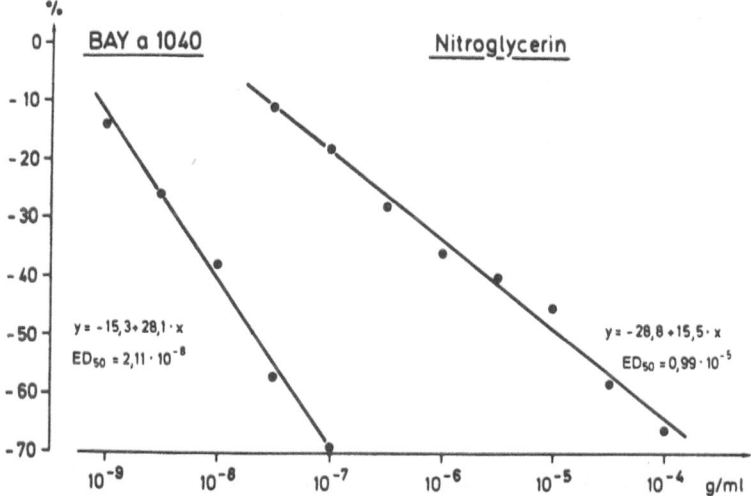

Fig. 3. Isolated papillary muscle of guinea pig. Action of nifedipine (BAY a 1040) and nitroglycerin on the velocity of the isometric tension development. The points represent mean values from 3 experiments. The curves are regression lines. *Ordinate:* decrease of the velocity of the isometric tension development in % of the initial value, *abscissa:* concentration in g/ml (VATER *et al.,* 1972)

In Fig. 3 experiments in the isolated papillary muscle of the guinea pig heart, carried out by Dr. STOEPEL [7] from our laboratories, are summarized showing the high inhibitory activity of nifedipine in the isolated preparation: The curves represent the decrease of velocity of the isometric contraction, otherwise expressed as *dk/dt* after increasing concentrations of nifedipine and nitroglycerin.

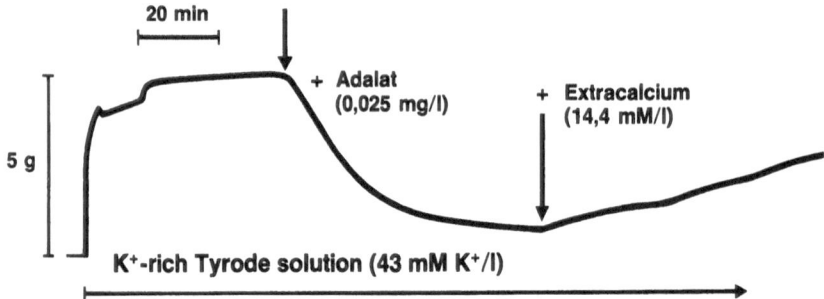

Fig. 4. Abolishment of the potassium contracture of the isolated coronary artery strip of cattle by nifedipine and restitution of the contractility by extra calcium (GRÜN and FLECKENSTEIN, 1972)

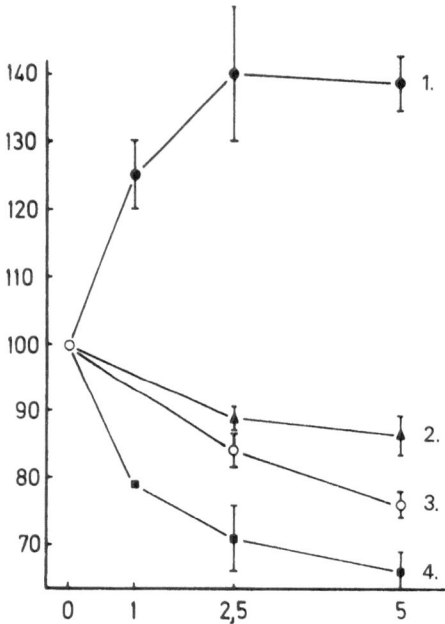

Fig. 5. Isolated guinea pig heart. *Ordinate:* changes in % of the initial value, *abscissa:* nifedipine, µg/l. *1* coronary flow. *2* oxygen consumption. *3* systolic pressure in the left ventricle, *4* left ventricle dp/dt_{max}, means of 24 experiments

While the ED_{50} of nifedipine is almost 10^{-8}, that of nitroglycerin is only 10^{-5}, in other words, nitroglycerin is 1000 times less active in this special isolated preparation. As has been demonstrated also in our laboratories, this high efficacy of nifedipine is diminished by the high protein binding properties of nifedipine. Thus in the heart-lung preparation of the guinea pig where blood instead of aqueous Tyrode solution is used as the drug-bearing medium, the cardio-inhibitory activity of nifedipine is nearly 100 times less due to the large percentage of protein binding.

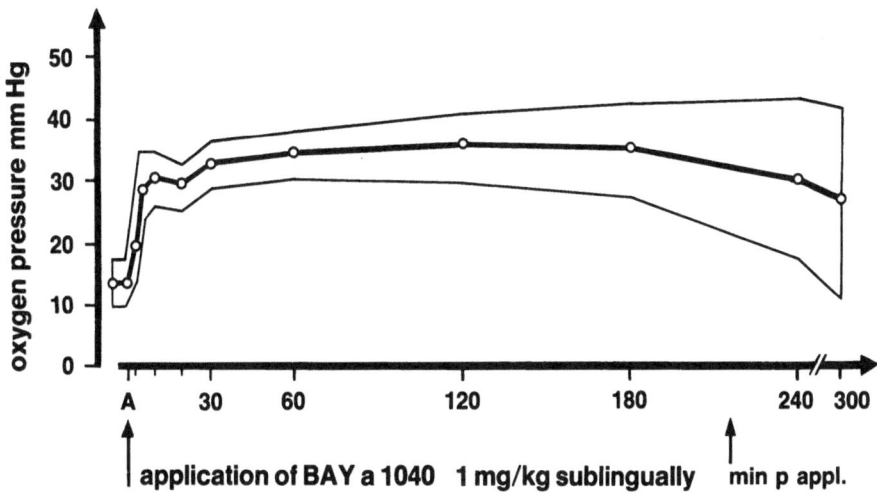

Fig. 6. Oxygen pressure in the coronary sinus of the dog after sublingual administration of nifedipine 1 mg/kg, urethane-chloralose i.v. ($n=7$), Phanodorm i.p. ($n=3$), $\bar{x}$ of 10 dogs. Mean values and fiducial limits $p=0.05$. *Abscissa:* min after administration, *ordinate:* mm Hg oxygen pressure (VATER et al., 1972)

Almost the same nifedipine concentration that is effective in the isolated heart muscle also relaxes the coronary vessel under isolated organ conditions. In the experiment published by GRÜN and FLECKENSTEIN [3] in 1972 (Fig. 4), 0.025 mg/l or 2.5×10^{-8} completely relaxes the potassium-induced contraction of the isolated coronary strip.

This means that the basic quantitative activity of nifedipine, due to its excitation-contraction coupling action, is practically the same in the cardiac muscle as in the muscle of the coronary vessel.

This conclusion may be drawn also from experiments published by RAFF et al. [4] in 1972, summarized in Fig. 5. Nifedipine in approximately similar concentrations as in the foregoing experiments, namely $0.25–0.5 \times 10^{-8}$, increases remarkably the coronary perfusion (upper curve No. 1) and simultaneously decreases the contractile force of the heart, as expressed by the decrease of the systolic pressure and the maximal pressure increase velocity in the left ventricle (curve No. 3 and 4) as well as by the oxygen consumption (No. 2).

The high efficacy of the drug (or its intrinsic activity) on the coronary vessel can also be seen from experiments in the classical Langendorff preparation. As Dr. STOEPEL [7] from our laboratories stated, nifedipine is 2700 times more potent than papaverine and the β-stimulating compound buphenine.

The duration of action in this perfusion test object is relatively short, showing that the binding of the drug at the sites of action is relatively weak.

In contrast to the more transient effect in the isolated perfused heart, the duration of the coronary action is extremely long, if the drug is given sublingually or orally. In Fig. 6, experiments of Dr. VATER [7] in dogs are summarized, indicating that several minutes after sublingual administration of 1 mg/kg nifedipine a rapid increase of the oxygen pressure in the coronary sinus blood occurs, mainly

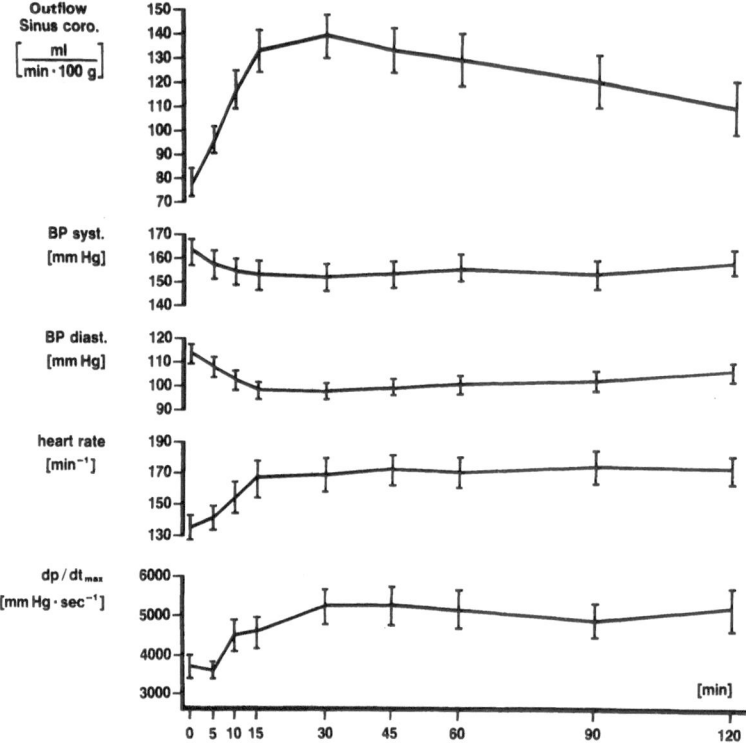

Fig. 7. Nifedipine action on cardiac function in the anesthetized dog ($n = 16$); means with standard deviation of coronary outflow, systolic (BP syst.) and diastolic (BP diast.) blood pressure, heart rate and dp/dt_{max}

due to an increased coronary perfusion. This drug-induced elevated perfusion lasts several hours, as can be seen from the right part of the figure.

Dr. PATZSCHKE will discuss in his paper results with radioactive labelled nifedipine, which demonstrate more clearly the kinetics of the absorption and the distribution of the drug in the animal body.

From a summary of all results concerning the orally- or sublingually-induced rapid onset and long duration of nifedipine action, one can conclude that at first relatively *small*, but *effective* amounts of nifedipine are quickly absorbed and that then a permanent and relatively slow absorption—relatively slowly compared to the total amount given—follows, which continuously provides the necessary dose to maintain a long-lasting effect without excessive intensity. Also the high protein binding of nifedipine in the blood plasma may be an additional factor in the complex mechanism of its long-lasting oral effects.

In comparison to the demonstrated parallelism between the action of nifedipine on the isolated heart muscle and on the isolated coronary vessel and the coronary perfusion, experiments in the *intact* animal produced different results: In experiments carried out by RAFF et al. [4] (Fig. 7), about 0.4 mg/kg nifedipine were given sublingually to only lightly anesthetized dogs. Similarly to the experiments in the isolated heart preparations, the coronary flow increased remarkably

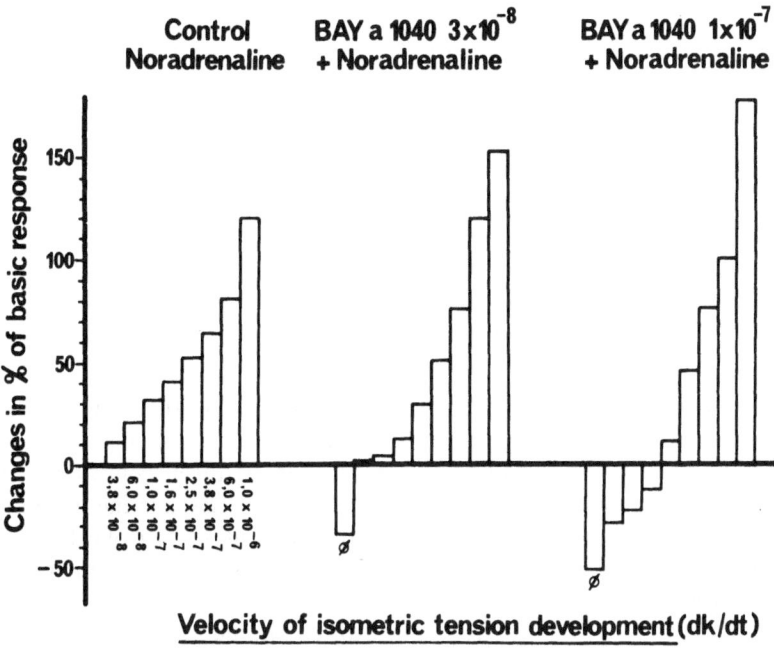

Fig. 8. Isolated papillary muscle of guinea pig heart (electrically stimulated)

(here to about 100%) (upper curve), but the contractile force of the heart, expressed as dp/dt, was not inhibited, as could be expected from the high inhibitory action in the isolated heart muscle preparation. Instead of a decrease, a certain increase of dp/dt was established, as can be seen from the lower curve. This cannot be due to a direct action of nifedipine because it is devoid of β-adrenergic stimulant properties.

In principle, FLECKENSTEIN and his group have already shown that β-adrenergic stimulation can easily abolish the cardio-inhibitory action of calcium antagonists and also of nifedipine.

Dr. STOEPEL [6] from our pharmacological laboratories studied the antagonism between nifedipine and noradrenaline at the cardiac muscle more quantitatively.

Preliminary results are shown in Fig. 8. If noradrenaline is added in increasing concentrations to an electrically stimulated isolated guinea pig heart muscle, the velocity of the isometric tension development increases continuously, as is demonstrated by the left group of columns in Fig. 8. In the presence of 3×10^{-8} nifedipine, but *without* noradrenaline, the response of the muscle is diminished (marked by $\varnothing$). If noradrenaline is added, the inhibiting effect of nifedipine is completely abolished. Increasing doses of noradrenaline are then as effective as without nifedipine.

A contribution to the question of how interactions of nifedipine at the vessel sites occur was given by experiments of Dr. GÖRLITZ in the laboratory of Prof. SCHÜMANN [5] in Essen. The numbers in Table 1 represent *relative* effects of papaverine and nifedipine on the isolated aorta and mesenteric artery strip. Two kinds

Table 1. Relative effects of papaverine and nifedipine on the aorta and the mesenteric artery calculated from the pD 2' values (SCHÜMANN, 1974)

	Aorta		Mesenteric artery	
	noradrenaline induced contraction	Ca^{++} induced contraction	noradrenaline induced contraction	Ca^{++} induced contraction
Papaverine	1	1	1	1
Nifedipine	0.7	2350	3.5	670

of contractions were induced, one with noradrenaline and the other with Ca^{++}-ions. As one can easily see, nifedipine is highly active against the Ca^{++}-induced contraction and far less against the noradrenaline-induced contraction. In the aorta preparation, nifedipine is practically as active as papaverine in the case of noradrenaline, but 2350 times as active as papaverine in the case of calcium. In the mesenteric artery the corresponding values are 3.5 and 670. Two conclusions can be drawn from these results:

1. It is much more difficult to dilate with nifedipine a vessel that has a predominant noradrenaline or sympathetic (or neurogenic) tone than to dilate a vessel with a predominant calcium or myogenic tone.

2. There are apparently sensitivity differences against nifedipine in the different kinds of vessels.

Considering these results one may suggest that regulatory mechanisms of the cardiovascular system are involved in the total hemodynamic action of nifedipine. These mechanisms are able to diminish or even abolish the negative inotropic effect of nifedipine in the heart in situ, particularly in the case of higher nifedipine doses. This suggestion would explain

1. why in the intact animal with reasonable doses, no or only slight negative inotropic effects on the heart are seen,

2. why nifedipine increases relatively specifically the coronary perfusion,

3. the differences in the hemodynamic effects of nifedipine in anesthetized and non-anesthetized animals and in man.

How far and to what extend cardiovascular regulations are involved depends certainly on the individual dose of nifedipine.

Abstract

The basic action of nifedipine is to relax the muscle fibre of the vessel wall and of the myocardium by an inhibition of the excitation contraction coupling. This leads to a vasodilation and a decreased contractility of the isolated cardiac muscle. In the intact organism these actions are influenced and modified by secondary mechanisms mainly due to reactions of the baroreceptor system. The resulting hemodynamic effects of nifedipine consist mainly in an increase of the coronary perfusion and a decrease of the peripheral vessel resistance.

The concept of a nifedipine induced vasodilation-baroreceptor interaction makes the differences of the pharmacological results in isolated preparations, in anesthetized and non anesthetized animals less inconsistent and the clinical effects of the drug better understandable.

References

1. BOSSERT,F., VATER,W.: Naturwissenschaften **58**, 578 (1971).
2. FLECKENSTEIN,A., TRITTHART,H., DÖRING,H.J., BYON,K.Y.: Arzneim. Forsch. (Drug Res.) **22**, 22 (1972).
3. GRÜN,G., FLECKENSTEIN,A.: Arzneim. Forsch. (Drug Res.) **22**, 334 (1972).
4. RAFF,W.K., KOSCHE,F., LOCHNER,W.: Arzneim. Forsch. (Drug Res.) **22**, 33 (1972).
5. SCHÜMANN,H.J.: personal communication (1974).
6. STOEPEL,K., KRONEBERG,G.: unpublished.
7. VATER,W., KRONEBERG,G., HOFFMEISTER,F., KALLER,H., MENG,K., OBERDORF,A., PULS,W., SCHLOSSMANN,K., STOEPEL,K.: Arzneim. Forsch. (Drug Res.) **22**, 1 (1972).

Discussion Remarks

KIRCHHEIM: In the unanesthetized dog we have studied "calciumantagonistic" agents on kidney blood flow and muscle blood flow. In the kidney we found an increase of 30% and in the muscle vasculature an increase of 600%. So there are differences; but if you mean by "specificity" that the coronary vasculature does dilate more than the integral of the peripheral vascular bed, indicated by total peripheral resistance, then we have different results. From our results we would not conclude that the coronary vessels behave differently than the integral of the peripheral vascular beds.

KRONEBERG: For me, as a pharmacologist, "specificity" means that you get the primary effect with the lowest dose. If you increase the dose you also get, of course, other effects so I understand that specificity is the relationship between the effect of the lowest dose in comparison with the effect of higher doses. You can define specificity only if you compare dose response curves.

KIRCHHEIM: I agree, but my comment on kidney and muscle blood flow is based on a comparison of dose response curves; we found a difference between the two vascular areas with supramaximal doses.

The Chemistry of Nifedipine

F. BOSSERT

Pharma Research Center, Bayer AG, Wuppertal, Fed. Rep. Germany

The increase in cardiovascular disorders during the last twenty years has lead, understandably, to an intensification of research in this field.

Of special interest were the various symptoms of coronary insufficiency, because no specifically active compound was available for the treatment of such cases.

The discovery of the coronary dilation activity of khellin in the Langendorff heart test was a great stimulus for further studies and investigations [4].

Many groups of workers, therefore, used khellin as the starting point in programs designed to develop synthetic compounds, that were more active. One possibility is the elimination of the furan ring and its replacement by a carboxy-ester group. This leads to readily obtainable chromone and coumarin derivatives of the general formulas shown in Fig. 1. Some compounds representative of this class have already been introduced into therapeutic practice. They have, however, the general disadvantage that satisfactory coronary dilation is achieved only by parenteral administration. Our own research target was therefore clear. In addition to improving the coronary activity, we had to develop a compound that could be taken orally in order to make reasonable prophylactic therapy possible.

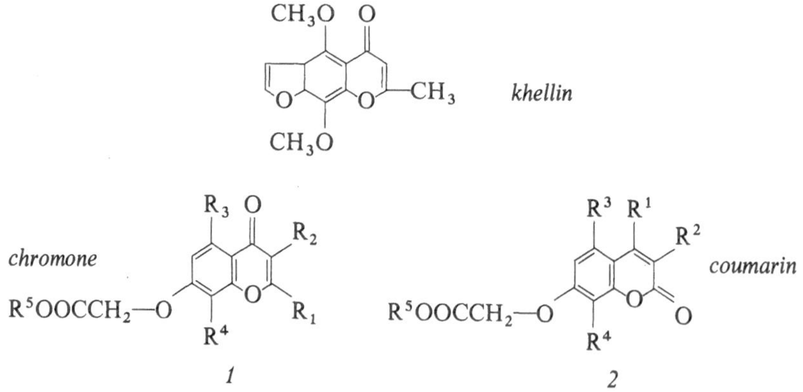

Fig. 1

We first tackled this problem by varying the heteroatom in the six-membered heterocyclic ring. By this means a favorable change in the metabolization of the compounds could follow. In Fig. 2, this scheme is presented more generally.

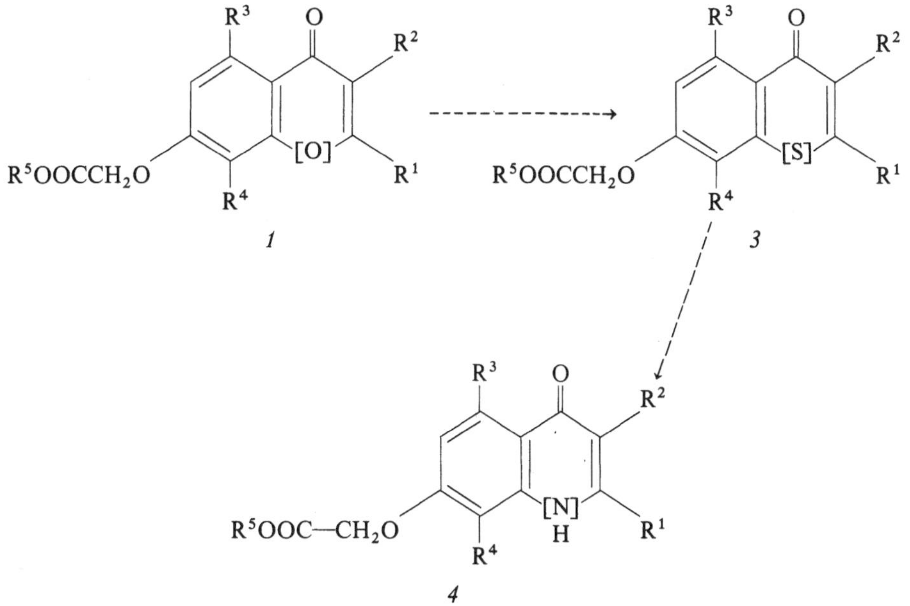

Fig. 2

Substitution of the oxygen atom by sulphur leads to the thiochromones (3); by nitrogen to the quinolones (4).

In both classes we obtained highly coronary-active compounds, which were, however, only effective on parenteral administration. Still, our initial presumption had been corroborated. The coronary activity was not restricted to chromone and coumarin derivatives but was probably a general property of a six-membered heterocyclic system with two double bonds, and a carboxyester group to aid adsorption and elimination.

More precise studies of the metabolization of these compound-classes showed clearly that the first step was the rapid saponification of the ester group yielding the inactive carboxylic acid. This reaction was so rapid that, by oral administration, no active serum levels could be obtained.

The next move in the synthetic program followed logically: the introduction into the molecule of such carboxylic ester functions as were known to be resistant to hydrolysis. Examples are shown in Fig. 3.

Sterically hindered esters of type (5) are known to be resistant to normal saponification conditions, the ester group being screened by the substituents R_1 und R_2. Also resistant are amido-carboxylic esters (6) where the electronic effect of the nitrogen hinders attack at the carbonyl carbon atom. This is also the case for the vinylogous esters (7).

Returning now to consider the general structure (4) (Fig. 4), we can see that both principles, namely steric hinderance by R_1 and the carbonyl group, and the presence of a vinylogous amide-carboxylic ester, may be realized if R_2 is a carboxylic ester group.

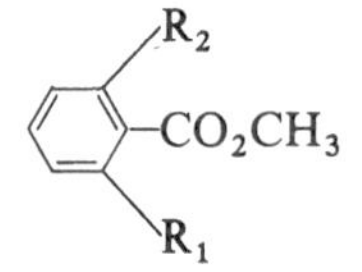

5

sterically hindered carboxylic ester

$-NH-CO_2CH_3$

6

amido-carboxylic ester

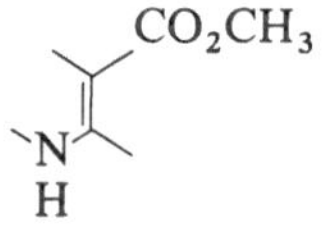

7

vinylogous amido-carboxylic ester

Fig. 3

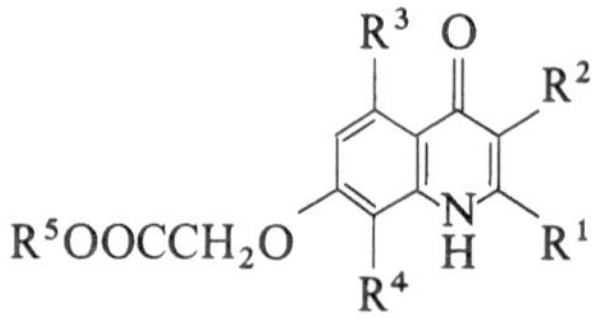

4

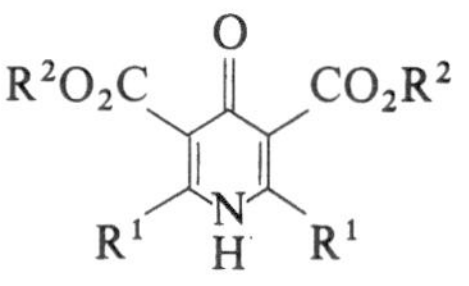

8

Fig. 4

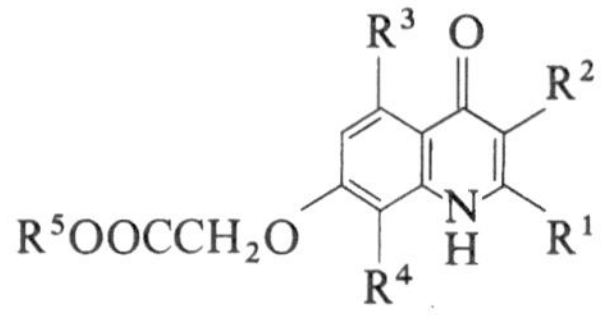

4

quinolone

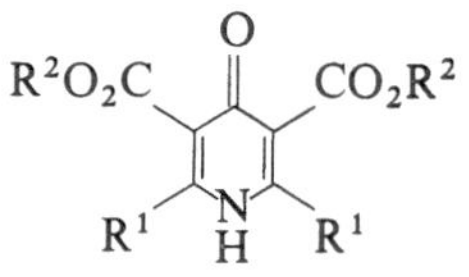

8

pyridone

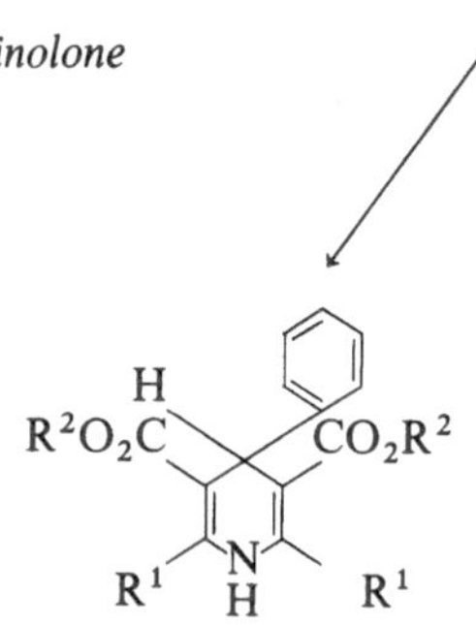

9

1,4-dihydropyridine

Fig. 5

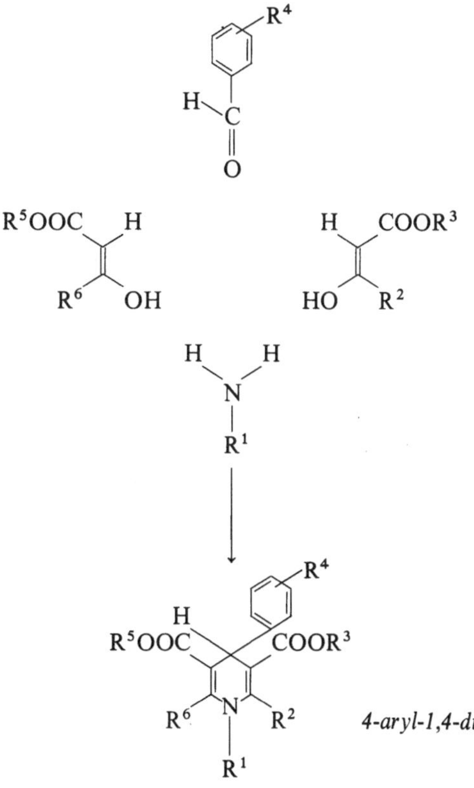

Fig. 6

At first we also removed the second ring and synthesized the readily available pyridone derivatives (8), which contained this "ester principle" twice over. These compounds were, however, totally inactive in the coronary test. Evidently the reduction of the molecular size had gone too far.

For an increase in the molecular size, the dihydropyridines (9) (Fig. 5) offered the opportunity to re-introduce in another position the aromatic residue removed from the quinolone (4). These dihydropyridines were synthesized according to the Hantzsch method [2, 3]—the reaction of a benzaldehyde with β-ketoesters and ammonia or an amine (Fig. 6).

In fact these 4-aryl-1,4-dihydropyridines had the desired properties: coronary activity and effectiveness also by oral administration.

Because the residues R_1–R_4 may be widely varied, the HANTZSCH synthesis allows the preparation of a very large number of different 1,4-dihydropyridines.

Of the 2000 derivatives synthesized to date, a great number have been more closely investigated. Of special interest was the 2-nitrophenyl derivative BAY a 1040—nifedipine [1] (Fig. 7).

It must be emphasized that the nitro group attached to the phenyl ring in this compound is in no way to be compared with the nitrates used in the treatment of angina pectoris, which are relatively labile esters of nitrous acid and are often falsely referred to as nitro compounds. The nitro group in nifedipine serves only

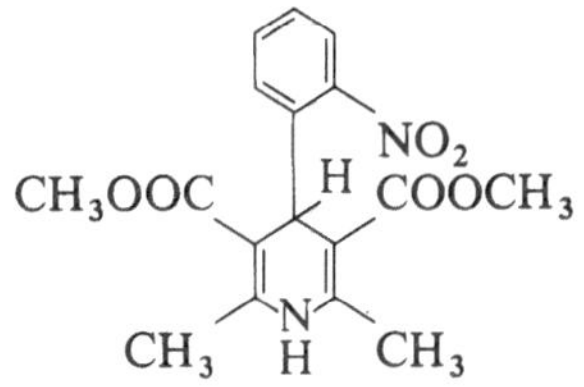

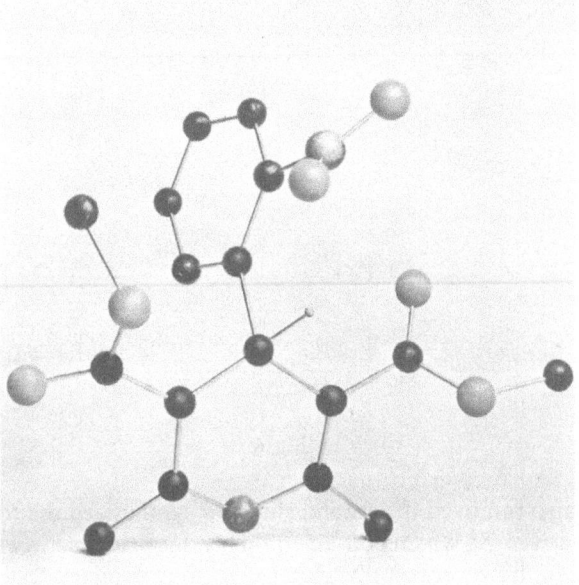

CH₃OOC, H, COOCH₃ (structure)

BAY a 1040 –*nifedipine-Adalat*

Fig. 7

Fig. 8

to optimize the physicochemical parameters and has nothing to do with the special pharmacological properties of the 1,4-dihydropyridine system. 1,4-dihydropyridines without the nitro group also have, of course, coronary activity.

The spatial proximity of the nitro group to the carboxylic ester group leads to the presumption that a fully planar arrangement of the whole molecule is impossible. This has been proved by X-ray analysis. As shown in Fig. 8 the dihydropyridine ring is planar, while the benzene ring is rotated so far that the ester and nitro groups are the maximum possible distance apart.

1,4-dihydropyridines are in many respects an interesting class of compounds. They are components of hydrogen transfer enzyme systems in biological processes, because the change from the 1,4-dihydropyridine to the pyridine system is easily effected. This property plays no part in the activity of nifedipine, however, although nifedipine irradiation *in vitro* forms the corresponding pyridine deriva-

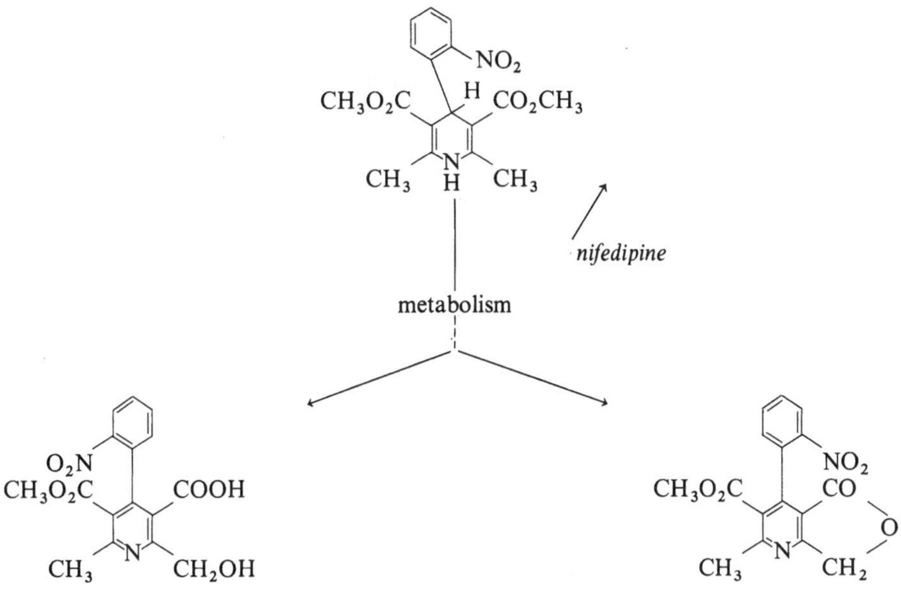

Fig. 9

.ive. This pyridine derivative is no longer biologically active, and therefore nifedipine must always be protected from light upon storage.

Nifedipine is also converted to the inactive pyridine system *in vivo*. However, the same degradation products are not obtained as *in vitro* (Fig. 9).

The main metabolites are a hydroxymethyl-pyridine carboxylic acid (*10*) and the corresponding lactone (*11*) [5]. The fact that only a carboxylic ester is saponified to the acid *in vivo* is in good agreement with our original concept of the introduction of hydrolysis-resistant ester groups.

The structure of both metabolites has been confirmed by synthesis.

Abstract

In 1,4-dihydropyridines the author found a potent coronary dilator. The chemically, readily available 1,4-dihydropyridines had until then not been pharmacologically or therapeutically studied. Due to their coronary dilatory effect they represent a completely new class of substances.

Methyl-1,4-dihydro-2,6-dimethyl-4-(2-nitrophenyl)-3,5-pyridine dicarboxylate (nifedipine) proved to be the most interesting and effective of those compounds.

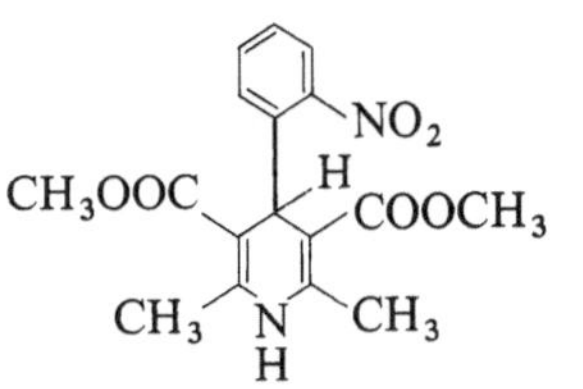

BAY a 1040 nifedipine

Chemically, there is no similarity between nifedipine and the other, already known coronary effective compounds, in particular nitrates.

Nifedipine is rapidly metabolized in the body and excreted mainly as a hydroxymethyl-pyridine-carboxylic acid.

References

1. Bossert, F., Vater, W.: Naturw. **58**, 578 (1971).
2. Eisner, U., Kuthan, J.: Chem. Reviews **72**, 1 (1972).
3. Hantzsch, A.: Liebigs Ann. Chem. **215**, 1 (1882).
4. Huttrer, C. P., Dale, E.: Chem. Reviews **48**, 543 (1951).
5. Medenwald, H., Schlossmann, K., Wünsche, C.: Arzneim. Forschung (Drug Res.) **22**, 53–56 (1972).

Pharmacokinetics of Adalat in Animal Experiments

K. PATZSCHKE, B. DUHM, W. MAUL, H. MEDENWALD, and L. A. WEGNER

Isotopen-Institut der Bayer AG, Wuppertal 1, Fed. Rep. Germany

The clinical efficacy and tolerance of a drug are closely related to its pharma-cokinetic behavior. This study investigated the pharmacokinetic properties of Adalat (nifedipine, BAY a 1040, dimethyl 1,4-dihydro-2,6-dimethyl-4-(o-nitro-phenyl)-3,5-pyridinedicarboxylate) in animal experiments [1].

For the detection of the substance and its metabolites in biological material radioactive methods were used. Figure 1 shows the chemical structure of Adalat. The positions of the labelled carbon ^{14}C atoms are marked by asterisks. During the biotransformation of the compound they remain part of the metabolites. By measuring the radioactivity we determined the amount of the unchanged radioac-tive compound and its metabolites simultaneously.

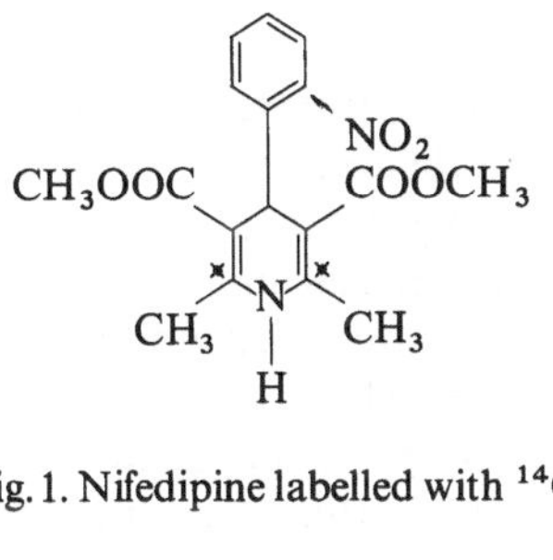

Fig. 1. Nifedipine labelled with ^{14}C

The animal experiments were carried out in rats and dogs. The rats received 0.03 to 3 mg labelled nifedipine per kg body weight either enterally or parenter-ally. This dose range covers the usual oral human dose.

In Fig. 2 the absorption and excretion processes are shown in the form of a block diagram: on the left is the digestive tract with stomach, small and large intestines and on the right, the sum of the other organs.

After oral administration via a stomach tube the absorption from the stomach was rather small. The substance was almost completely absorbed from the small intestine. Of the absorbed activity or the intravenously administered activity, 50 to 60% was excreted via the liver and bile into the intestinal tract.

A portion of approx. 20% was reabsorbed. Thus an enterohepatic circulation was present. The greater part of the activity eliminated via the bile was excreted with the feces. The portion not absorbed after oral administration was less than 10%.

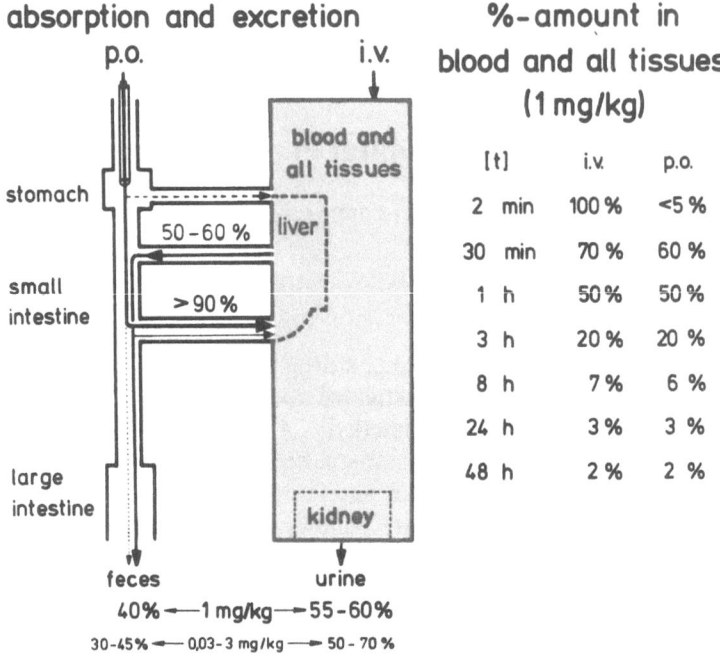

Fig. 2. Absorption and excretion of nifedipine-^{14}C in the rat (block diagram)

After oral or intravenous administration of 1 mg/kg nifedipine-^{14}C, a total of approx. 40% was excreted via the feces and approx. 60% via the kidneys. Within the dose range of 0.03 to 3 mg/kg the renal excretion varied between 50 and 70% while fecal excretion varied between 30 and 45%.

After intravenous administration the amount of activity in all tissues decreased rapidly due to renal and biliary excretion. Following oral administration the activity measured in the body, excluding the gastro-intestinal tract, was approx. 60% after 30 min. Because, at this time, a portion of the activity had already been excreted via the liver and kidneys, the absorption rate must have been higher. At 1 h after administration and later, the amounts of activity present were the same for each application route. The absorption was more than 90%. Forty-eight h after treatment, the activity-content in the animals was only approx. 2%.

In Fig. 3 the courses of concentrations of activity are shown for various organs in relation to time covering a period of 4 h. The ordinate axis represents the relative activity concentration. A "P" value of 1 corresponds to an equivalent concentration of 1 µg/g tissue.

The courses of the concentration curves were similar for all organs. Due to the rapid start of the absorption, maximal values were already achieved 10 to 30 min after oral administration. According to these curves the half-life for the elimination was 1 to 2 h.

The whole-body autoradiograms in Fig. 4 demonstrate the distribution of the activity after intravenous administration of nifedipine-^{14}C. The intensity of the darkening on the autoradiograms represents the activity in the organs and tissues

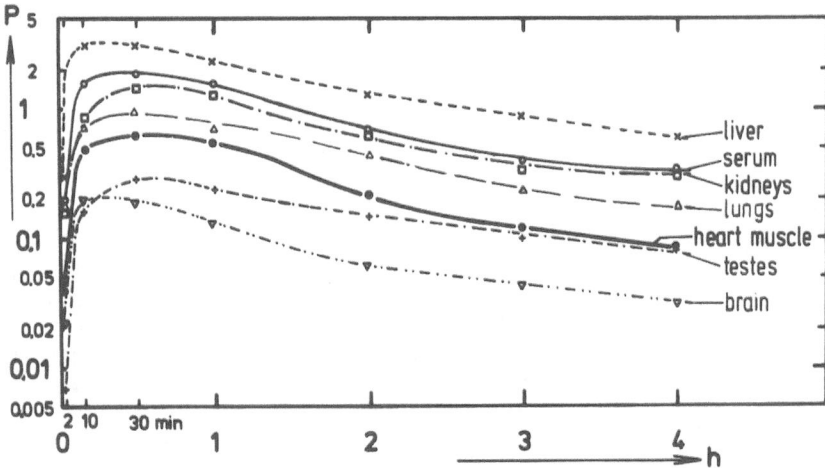

Fig. 3. Relative concentrations "P" in the organs of the rat after oral administration of 1 mg/kg nifedipine-[14]C

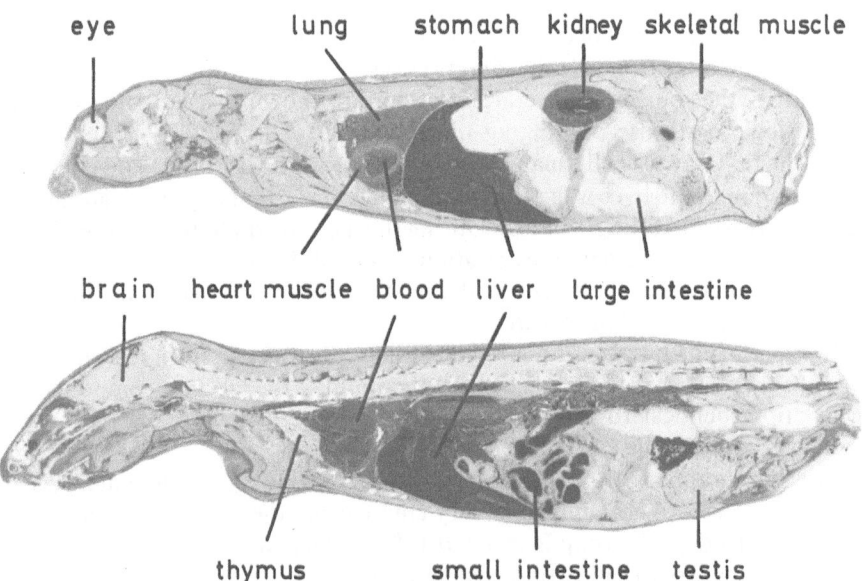

Fig. 4. Whole-body autoradiograms 1 h after intravenous administration of 3 mg/kg nifedipine-[14]C

of the animal. Increased concentrations—such as shown in the curves in Fig. 3 after oral administration—were present in liver, kidneys and blood. The high concentrations in some parts of the small intestine and in the urinary bladder were induced by biliary and renal excretion. It is remarkable that the concentration in the heart muscle was higher than in the skeletal muscles. By measuring the blood-content of the heart muscle using ^{51}Cr-labelled erythrocytes, one can esti-

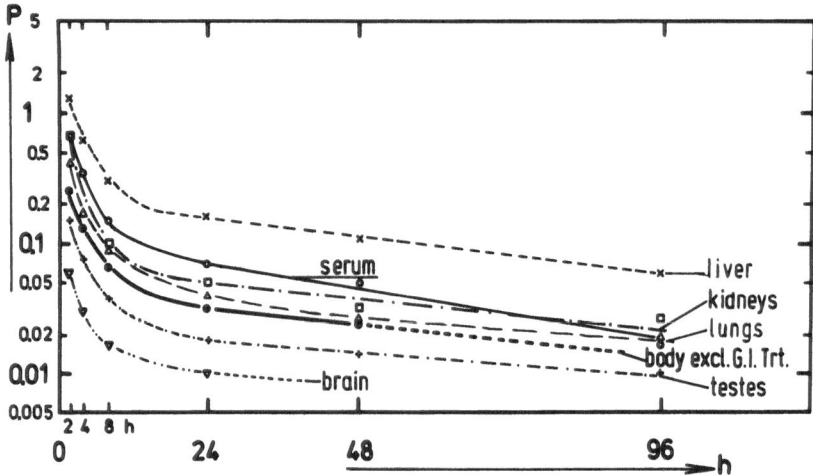

Fig. 5. Relative concentrations "P" in the organs of the rat after oral administration of 1 mg/kg nifedipine-^{14}C

mate that more than half of the carbon-^{14}C activity in the heart was located in the tissue of the heart, i.e. outside the blood vessels.

In Fig. 5, the courses of the concentrations are shown over a period of 4 days after a single oral dose of 1 mg/kg nifedipine-^{14}C. The activity not eliminated within the first day was eliminated with a half-life of 2 to 3 days. The equivalent concentration in the liver was rather high. However, 2 to 4 days after administration, it decreased to 0.1 µg/g or less. During this period whole-body autoradiography did not reveal a higher concentration in any of the other tissues. Therefore it may be concluded that there is no evidence of a selective storage of nifedipine and its metabolites in any of the organs.

In experiments on dogs, 1 mg/kg nifedipine-^{14}C was administered orally. The dogs of group A received gelatin capsules containing the labelled compound in a formulation identical to that used in clinical trials. Group B received gelatin capsules containing the crystalline compound.

In group A approx. 70% of the administered activity was eliminated via the kidneys. Taking into account the biliary elimination, the absorption was greater than 90%. The dogs of group B excreted 15% of the administered activity via the kidneys. In this case the absorption was approx. 20%.

The curves in Fig. 6 show the equivalent plasma concentrations of both groups. After administration of the optimal formulation, maximal values were achieved earlier and were 10 times higher than those obtained after administration of the crystalline substance. The areas below the curves representing a relative measure of the amount of absorption differ by a factor of 5 to 6. These results clearly show the influence of the formulation on the bioavailability of the substance.

In another experiment on 3 dogs [2], the coronary effect of the substance was recorded by measuring the oxygen tension in the coronary sinus blood. Simultaneously, the equivalent concentrations were determined in the arterial plasma.

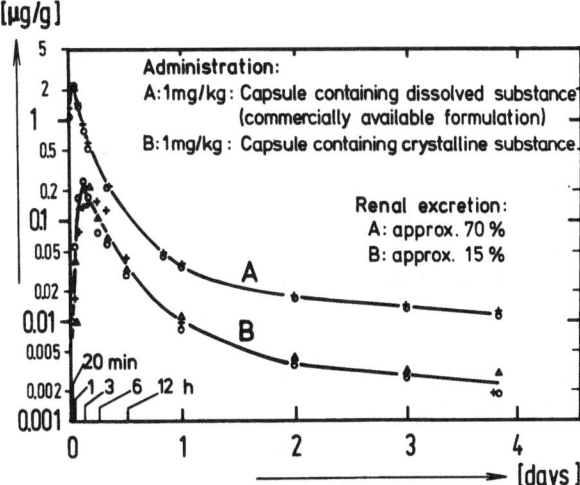

Fig. 6. Equivalent concentrations in plasma and renal excretion in rats after oral administration of 1 mg/kg nifedipine-^{14}C in two different formulations

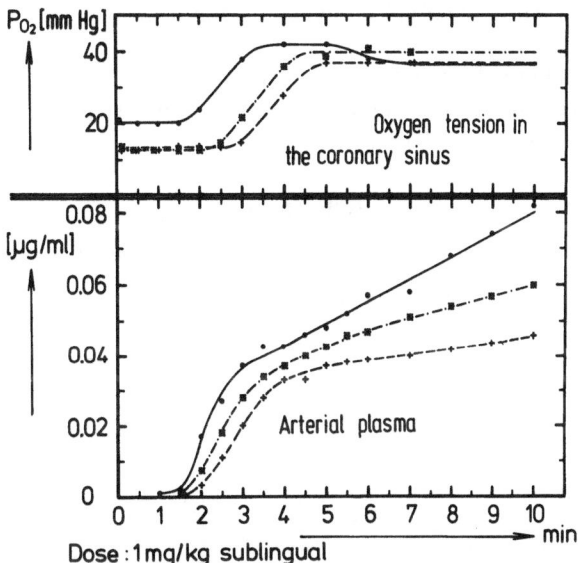

Fig. 7. Coronary oxygen tension and equivalent concentration in the plasma of 3 dogs after sublingual administration of 1 mg/kg nifedipine-[14]C

In this case the animals received a sublingual dose of 1 mg/kg labelled nifedipine (Fig. 7). As early as 2 to 3 min after administration, the coronary oxygen tension increased. During this time an equivalent concentration of approx. 0.02 µg/ml was present in the arterial plasma. When maximal oxygen tension was reached the equivalent concentration was 0.04 to 0.05 µg/ml. That means that even very small concentrations of drug are sufficient to produce a pharmacody-namic effect.

Abstract

The pharmacokinetics of Adalat labelled with carbon-^{14}C were studied in rats (0.03 to 3 mg/kg) and dogs (1 mg/kg).

In rats more than 90% of the orally administered substance was absorbed. Of the orally or intravenously administered activity, 50 to 70% was excreted via the kidneys and 30 to 50% via the feces. The activity-content in the tissues (body excluding gastro-intestinal tract), 48 h after administration, was approx. 2%.

In the organs, maximal concentrations were determined 10 to 30 min after oral administration. One hour after oral or intravenous administration the courses of the concentration curves for the various organs were similar. Temporarily increased concentrations were detected in the liver, serum and kidneys. Low concentrations were found in the brain, testes and skeletal muscles. At later times after administration, whole-body autoradiography revealed no evidence of a selective storage of Adalat or its metabolites.

In dogs, approx. 70% of the orally administered activity was excreted via the kidneys. In the plasma, maximal equivalent concentrations were achieved after approx. 30 min.

Two minutes after sublingual administration, measurable concentrations were present in the arterial plasma. The concentration range required to increase the coronary oxygen tension was 0.02 to 0.05 µg/ml.

References

1. DUHM, B., MAUL, W., MEDENWALD, H., PATZSCHKE, K., WEGNER, L. A.: Arzneim.-Forsch. (Drug Res.) **22**, 42–53 (1972).
2. VATER, W., PATZSCHKE, K., WEGNER, L. A.: in press.

Investigations on the Metabolism
and Protein Binding of Nifedipine

K. Schlossmann, H. Medenwald, and H. Rosenkranz

Forschungslaboratorien der Bayer AG, Leverkusen und Wuppertal-1, Fed. Rep. Germany

Introduction

Studies in man, dog, and rat showed that nifedipine is almost completely absorbed [2, 3]. Excretion is mainly renal. The urine contains only traces of the unchanged substance, which means that nifedipine is transformed in the body and eliminated in metabolized form.

The aim of the present study was to analyze the metabolism of nifedipine and to assess the protein binding of the drug.

Methods

All experiments were carried out with daylight excluded, using sodium vapor lamps. Urine was collected from rats and dogs treated with ^{14}C-labelled or non-radioactive substance [4].

High-voltage electrophoresis was carried out on the "Original Frankfurt"-equipment, Fa. Hormuth-Vetter, using paper Nr. 2043b (Schleicher u. Schüll) and the buffer "pyridine-acetic acid-water 10:1:89 (pH 6.2)".

The mobile phase for thin-layer chromatography on silica gel was toluene-acetic acid-water 5:5:1 (organic phase). R_f values: nifedipine 0.40; "free acid" 0.10; lactone 0.50.

Urine and plasma were extracted with ethyl acetate.

The determination of ^{14}C-nifedipine in plasma of rats was conducted as follows:

After extraction by organic solvent and evaporation of the solvent, the residue was taken up in 0.2 ml ethanol. An aliquot of 0.1 ml was used for thin-layer chromatography. The spots detected by autoradiography were scraped off, and the substances were eluted from the silica gel by leaving over night with 1.3 ml ethanol. Subsequently 5 ml water and 10 ml "Insta Gel" (Packard Instrument Comp.) were added, and the radioactivity was measured in liquid scintillation counter.

The efficacy of the metabolites was investigated in mongrel dogs (15–18 kg). After intravenous administration of the substances, the oxygen saturation was estimated in the coronary sinus [9].

The extent of protein binding of nifedipine and its main metabolite was assessed by the ultracentrifuge method [8] (ultracentrifuge L 50, Beckman Instruments Inc.; rotor 40/3; 40 000 U/min $= 142 000$ g; temp. $20°$ C; 15 h). The concentrations of unbound nifedipine were estimated fluorometrically [6] or by liquid scintillation counting (^{14}C-nifedipine).

Results and Discussion

Studies on the metabolism of nifedipine were performed by evaluating the concentrations of the unchanged substance and its metabolites occurring in the rat plasma and in the urine of rats and dogs.

High-voltage electrophoresis of the original urine or of organic solvent extracts of the urine showed that, whatever the dose, the main renal metabolite eliminated is an acid. Thin-layer chromatography revealed the presence of a second metabolite.

To clarify their structures, the metabolites were concentrated and purified by thin-layer chromatography, and examined spectroscopically. The final structures of the two metabolites were defined by means of mass spectrography as well as by IR spectra and NMR spectra [4].

In contrast to nifedipine, which is a dihydropyridine derivative, both metabolites were identified as pyridine derivatives (Fig. 1). The main metabolite is is a hydroxycarboxylic acid, the second metabolite has a lactone structure. In aqueous solution a pH-dependent equilibrium exists between the two metabolites. At acid pH the formation of the lactone is favored whereas in alkaline medium the acid form predominates.

The lactone was synthesized in order to confirm the structure of this metabolite and its hydrolytic product, the "free acid" [1]. The synthetic compound was found to be identical with the metabolite isolated from the urine of rats and dogs.

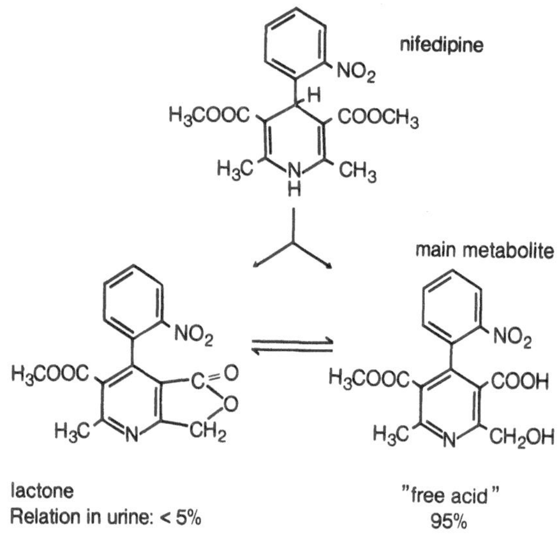

Fig. 1. Structure of nifedipine and its metabolites

Table 1. Concentration of nifedipine and the sum of its metabolites ("free acid" and lactone) in plasma of rats. Dose: 5 mg ^{14}C-nifedipine/kg P. O.

time p. appl. [min]	nifedipine [μg/ml]	metabolites "free acid" + lactone [μg/ml]
30	2.5	1.6
120	1.0	1.2

In investigations with ^{14}C-labelled nifedipine, MEDENWALD et al. [4] have shown that the rat and dog urine collected over a period of 24 h contains very small amounts of the unchanged substance.

Our experiments demonstrated that in contrast to urine the rat plasma contains considerable amounts of unchanged nifedipine after oral administration. Thirty minutes after administration of 5 mg/kg, the plasma concentration of the unchanged nifedipine was 2.5 μg/ml (Table 1), representing 60% of the determined substances (nifedipine plus metabolites). Two hours after oral administration, the unchanged nifedipine represented only 45% of the determined substances.

Since rat and dog form the same metabolites, a similar metabolic pathway is to be expected for nifedipine in *man*. In studies in human subjects, an acid has been found which, according to high-voltage-electrophoresis and thin-layer chromatography, showed the same characteristics as the main metabolite isolated from the urine of dog and rat.

An essential question in studies of the biotransformation of drugs is whether metabolites exhibit pharmacologic activity. Both the metabolites isolated from urine and the synthetic product were investigated in dogs. The dose required for an increase of oxygen in the coronary sinus blood of the dogs by 30 saturation-percent (ED) was measured [10]. After intravenous administration the efficacy of the "free acid" and the lactone is 1000-fold weaker, as compared to nifedipine (Table 2).

It is of interest that oxidation of nifedipine to the respective pyridine-derivative leads to a remarkable diminution of the pharmacologic potency (Table 2, substance BAY b 4759). Since the main metabolite is also a pyridine derivative the loss of activity during metabolization is probably due to oxidation of the dihydropyridine ring to the pyridine ring rather than to ester hydrolysis.

Because polarographic investigations *in vitro* [7] have demonstrated that the dihydropyridine derivative nifedipine and its oxidation product, the pyridine derivative BAY b 4759, are not considered to be a reversible redox pair, the reduction of the pyridine to the dihydropyridine structure seems to be unlikely under *in vivo* conditions.

Apart from the metabolic fate, the pharmacodynamics of a drug are influenced by the extent of protein binding. The protein binding of nifedipine was determined over a concentration range covering 4 powers of ten [5]. In Fig. 2 the concentration of bound substance (c_g) is plotted against the concentration of free, unbound substance (c_f) on a double logarithmic scale for human and dog serum.

Table 2. Efficacy of nifedipine, its metabolites and the oxidation product of nifedipine. Dose required to increase the oxygen saturation by 30% absolute (ED) in the coronary sinus blood

	structure	ED [mg/kg] i. v.
nifedipine		0.005
main metabolite		
"free acid"		> 5
lactone		5
BAY b 4759		>3

If the gradient of the straight line had a value of $m = 1$, the binding would be independent of the drug concentration. Because the m-values calculated from Fig. 2 differ from unity ($m = 0.78$ and 0.89), this indicates that the extent of protein binding depends on the nifedipine concentration. At a total nifedipine concentration of 2 mg/100 ml, 92% of the substance is bound to the proteins of the human serum and 89% to those of dog serum. At a nifedipine concentration of 0.02 mg/100 ml, 98 and 93% respectively are bound to human or dog serum.

Further experiments were carried out using serum albumin. With a 4% solution of human serum albumin and a nifedipine concentration of 2 mg/100 ml, 88% of the substance was bound, indicating that in human serum the substance is mainly bound by the albumin.

However, other protein fractions also have a relatively intense binding capacity for nifedipine. At a protein concentration of 1%, nifedipine is more strongly bound by α_1-lipoprotein than by albumin (Table 3).

The binding of nifedipine to β-globulin was determined at the β-globulin concentration of 0.1%, due to the low solubility of this protein fraction. Even at this low protein concentration, 42% of nifedipine is bound to β-globulin.

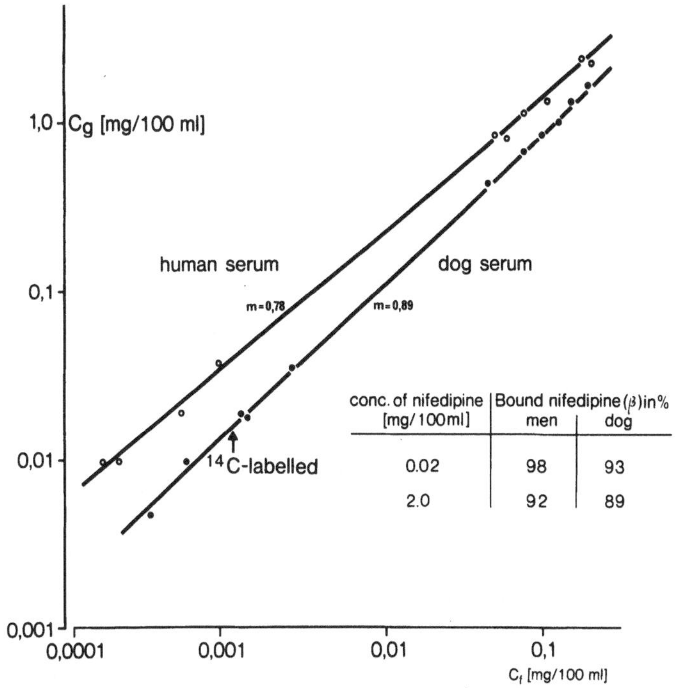

Fig. 2. Binding capacity of human and dog serum for nifedipine. c_g = bound nifedipine. c_f = free, unbound nifedipine [mg/100 ml]. m = the gradient. $\beta = \frac{c_g}{c_g + c_f}$ [%]

Table 3. Binding capacity of protein fractions of human and dog serum for nifedipine. nifedipine conc.: 2 mg/100 ml. β = percentage of bound nifedipine. K_1 = binding constant = $1/c_p \times (c_g/c_f) c_g \rightarrow 0$. c_p = protein concentration [mol/l]

Protein	Protein conc. [g/100 ml]	Man		Dog	
		β [%]	$K_1 \cdot 10^{-3}$ [l/mol]	β [%]	$K_1 \cdot 10^{-3}$ [l/mol]
albumin	1	51	6.9	51	6.9
α_1-lipoprotein	1	86	126	82	100
β-lipoprotein	1	46	320	35	212
β-globulin	0.1	42	132	42	120
γ-globulin	1	10	1.6	10	1.6

There is no difference between the binding capacity of human and dog serum albumin. However, the β-lipoprotein fraction of human serum has a stronger binding capacity than the respective fraction of the dog serum (Table 3).

The fact that nifedipine is extensively bound to serum proteins probably contributes to the drug's long duration of action. The main metabolite in its acid form is bound to a lesser extent than the unchanged substance. As can be seen from Fig. 3, 92% of nifedipine but only 54% of the metabolite is bound to human serum.

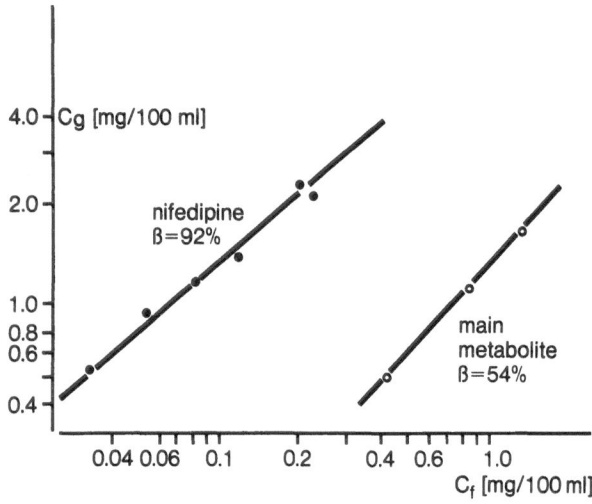

Fig. 3. Protein binding of nifedipine and its main metabolite in human serum. c_g and c_f, see

$$\text{Fig. 2 [mg/100 ml]. } \beta = \frac{c_g}{c_g + c_f} [\%]$$

Conclusions

Nifedipine is transformed to one main metabolite, which occurs in two forms: a hydroxycarboxylic acid and the corresponding lactone. The acid form is mainly excreted by the urine. Protein binding of nifedipine exceeds 90%, whereas binding of the metabolite is 54%. The metabolite, a pyridine derivative, exhibits no pharmacologic activity.

Abstract

Nifedipine is almost completely metabolized in rat, dog and man. The main metabolite, 2-hydroxymethyl-5-methoxycarbonyl-6-methyl-4-(o-nitrophenyl)-pyridine-3-carboxylic acid (referred to as "free acid") was isolated from the urine of rats and dogs. A second excretory product is the corresponding lactone. A pH-dependent equilibrium exists between the "free acid" and the lactone. The two metabolite forms were subsequently synthesized and their structures thereby confirmed.

The amounts of the unchanged nifedipine and its metabolites were measured in rat plasma 30 min and two hours after administration. At those times a considerable part of the administered substance remained unchanged (60%, 30 min and 45%, two hours after administration).

Both the "free acid" and the lactone are pharmacologically inactive.

Nifedipine is strongly bound to serum proteins. This binding is dependent on the drug concentration. In concentrations ranging from 0.02 mg/100 ml to 2 mg/100 ml, 98–92% of the nifedipine is bound to the proteins of human serum and

93–89% to the proteins of dog serum. The binding capacity of serum is mainly due to albumin.

The "free acid" is not bound to the same extent (54% at a concentration of 2 mg/100 ml human serum).

References

1. BOSSERT, F.: Vortragstagung der Gesellschaft Deutscher Chemiker, Fachgruppe Medizin, Bad Nauheim, Nov. 1972.
2. DUHM, B., MAUL, W., MEDENWALD, H., PATZSCHKE, K., WEGNER, L.: Arzneim.-Forsch. (Drug Res.) **22**, 42 (1972).
3. HORSTER, F. A., DUHM, B., MAUL, W., MEDENWALD, H., PATZSCHKE, K., WEGNER, L.: Arzneim.-Forsch. (Drug Res.) **22**, 330 (1972).
4. MEDENWALD, H., SCHLOSSMANN, K., WÜNSCHE, C.: Arzneim.-Forsch. (Drug Res.) **22**, 53 (1972).
5. ROSENKRANZ, H., SCHLOSSMANN, K., SCHOLTAN, W.: Arzneim.-Forsch. (Drug Res.) **24**, 455 (1974).
6. SCHLOSSMANN, K.: Arzneim.-Forsch. (Drug Res.) **22**, 60 (1972).
7. SCHLOSSMANN, K., HARZDORF, C.: unpublished results (1972).
8. SCHOLTAN, W.: Arzneim.-Forsch. (Drug Res.) **15**, 1433 (1965).
9. VATER, W., KRONEBERG, G., HOFFMEISTER, F., KALLER, H., MENG, K., OBERDORF, A., PULS, W., SCHLOSSMANN, K., STOEPEL, K.: Arzneim.-Forsch. (Drug Res.) **22**, 1 (1972).
10. VATER, W.: unpublished results (1974).

Discussion Remarks

KERN: You mentioned in the last part of your paper that the metabolite had no pharmacologic action. Would this mean that there is perhaps a possibility of going to the molecular action of these compounds? For example, to the molecular action on the membrane of the heart muscle cells? There must be a stereochemical arrangement for receptor and drug reaction on this calcium level.

SCHLOSSMANN: We have found that the dihydropyridine structure is typical for the effect of this compound and we have found no effects with pyridine compounds. Only with very high doses are there slight effects with the metabolites.

Experimental Pharmacological Investigations of Effects of Nifedipine on Atrioventricular Conduction in Comparison with Those of Other Coronary Vasodilators

N. Taira, S. Motomura, A. Narimatsu, and T. Iijima

Department of Pharmacology and Experimental Therapeutics, Tohoku University School of Medicine, Sendai, Japan

Introduction

Pharmacological investigations carried out so far on the cardiovascular actions of nifedipine (Adalat) (Vater et al. [10]; Hashimoto et al. [6]) have revealed that nifedipine is the most potent coronary vasodilator ever synthesized. The mechanism of its vasodilator action has been ascribed to the calcium antagonistic action: inhibition of the transmembrane calcium influx of the vascular smooth muscle to reduce the tone (Fleckenstein et al. [3]; Grün and Fleckenstein [4]). On the other hand, it has been suggested that the ionic channel operative in excitation of cells in the atrioventricular (A-V) junctional area concerned in the major delay of A-V conduction is a slow channel which allows the transmembrane inflow of calcium, sodium ions or both (Zipes and Mendez [12]). A coronary vasodilator, verapamil, the mechanism of action of which has also been described as that of calcium antagonism (Grün and Fleckenstein [4]), is able to block this slow channel and cause impairment of A-V conduction (Zipes and Fischer [11]). From a therapeutic point of view, however, the impairment of A-V conduction by coronary vasodilators is one of their untoward effects. Thus, it is worthy to examine whether nifedipine as a potent calcium antagonist might impair A-V conduction. The present study was carried out in an attempt to elucidate this point. To characterize the effect of nifedipine on A-V conduction, comparison was made with those of other coronary vasodilators—verapamil, diltiazem (Sato et al. [9]), dipyridamole and dilazep. Diltiazem is thought to dilate the coronary vascular bed probably by a calcium antagonistic action (Kiyomoto, personal communication), whereas dilazep is thought to do so by potentiation of the action of endogenous adenosine (Buyniski et al. [2]) like dipyridamole (Bretschneider et al. [1]).

Materials and Methods

Experiments were carried out on *in situ* hearts of open-chest dogs weighing about 10 kg, anesthetized with sodium pentobarbital, 30 mg/kg i.v., and maintained on artificial respiration. After the sinus node area had been destroyed, the right atrium was paced at a rate of 150 beats/min with rectangular pulses of 2–6 V (3 times threshold voltage) and of 1 msec duration through bipolar stimulating electrodes sutured on the right auricle. Atrial (A) and ventricular (V) bipolar elec- trograms were picked up with recording electrodes sutured on the right auricle and ventricular apex. The atrial and ventricular electrograms were fed to an A-V interval counter (Data-Graph, NH-110) and to an electronic apparatus (Data- Graph, HT-11) which measures automatically the functional refractory period of the A-V conduction system (FRP). Both apparatuses were developed originally in our laboratories in collaboration with Data-Graph Co. Ltd., Tokyo. The A-V interval counter measures the A-V conduction time with an analysis pitch of 1 msec, indicates values digitally every minute, and has an analogue output for a pen-recorder. The apparatus for the measurement of the FRP consists of the programmed stimulator, the counter and display units. The programmed stimula- tor generates a sequence of test stimuli S′ in every 7 regular stimuli S, and the counter unit measures A-A′ and V-V′ intervals with an analysis pitch of 1 msec, indicates the two values digitally and displays A-A′ interval versus V-V′ interval relations graphically on a cathode ray oscilloscope screen of the display unit. A′ and V′ are atrial and ventricular electrograms elicited by a test stimulus S′. The image of an A-A′ interval versus V-V′ interval curve displayed as a curved line of dots was recorded by means of a Polaroid camera. Figure 1 shows diagrammati- cally the devices for measuring the two parameters. Triangular excursions of records of the A-V conduction time on a chart in the lower right corner of Fig. 1 and in the following figures were caused by test stimuli delivered for the measure- ment of the FRP. The FRP is defined as the minimum V-V′ interval (KRAYER et al. [8]). Drug effects on A-V conduction were evaluated from changes in the A-V conduction time and the FRP. The FRP was measured when the effect of a given dose of a drug on the A-V conduction time reached a peak.

Nifedipine (Bayer AG, solution in ampule), verapamil hydrochloride (Knoll AG), diltiazem hydrochloride (Tanabe Pharmaceutical Co.), dipyridamole (C.H. Boeringer Sohn, Ingelheim, solution in ampule) and dilazep dihydrochlo-

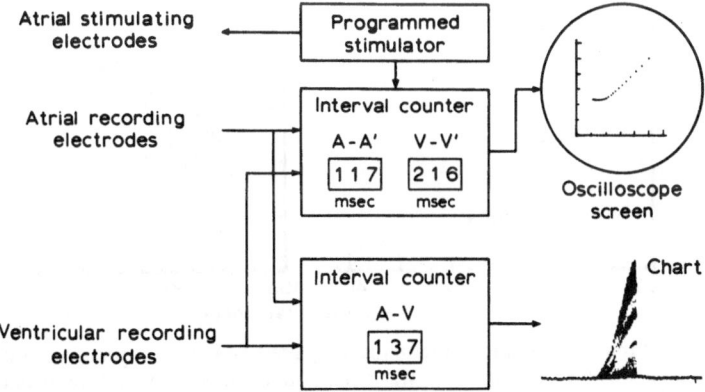

Fig. 1. Schematic diagram of the devices for measuring the A-V conduction time and the functional refractory period of the A-V conduction system (FRP). Further explanation is in text

ride monohydrate (Asta AG) were used. All drugs except nifedipine and dipyridamole were dissolved in 0.9% saline and all drug solutions were diluted with 0.9%
saline. The drug solutions were injected into a rubber cannula inserted into the
femoral vein and flushed in with 2 ml of 0.9% saline for 8 sec. Doses are expressed
in terms of bases.

Results

1. Nifedipine

The A-V conduction time and the functional refractory period of the A-V
conduction system (FRP) of the *in situ* heart with the intact vagus and cardiac
nerves were about 120 msec and 220 msec, respectively. A single i.v. injection of

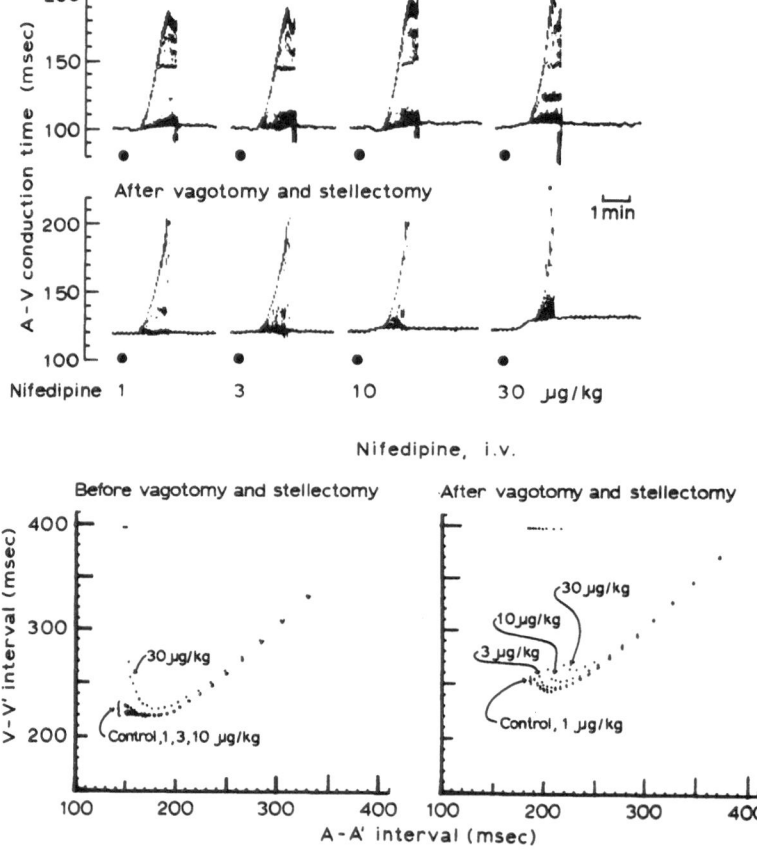

Fig. 2. Records of the A-V conduction time (upper panel) and superimposed records of A-A'
interval versus V-V' interval relations (lower panel) obtained with i.v. injections of nifedipine
given to a dog before and after vagotomy and stellectomy. Triangular excursions of traces in
the records of the A-V conduction time were caused by test stimuli delivered for the measurement of the FRP. The minimum V-V' interval in each curved line of dots in the lower panel is
the FRP at an indicated dose of nifedipine

$3 \mu g/kg$ of nifedipine, a dose almost doubling the coronary sinus outflow in the anesthetized dog (CF-ED$_{100}$) (VATER et al. [10]; HASHIMOTO et al. [6]) exerted no effect on the A-V conduction time and the FRP in some dogs (Fig. 2) or shortened the two parameters transiently in others (Fig. 3). At $30 \mu g/kg$ i.v., 10 times CF-ED$_{100}$, nifedipine prolonged slightly both the A-V conduction time and the FRP (Figs. 2 and 3). Dose-effect curves of nifedipine on the A-V conduction time ($\circ - \circ - \circ$) and the FRP ($\bullet - \bullet - \bullet$) obtained as the mean from 7 dogs before vagotomy and stellectomy are shown in Fig. 4.

After the heart had been deprived of the sympathetic tone by bilateral stellectomy plus vagotomy, the A-V conduction time and the FRP were increased by about 20 msec, being about 140 msec and 240 msec, respectively. Even in this state, $3 \mu g/kg$ i.v. of nifedipine, CF-ED$_{100}$, exerted almost no effect on the A-V conduction time and the FRP (Figs. 2 and 3). An increase in doses of nifedipine up to $30 \mu g/kg$ i.v. prolonged both the A-V conduction time and the FRP in a dose-dependent manner. However, even with $30 \mu g/kg$ i.v., 10 times CF-ED$_{100}$, increases

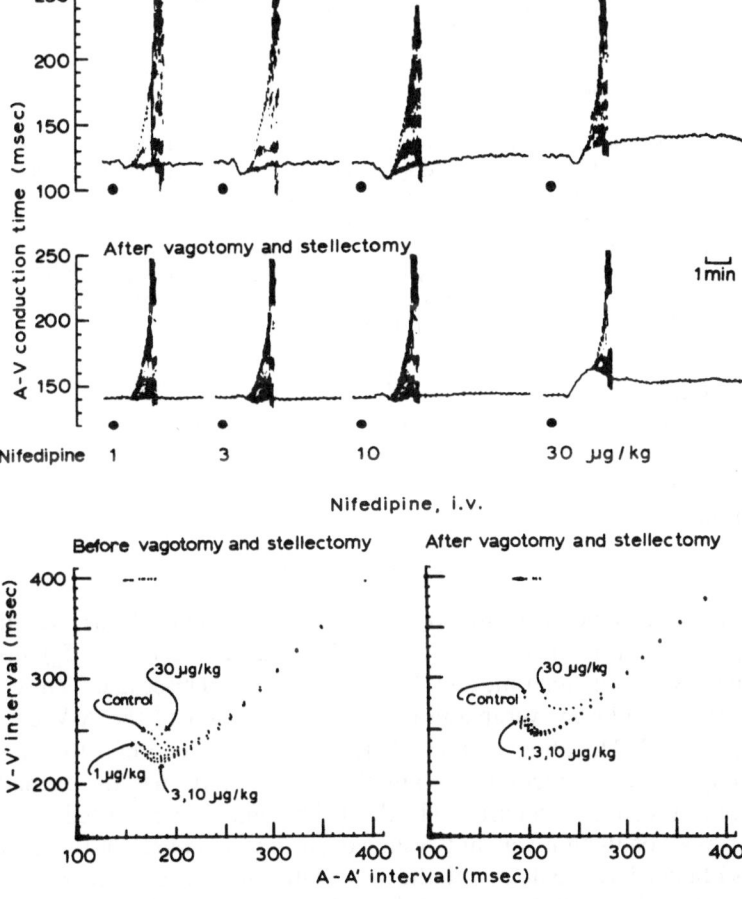

Fig. 3. Records similar to those in Fig. 2, obtained in a dog in which shortening of the A-V conduction time and the FRP by nifedipine was marked before vagotomy and stellectomy

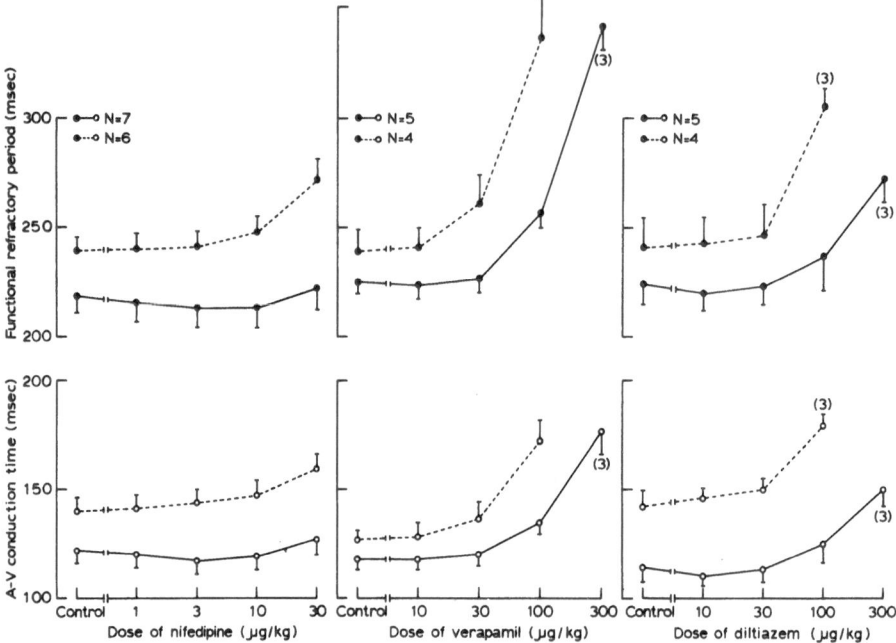

Fig. 4. Dose-effect curves of nifedipine, verapamil and diltiazem on the A-V conduction time and the FRP. N refers to the number of dogs. Solid or open circles connected with continuous lines for nifedipine and diltiazem refer to the results obtained before vagotomy and stellectomy, whereas those connected with broken lines were obtained after vagotomy and stellectomy in the same animals. Solid or open circles connected with continuous lines for verapamil refer to the results obtained in dogs with the nerve-intact heart, whereas those connected with broken lines were obtained in other vagotomized and stellectomized dogs. Vertical bars are standard errors of the mean

in the A-V conduction time and the FRP remained about 20 and 30 msec respectively, and there occurred no second-degree block of A-V conduction (Table 1). Figure 4 shows dose-effect curves of nifedipine on the A-V conduction (o---o---o) and the FRP (●---●---●) obtained as the mean of 6 dogs after vagotomy and stellectomy.

2. Verapamil and Diltiazem

Unlike nifedipine, even in dogs with the nerve-intact heart, verapamil at 100 µg/kg i.v., approximately CF-ED$_{100}$ (HAAS and HÄRTFELDER [5]), prolonged both the A-V conduction time and the FRP by about 20 msec and 30 msec respectively. At 300 µg/kg i.v. verapamil caused prolongation of the A-V conduction time and the FRP by about 50 and 70 msec respectively in 3 of 5 dogs, and in the remaining 2 A-V conduction was impaired so severely that the second-degree block of A-V conduction ensued (Table 1). This impairment lasted so long that normal A-V conduction was not resumed during the course of the experiment. Results obtained from 5 dogs with the nerve-intact heart are summarized in Fig. 4. In vagotomized and stellectomized dogs the detrimental effect of verapamil on A-V conduction was more marked, and with 100 µg/kg i.v. increases in the A-V

Table 1. Effects of coronary vasodilators on A-V conduction in the *in situ* heart of the dog

	CF-ED$_{100}$[a] (µg/kg)		Number of dogs	Incidence of second-degree conduction block			
				$^1/_3 \times$ CF-ED$_{100}$	CF-ED$_{100}$	$3 \times$ CF-ED$_{100}$	$10 \times$ CF-ED$_{100}$
Nifedipine	3	1	7	0	0	0	0
		2	6	0	0	0	0
Verapamil	100	1[b]	5	0	0	2	—
		2[b]	4	0	0	4	—
Diltiazem	100	1	5	0	0	2	5
		2	4	0	1	4	—
Dipyridamole	100	1	5	0	0	0	0
		2	5	0	0	0	0
Dilazep	100	1	5	0	0	0	0
		2	4	0	0	0	0

1, before vagotomy and stellectomy.
2, after vagotomy and stellectomy.
[a] Intravenous dose causing about 100% increase in the coronary sinus outflow.
[b] Different animals.
— Not examined.

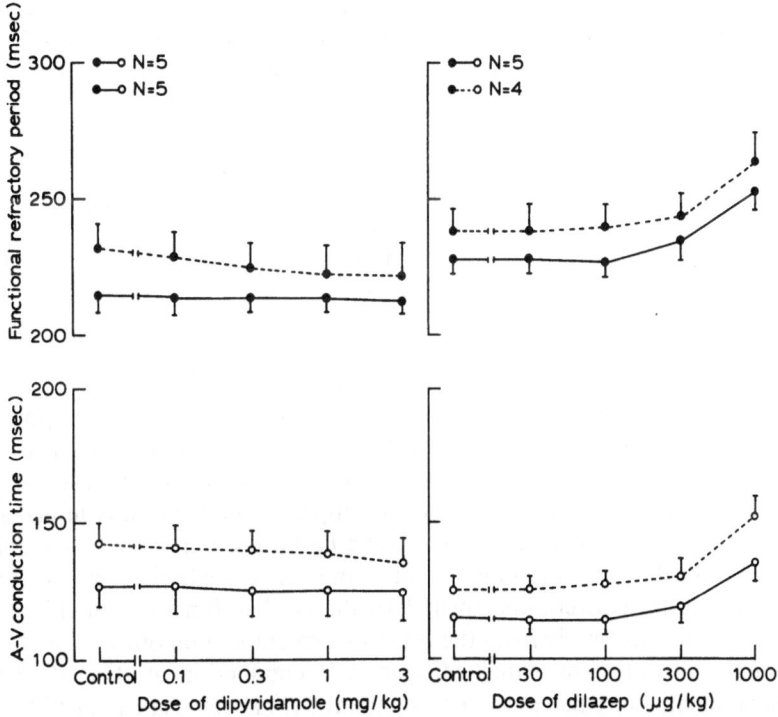

Fig. 5. Dose-effect curves of dipyridamole and dilazep on the A-V conduction time and the FRP. Solid or open circles connected with continuous lines refer to the results obtained before vagotomy and stellectomy and those connected with broken lines were obtained after vagotomy and stellectomy in the same animals. Otherwise, the same as in Fig. 4

conduction time and the FRP amounted to about 50 and 70 msec respectively. Results obtained from 4 dogs are summarized in Fig. 4. With 300 μg/kg i.v. of verapamil, a second-degree block of A-V conduction occurred in all 4 dogs (Table 1).

The effect of diltiazem on A-V conduction was similar to that of verapamil except for the duration of the effect. As shown in Fig. 4, diltiazem at 100 μg/kg i.v., approximately CF-ED$_{100}$ (SATO *et al.* [9]), increased the A-V conduction time and the FRP by about 10 and 15 msec respectively. However, after vagotomy and stellectomy the same dose of diltiazem impaired A-V conduction so severely that the second-degree block of A-V conduction occurred in 1 of 4 dogs. At 300 μg/kg i.v. diltiazem produced the second-degree block of A-V conduction in 2 of 5 dogs before and in all 4 dogs after vagotomy and stellectomy (Table 1). However, A-V conduction was resumed in about 5 min before, and in about 20 min after vagotomy and stellectomy.

3. Dipyridamole and Dilazep

Dipyridamole, of which CF-ED$_{100}$ is about 0.1 mg/kg i.v. (BRETSCHNEIDER *et al.* [1]), in a wide range of doses (0.1–3 mg/kg i.v.), had no effect on A-V conduction and facilitated somewhat A-V conduction in the heart deprived of the sympathetic tone (Fig. 5 and Table 1). Dilazep at 100 μg/kg i.v., approximately CF-ED$_{100}$ (HENSEL *et al.* [7]), had virtually no detrimental effect on A-V conduction. Even with increasing doses up to 1 mg/kg i.v., dilazep failed to produce the second-degree block of A-V conduction although it increased both the A-V conduction time and the FRP by about 20 msec (Fig. 5 and Table 1).

Discussion

As clearly demonstrated in the present experiments, nifedipine at 3 μg/kg i.v., CF-ED$_{100}$, facilitated A-V conduction in the nerve-intact heart, and had no detrimental effect at all even in the heart deprived of a compensatory sympathetic mechanism by bilateral stellectomy. Since the facilitating effect on A-V conduction observed with 3–10 μg/kg i.v. of nifedipine was abolished by bilateral stellectomy, it is probably due to a sympathetic mechanism triggered by hypotension, but it cannot be ascribed to the direct action. Even with increasing doses of nifedipine up to 30 μg/kg i.v., 10 times CF-ED$_{100}$, A-V conduction was scarcely affected as long as the sympathetic nerve supply to the heart was intact. In the heart deprived of sympathetic control, 30 μg/kg i.v. prolonged both A-V conduction time and the FRP to some extent. However, a slight increase in the two parameters is not entirely detrimental to the cardiac function. In this respect, nifedipine differs distinctly from the other two calcium antagonistic vasodilators, verapamil and diltiazem, which affected A-V conduction at their CF-ED$_{100}$, although nifedipine is also a calcium antagonist (FLECKENSTEIN *et al.* [3]; GRÜN and FLECKENSTEIN [4]). The virtual absence of a detrimental effect of nifedipine in a wide range of doses can be ascribed to its greater preference to the vasculature. From a therapeutic point of view nifedipine is the safest on A-V conduction among the calcium antagonistic coronary vasodilators.

Abstract

Effects of nifedipine on A-V conduction were investigated in the *in situ* paced hearts of open-chest dogs anesthetized with pentobarbital in comparison with those of 4 other coronary vasodilators. All drugs were given i.v. Drug effects on A-V conduction were evaluated from those on the A-V conduction time and the functional refractory period of the A-V conduction system (FRP), both of which were measured with completely automated devices. Nifedipine from 3 µg/kg i.v., a dose almost doubling the coronary sinus outflow (CF-ED$_{100}$), to 30 µg/kg i.v. had virtually no detrimental effect on A-V conduction. Verapamil and diltiazem at 100 µg/kg i.v., CF-ED$_{100}$, prolonged the A-V conduction time and the FRP, and at 300 µg/kg i.v. produced a second-degree block of A-V conduction in some dogs. This detrimental effect was aggravated by deprivation of the sympathetic inflow to the heart. Dipyridamole in a wide range of doses and dilazep at 100 µg/kg i.v., CF-ED$_{100}$, were devoid of a detrimental effect on A-V conduction.

Acknowledgement. This study was supported by a grant from Bayer Yakuhin Ltd., Osaka, Japan. The invaluable advice given by Professor Emeritus K. HA-SHIMOTO in the course of the study is gratefully acknowledged.

References

1. BRETSCHNEIDER, H. J., FRANK, A., BERNARD, U., KOCHSIEK, K., SCHELER, F.: Die Wirkung eines Pyrimidopyrimidin-Derivates auf die Sauerstoffversorgung des Herzmuskels. Arzneim.-Forsch. (Drug Res.) **9**, 49–59 (1959).
2. BUYNISKI, J. P., LOSADA, M., BIERWAGEN, M. E., GARDIER, R. W.: Cerebral and coronary vascular effects of a symmetrical N,N'-disubstituted hexahydrodiazepine. J. Pharmacol. Exp. Ther. **181**, 522—528 (1972).
3. FLECKENSTEIN, A., TRITTHART, H., DÖRING, H.-J., BYON, K. Y.: BAY a 1040 — ein hochaktiver Ca^{++}-antagonistischer Inhibitor der elektro-mechanischen Koppelungsprozesse im Warmblüter-Myokard. Arzneim.-Forsch. (Drug Res.) **22**, 22–33 (1972).
4. GRÜN, G., FLECKENSTEIN, A.: Die elektromechanische Entkoppelung der glatten Gefäß-muskulatur als Grundprinzip der Coronardilatation durch 4-(2'-Nitrophenyl)-2,6-dime-thyl-1,4-dihydropyridin-3,5-dicarbonsäure-dimethylester (BAY a 1040, Nifedipine). Arzneim.-Forsch. (Drug Res.) **22**, 334–344 (1972).
5. HAAS, H., HÄRTFELDER, A.: α-Isopropyl-α-[(N-methyl-N-homoveratryl)-γ-amino-pro-pyl]-3,4-dimethoxyphenylacetonitryl, eine Substanz mit coronargefäßerweiternden Eigenschaften. Arzneim.-Forsch. (Drug Res.) **12**, 549–558 (1962).
6. HASHIMOTO, K., TAIRA, N., CHIBA, S., HASHIMOTO, K., ENDOH, M., KOKUBUN, M., KOKU-BUN, H., IIJIMA, T., KIMURA, T., KUBOTA, K., OGURO, K.: Cardiohemodynamic effects of BAY a 1040 in the dog. Arzneim.-Forsch. (Drug Res.) **22**, 15–21 (1972).
7. HENSEL, I., BRETSCHNEIDER, H. J., KETTLER, D., KNOLL, D., KOCHSIEK, K., REPLOH, H. D., SPIECKERMANN, P. G., TAUCHERT, M.: Die Wirkung von 1,4-Bis[3-(3,4,5-trimethoxyben-zoyloxy)-propyl]-perhydro-1,4-diazepin-dihydrochlorid auf Herzstoffwechsel, Haemody-namik, Koronar- und Nierendurchblutung. Arzneim.-Forsch. (Drug Res.) **22**, 652–663 (1972).
8. KRAYER, O., MANDOKI, J. J., MENDEZ, C.: Studies on veratrum alkaloids. XVI. The action of epinephrine and of veratramine on the functional refractory period of the auriculo-ventricular transmission in the heart-lung preparation of the dog. J. Pharmacol. Exp. Ther. **103**, 412–419 (1951).
9. SATO, M., NAGAO, T., YAMAGUCHI, I., NAKAJIMA, H., KIYOMOTO, A.: Pharmacological stu-dies on a new 1,5-benzothiazepine derivative (CRD-401). I. Cardiovascular actions. Arzneim.-Forsch. (Drug Res.) **21**, 1338–1343 (1971).

10. VATER, W., KRONEBERG, G., HOFFMEISTER, F., KALLER, H., MENG, K., OBERDORF, A., PULS, W., SCHLOSSMANN, K., STOEPEL, K.: Zur Pharmakologie von 4-(2'-Nitrophenyl)-2,6-dimethyl-1,4-dihydropyridin-3,5-dicarbonsäuredimethylester (Nifedipine, BAY a 1040). Arzneim.-Forsch. (Drug Res.) **22**, 1–14 (1972).
11. ZIPES, D. P., FISCHER, J. C.: Effects of agents which inhibit the slow channel on sinus node automaticity and atrioventricular conduction in the dog. Circulation Res. **34**, 184–192 (1974).
12. ZIPES, D. P., MENDEZ, C.: Action of manganese ions and tetrodotoxin on atrioventricular nodal transmembrane potentials in isolated rabbit hearts. Circulation Res. **32**, 447–454 (1973).

Discussion Remarks

FLECKENSTEIN: In our experiments on anesthetized guinea pigs, we injected verapamil, D 600, and nifedipine and could not detect principal differences in their influence on the atrioventricular (A-V) node. Moreover, Dr. Landmark has carried out similar studies on the A-V node of rats. He also found that nifedipine as well as verapamil increases A-V conduction time. The difference between nifedipine and verapamil is possibly due to a differential degree of reflex activation of the sympathetic system. Because nifedipine seems to exert a stronger hypotensive action than verapamil it should also induce a more pronounced reflex release of sympathetic transmitters. This could protect A-V conduction in the case of nifedipine more than in the case of verapamil, in spite of the fact that the basic calcium-antagonistic action of both substances on the A-V node is possibly identical. Professor Kroneberg has already pointed out how much the basic nifedipine effects can be altered by an increase in the endogenous β-adrenergic drive. In addition, there are perhaps species differences in that A-V conduction might be more susceptible to nifedipine in guinea pig and rat hearts than in dog (or human) hearts. In any case, Professor Taira's results are important and stimulating.

TAIRA: I have not found my effects on an intact heart preparation. So I do not think nifedipine has a negative dromotropic factor on A-V conduction time. The fact that I obtained different results cannot be explained as being due to an adrenergic drive. Of course, if you give high doses of nifedipine in the dog you can get an A-V block, but I would like to stress that I carried out my experiments from a therapeutical point of view.

Studies on the Extracardial Effects of Nifedipine in Anesthetized Dogs

K. Hagemann, W. Lochner, and B. Niehues

Physiologisches Institut I, Universität Düsseldorf, Fed. Rep. Germany

In the mechanism of action of antianginal drugs like nifedipine, we have to distinguish between two components: effects on the heart itself—consisting of coronary and myocardial effects—on the one hand, and extracardial effects on the systemic and pulmonary circulation on the other. To a certain extent both components may improve the disproportion between oxygen supply and oxygen demand of the myocardium in coronary artery or primary myocardial disease [1, 2].

The studies on nifedipine presented here deal mainly with the extracardial effects on precapillary resistance and capacitance function of the peripheral circulation. These two working points play an important role in the regulation of mean arterial pressure, which constantly is found to be decreased after the administration of nifedipine and other antianginal drugs. This effect may be due firstly to reduced precapillary arterial resistance and secondly to an augmented volume of the capacitance system resulting in decreased venous return [3]. In fact, a certain, numerically so far unknown, combination of these two variables is assumed.

From this point of view, we analyzed the extracardial effects of nifedipine. The drug was given in a dose that produced a standardized decrease in mean arterial pressure. Then under continuous administration of the drug, changes in arterial resistance to flow and in intravascular volume were measured.

The experiments were performed on 6 closed chest dogs. Anesthesia was started by thiobarbital and continued with chloralose-urethane. Ventilation was maintained artificially by a Starling pump, keeping endexpiratory carbon dioxide tension at about 40 mm Hg. Blood clotting was prevented by heparin. Prior to the measurements, we ligated the spleen.

Both femoral arteries were connected to a reservoir containing heparinized blood of a donor dog. Using variable pressures in the reservoir we were able to adjust intravascular arterial pressure to any desired level (Fig. 1). The following parameters were recorded or calculated: the pressure in the aorta, right and left ventricle, rate of rise of left ventricular pressure (dp/dt), and heart rate. Cardiac output was determined by dye dilution technique. Total blood volume was measured using radioactive iodine as indicator. Peripheral resistance was calculated. Hematocrit and body temperature were kept constant, and blood gases were monitored frequently.

When a steady state was reached after having finished the operation procedure, the first measurement of all parameters was performed as a control and

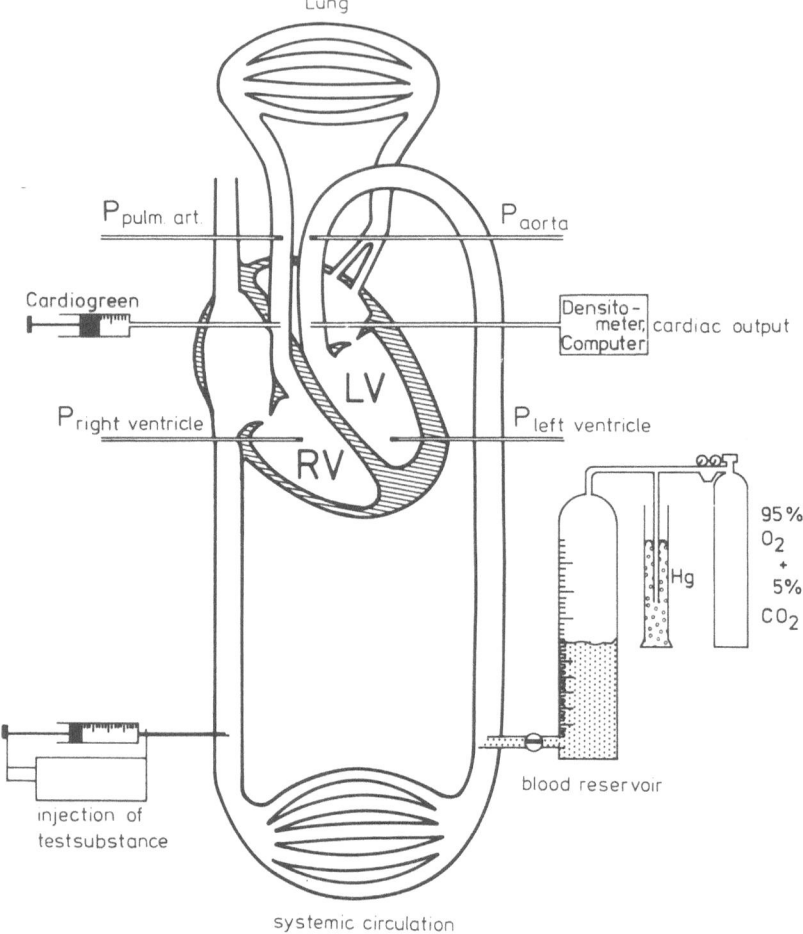

Fig. 1. Experimental set-up in the study of vasoactive drugs; see text

called period I (Table 1). Then an intravenous infusion of nifedipine was started and continued until mean arterial pressure decreased by 20 mm Hg. Under these conditions the second measurement was performed and called period II (see Table 1). At this time mean arterial pressure was decreased, and blood volume was still normal. Then, under continuous infusion of the drug, mean arterial pressure was returned to the control value by transfusion and kept at that level. After that a third measurement was performed and called period III. The change in blood volume was read from the calibrated extracorporeal reservoir.

The mean dose of nifedipine that lead to a decrease in mean arterial pressure by 20 mm Hg was 2.0 µg/kg·min.

The hemodynamic changes after the administration of nifedipine alone with mean arterial pressure decreased correspond to the results of previous investigations by RAFF *et al.* in our laboratory [4]. They are summarized as follows: an

Table 1. Experimental conditions in the study of vasoactive drugs; see text

control period	continuous infusion of the drug	
I	II	III
art. pressure normal blood vol. normal	art. pressure decreased blood vol. normal	art. pressure normal blood vol. increased

Table 2. Results of measurements during period III (mean arterial pressure normal); $\Delta CO\%$ = percent change in cardiac output, $\Delta R\%$ = percent change in arterial resistance, $\Delta BV\%$ = percent change in blood volume, $\Delta dp/dt_{max}\%$ = percent change in peak rate of rise of intraventricular pressure

	$\Delta CO\%$	$\Delta R\%$	$\Delta BV\%$	$\dfrac{\Delta BV}{\Delta R}$	$\Delta dp/dt_{max}\%$
papaverine	+ 55	−48	+19	0.386	+110
isoproterenol	+132	−61	+20	0.332	+110
nitroglycerin	+ 17	−13	+12	0.970	± 0
nifedipine	+194	−65	+26	0.394	+ 15

increase in cardiac output caused by a fall in arterial resistance to flow; a decrease in left ventricular enddiastolic pressure and in rate of rise of left ventricular pressure. Heart rate was nearly unchanged.

The effects of nifedipine on intravascular volume and resistance to flow can be evaluated from the results obtained in period III when the decreased mean arterial pressure had been compensated by transfusion (Table 2). The data for nifedipine are listed together with those for papaverine, isoproterenol and nitroglycerin, which were studied in previous experiments in our laboratory under the same conditions [2]. Cardiac output was excessively increased; the rate of rise of left ventricular pressure showed only a nonsignificant tendency to increase; heart rate was unchanged. Arterial resistance to flow was decreased by 65% from the control value. Furthermore we observed a significant increase in intravascular volume of 26%.

If we compare the overall hemodynamic effects of the four agents listed in Table 2 we can state that all of them cause a decrease in arterial resistance and an augmentation in cardiac output with the exception of nitroglycerin, which does not change these parameters significantly. Intravascular volume is consistently increased, with the greatest change occurring after nifedipine. Positive inotropic effects on the heart are strongest after the administration of papaverine and isoproterenol, small after nifedipine and almost absent after nitroglycerin.

In order to work out the specific effects on the peripheral circulation we established the ratio between the percent change in intravascular volume and arterial resistance to flow.

In addition, this quotient permits the comparison of the different pharmacologic agents. As you can see from Table 2 the value for nifedipine amounts to 0.394, which means that this drug has a relatively strong effect on arterial resis-

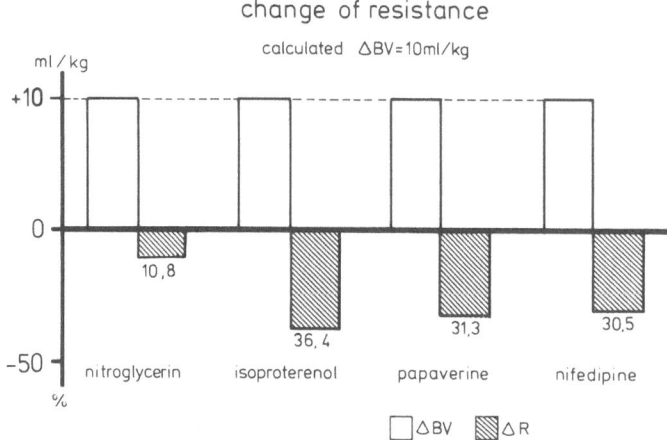

Fig. 2. Relationship between changes in arterial resistance (ΔR, shaded areas) an blood volume (ΔBV, blank areas) when blood volume was increased by 10 ml/kg under the influence of various drugs

tance in comparison to its effect on intravascular capacity. Papaverine and isoproterenol show similar results, with values of 0.386 and 0.332 respectively, despite their quite different effects on the heart itself.

The pattern of action of nitroglycerin is characterized by a very small effect on arterial resistance combined with a relatively strong influence on the capacitance function of the peripheral circulation. This leads to a quotient of 0.970 representing the special properties of this drug.

In Fig. 2 our results are presented in a different way, i.e., as a graphical representation of the blood volume-resistance ratio. The blank areas in the upper part of the diagram represent the changes in intravascular volume. It was assumed that each drug had caused a change of 10 ml/kg body weight. Then the corresponding percent changes in arterial resistance observed in our experiments were calculated and plotted as shaded areas in the lower part of the diagram. Related to the same change of volume, the change of resistance after nifedipine is about the same as after isoproterenol and papaverine. Here again nitroglycerin contrasts with the other drugs by its predominating effect on the capacitance vessels.

If we summarize the results of our investigations on nifedipine and compare them to those of papaverine, isoproterenol and nitroglycerin, we can distinguish between three different patterns of action on the peripheral circulation:

The first one is represented by the beta-receptor stimulating agents *isoproterenol* and *papaverine*. They predominantly lower arterial resistance and cause venous pooling too. Furthermore they have powerful positive inotropic and chronotropic effects on the heart.

The second is that of *nitroglycerin*, which produces only slight effects on both the arterial resistance and the myocardium. Its main effect is the dilation of capacitance vessels, thus leading to diminished venous return.

The third pattern of action is represented by the Ca-antagonistic agent *nifedipine*. It exhibits a marked overall vasodilating effect, especially on arterial resistance vessels—similar to isoproterenol and papaverine. But in contrast to the latter two drugs, positive inotropic and chronotropic effects cannot be observed. In comparison to the other drugs, nifedipine causes the largest venous pooling effect related to the same change in mean arterial pressure. The ability of this agent to reduce pre- and afterload of the heart may contribute considerably to its beneficial effect in the treatment of ischemic heart disease.

It is our opinion that in general extracardial effects of antianginal drugs are as important as the effects on the heart itself. Further investigations with the quantitative method used in this study can add to a better understanding of the overall mechanism of action of vasoactive drugs.

Abstract

In anesthetized dogs the relative effects of nifedipine on peripheral resistance and intravascular volume were studied. The drug was administered in a dose that produced a standardized decrease in mean arterial pressure of 20 mm Hg. Then, under continuous infusion of the drug, the control value of mean arterial pressure was reestablished by transfusion. The amount of blood required was determined. The pressure in aorta and both ventricles, cardiac output, heart rate, dp/dt_{max}, and total blood volume were measured.—In all experiments intravascular volume was significantly increased ($+26\%$). Peripheral resistance was diminished (-65%), and heart rate was unchanged. The effects of nifedipine are discussed in comparison to those of papaverine, isoproterenol and nitroglycerin studied under the same experimental conditions. The technique described in this study permits the assessment of extracardial actions of vasoactive drugs.

References

1. CHARLIER,R.: Antianginal drugs. In: Handbuch der experimentellen Pharmakologie, Vol.XXXI. Berlin-Heidelberg-New York: Springer 1971.
2. HAGEMANN,K., NIEHUES,B., SCHWANITZ,V., ARNOLD,G., LOCHNER,W.: Untersuchungen zur extracardialen Komponente der Wirkung vasoaktiver Substanzen am Gesamtkreislauf des Hundes. Res. exp. Med. **161**, 203 (1973).
3. MELLANDER,S., JOHANSSON,B.: Control of resistance, exchange and capacitance functions in the peripheral circulation. Pharmacolog. Rev. **20**, 117 (1968).
4. RAFF,W.K., KOSCHE,F., LOCHNER,W.: Untersuchungen mit Nifedipine, einer coronargefäßerweiternden Substanz mit schneller sublingualer Wirkung. Arzneim. Forsch. (Drug Res.) **22**, 1376 (1972).

Discussion Remarks

KRAUPP: In your experiment there was, after nifedipine, a considerable increase of cardiac output but only a very small increase of dp/dt_{max}. How is this increase in cardiac output brought about if, at the same time, the frequency does not change significantly. Unfortunately no heart rate values were included in the final table.

HAGEMANN: The lack of increase in heart rate has its origin in reflex mechanisms. First, there is, in the compensation period, a loading of circulation and we have to assume that via reflex mechanisms there is no increase in heart rate; second, there is the negative inotropic effect induced by nifedipine on the heart itself.

KRAUPP: How is cardiac output brought about?

HAGEMANN: The increase in cardiac output is brought about by an augmentation of end-diastolic pressure in the right ventrical which leads to better filling of the heart and an increase in cardiac output.

LOCHNER: When we have an increase in end-diastolic pressure we can expect, as you say, an increase in dp/dt_{max}. At the same time we have a negative inotropic effect because of the calcium antagonism of nifedipine; furthermore the arterial pressure has come back to normal. Therefore, it is understandable that the increasing effect on dp/dt_{max}, which usually can be seen when pressure falls, does not come through because the three factors compensate, for each other.

Session II

Experimental Pharmacology

Chairmen: H. A. Snellen (Leiden), N. Taira (Tohoku)

Adalat, a Powerful Ca-Antagonistic Drug

A. FLECKENSTEIN

Physiological Institute, University of Freiburg, Fed. Rep. Germany

1. The Physiological Role of Ca-Ions in Excitation-Contraction Coupling

There is overwhelming evidence that during excitation of mammalian myo-cardial fibers or smooth muscle cells an increased transmembrane Ca influx takes place simultaneously with liberation of Ca from certain endoplasmic stores. The rapid rise in free intracellular Ca during excitation initiates the splitting of ATP by the Ca-dependent ATPase of the myofibrils so that phosphate-bond energy is transformed into mechanical work. This means, in other words, that the Ca ions act as mediators in excitation-contraction coupling between the bioelec-tric events at the sarcolemma membrane and the intracellular biochemical pro-cesses which utilize ATP for contraction. Therefore, contractility is lost in a Ca-deficient medium.

Figure 1 shows the results of a fundamental experiment in which an electri-cally stimulated rabbit papillary muscle was put into a Ca-free Tyrode solution. Single fiber action potentials and isometric mechanograms were continuously recorded. As expected, isometric peak tension falls to almost zero within 14 min in a Ca-free environment, whereas the action potentials do not appreciably change. So, after the loss of mechanical responses, the Ca-deficient myocardium behaves like a nerve in which only action potentials are conducted. However, the mechan-ical function of the cardiac fibers is rapidly restored upon return to a normal Ca-

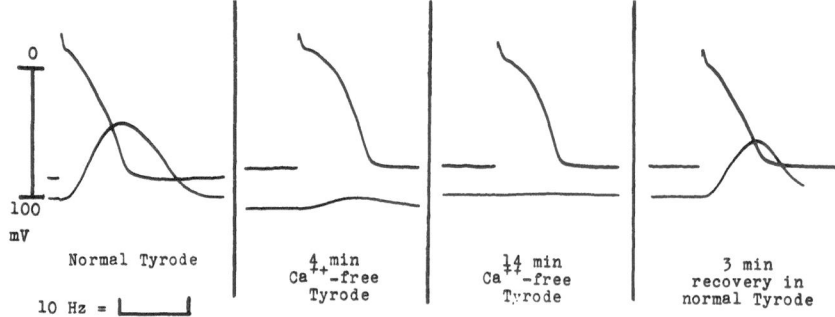

Fig. 1. Complete loss of contractility of an isolated rabbit papillary muscle in a Ca-free Tyrode solution at 37° C. Rapid recovery in ordinary Tyrode solution. Rate of stimulation: 3 shocks/min. Potentials were measured with intracellular microelectrodes of conventional type. Isometric tensions were recorded with a transducer valve (RCA 5734)

containing medium. Biochemically, the Ca-deficient myocardium exhibits a striking insufficiency in splitting its high-energy phosphate compounds in the state of excitation. But after addition of Ca, the high-energy phosphate utilization is normalized. If, on the other hand, the extracellular Ca concentration is increased above normal, more Ca is taken up by the beating heart so that both splitting of high-energy phosphates and contractility are potentiated. All these observations clearly show that Ca-ions not only trigger the contractile process but also control quantitatively the output of mechanical tension in regulating the amount of ATP that is metabolized during activity.

2. Specific Inhibition of Excitation-Contraction Coupling by Ca-Antagonistic Substances

From our studies on myocardial fibers we found, 10 years ago, that the Ca supply to the contractile system can also be selectively reduced by pharmacological means[1]. So it turned out that the negative inotropic effects of numerous compounds are due to an interference with the Ca action in excitation-contraction coupling. Among these substances prenylamine, verapamil, D 600 and nifedipine are probably the most interesting ones (see Table 1). The first drug on this list, prenylamine, was still relatively weak and of modest specificity. The other compounds, however, namely verapamil, D 600 (a methoxy-derivative of verapamil) and nifedipine (code number BAY a 1040) are very powerful.

As to nifedipine, Dr. KRONEBERG had first expressed the idea that, possibly, this compound might also belong to the new family of Ca-antagonistic inhibitors of excitation-contraction coupling. This was, in fact, proved by our subsequent studies, which led us to the conclusion that nifedipine exhibits an outstanding Ca-antagonistic efficacy. Figure 2 shows, for instance, the depression of contractility of a rabbit papillary muscle in Tyrode solution with increasing concentrations of nifedipine, i.e. 10, 20, 50, and 100 µg/l. With 100 µg/l, contractility was nearly abolished. But this effect could be easily neutralized by addition of extra Ca, so that the isometric peak tension returned practically to normal in the lowest part of the picture after the Ca concentration had been increased up to 16 mM.

As mentioned previously the specific inhibitors of excitation-contraction coupling reduce the contractile response of the ventricular myocardium without inhibiting the electrical excitation process. Figure 3 shows experiments on 2 cat papillary muscles in which an 80% loss of contractility was obtained with 400 µg of nifedipine/l, whereas the height and the shape of the single fiber action potentials remained practically the same. In the right part of the picture contractility was restored by extra Ca, as shown in the upper graph, or by isoproterenol, as can be seen from the lower record. The graphs in Fig. 4 represent a quantitative evaluation of such an experiment with nifedipine on an isolated papillary muscle.

Obviously resting potential, as well as the action potential parameters, upstroke velocity and height of the overshoot, which indicate the transmembrane

---

[1] A comprehensive report about the fundamental actions of Ca-antagonistic compounds on the mammalian myocardium has been presented in previous papers [2–5].

Table 1. Specific Ca-antagonistic inhibitors of excitation-contraction coupling of mammalian myocardium

Prenylamine (Segontin) Farbwerke Hoechst	
Verapamil (Isoptin, Iproveratril) Knoll AG Ludwigshafen	
Compound D 600 Knoll AG Ludwigshafen	
Nifedipine (BAY a 1040, Adalat) Bayer AG Leverkusen	

Na influx, remain at a consistently high level whereas the Ca-dependent contractile response drastically diminishes.

3. Mechanism of Action of Ca-Antagonistic Drugs: Selective Restriction of Myocardial Transmembrane Ca Conductivity

In a further attempt to clarify the specific mechanism of action of these powerful drugs, separate measurements of the transmembrane Na and Ca currents were performed on ventricular trabeculae of cats, using a special voltage clamp technique developed by KOHLHARDT et al. [7, 8]. The following results were obtained: The negative inotropic action of the Ca-antagonistic inhibitors of excitation-contraction coupling is due to a drastic reduction in the transmembrane Ca conductivity. In some experiments the transmembrane Ca currents were blocked completely. This effect can be neutralized by addition of excess Ca to the bathing fluid even in the presence of the inhibitors. In contrast to their strong inhibitory effect on the passive transmembrane Ca movements, however, the fast Na current that

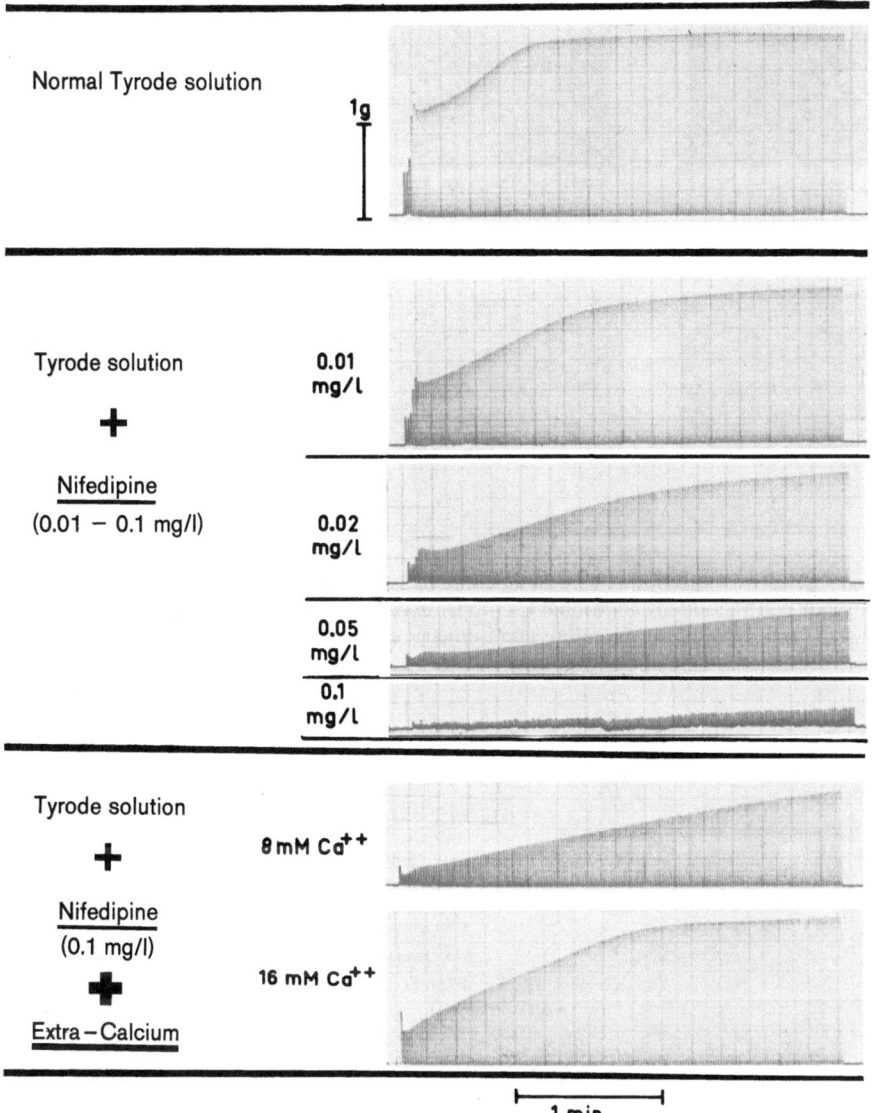

Fig.2. Depression of contractility of a rabbit papillary muscle (1.7 mg wet weight) in Tyrode solution containing 2 mM CaCl$_2$ by increasing concentrations of nifedipine (0.01–0.1 mg/l). Neutralization of the drug effect by additional Ca. Isometric tension measurements at a stimulation frequency of 60/min each time for 3 min at 30° C (FLECKENSTEIN *et al.* [5])

initiates the action potential is much less affected. The selective depression of the Ca conductivity by specific inhibitors indicates that during excitation the influxes of Na and Ca are independent of each other. Therefore, in the mammalian myocardium the existence of two separate channels for Na and Ca has to be assumed. As a functional consequence of this dual membrane transport system, it is possible to change the contractile force by inotropic substances that act on the Ca conductivity without a corresponding influence on Na-dependent excitation.

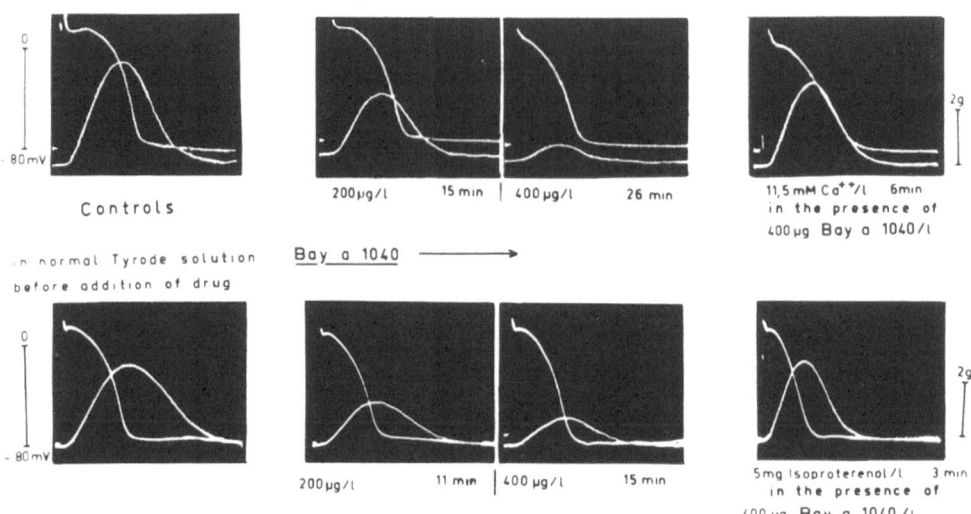

Fig. 3. Selective inhibition of contractile force of 2 cat papillary muscles by nifedipine. Restoration of contractility by additional Ca (upper experiment) or by isoproterenol (lower experiment). Single fiber action potentials and isometric contractions were measured using the same techniques as in Fig. 1 (FLECKENSTEIN et al. [5])

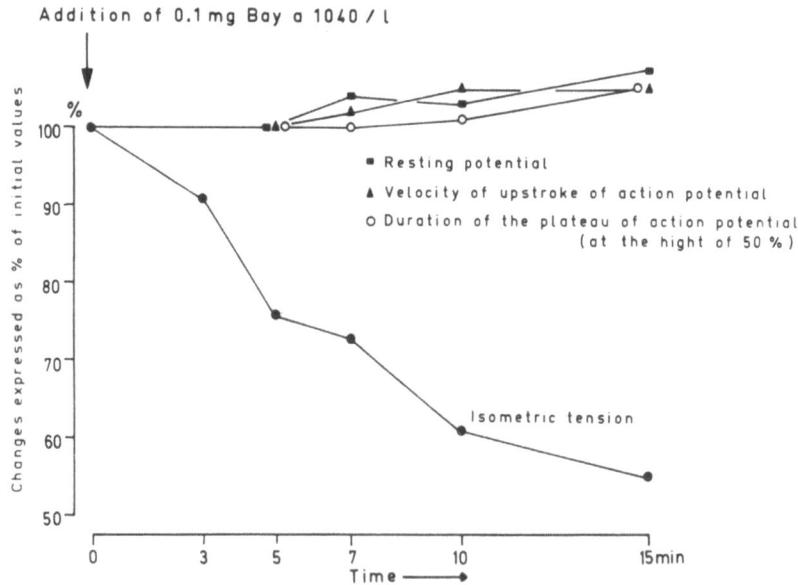

Fig. 4. Selective restriction by nifedipine of the contractile force of a cat papillary muscle without reduction of resting potential and without influence on velocity of rise, and duration of the plateau, of action potential. Experimental procedure as in Fig. 3 (FLECKENSTEIN et al. [5])

4. Neutralization of Ca-Antagonistic Drug Effects on Heart Muscle by Extra-Calcium, β-Adrenergic Catecholamines or Cardiac Glycosides

The specific Ca-antagonistic inhibitors of excitation-contraction coupling influence the Ca conductivity of the cardiac fiber membranes in exactly the opposite sense as the sympathomimetic catecholamines. In fact the positive inotropic action of sympathomimetic amines is caused by a potentiation of the Ca influx through the excited cardiac fiber membranes. Among the sympathomimetic amines tested, isoproterenol was by far the most potent Ca promoter. Even in the case of a nearly complete experimental block of contractility by Ca-antagonistic compounds, the mechanical function of the heart is restored as soon as the Ca supply to the contractile system is normalized with the help of isoproterenol.

Figure 5 shows as an example the development of severe contractile failure of a guinea pig heart after intravenous infusion of a large overdose of nifedipine. There was an increase in central venous pressure and a decrease in the aortic pressure while the heart was more and more dilated and the contraction ampli-

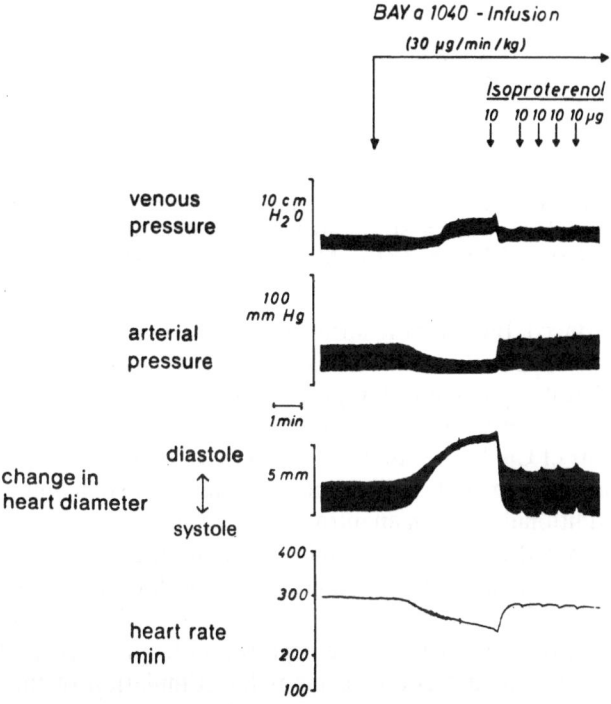

Fig. 5. Acute contractile failure of a guinea pig heart (open chest preparation with the pericardium removed) after intravenous infusion of relatively large amounts of nifedipine (BAY a 1040: 30 µg/min/kg). Rapid restoration of contractility (contraction amplitude, heart diameter) and of the original arterial and venous pressures by isoproterenol within 20 sec. Suitable Statham elements were used for the blood pressure registration in the left jugular vein (P 23 BB) and in the right carotid artery (P 23 Db) under nembutal-ether anesthesia. Continuous records of heart diameter were made using the method of KAMMERMEIER and DÖRING [6]

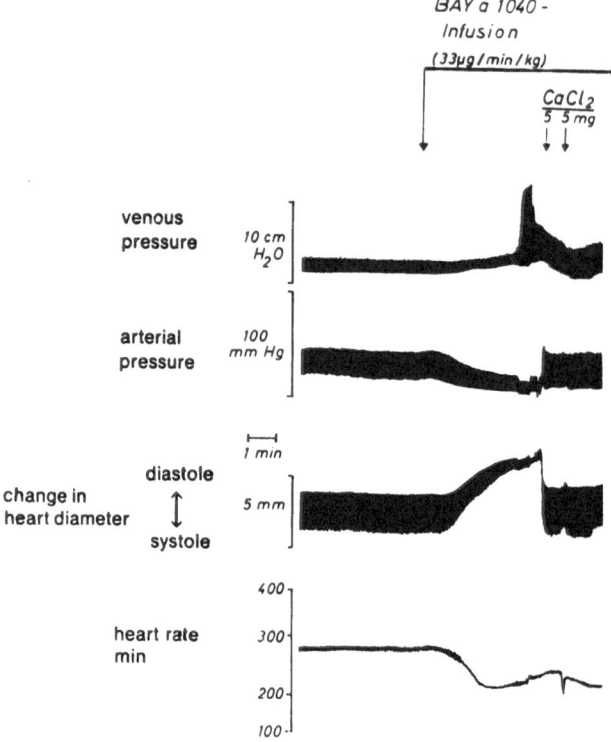

Fig. 6. Acute contractile failure of a guinea pig heart after intravenous infusion of relatively large amounts of nifedipine (BAY a 1040). Rapid neutralization of the drug effects by intravenous administration of 2×5 mg $CaCl_2$. Methods as in Fig. 4 (FLECKENSTEIN et al. [5])

tude severely reduced. But after the intravenous injection of a single dose of 10 µg isoproterenol the contractile function of the heart returned to normal within 20 sec. It is undoubtedly of clinical importance that even large overdoses of a Ca-antagonistic compound can be almost immediately neutralized in this way. Intravenous injections of $CaCl_2$ are similarly useful (see Fig. 6). Cardiac glycosides are also capable of restoring contractility but with a delay of some minutes. They act by liberating additional Ca from an intracellular pool.

It should be noted in this connection that the natural adrenergic transmitter substances adrenalin and noradrenalin are also very efficient in antagonizing the negative inotropic nifedipine effects. From this it is easily understood that the heart *in situ* does not necessarily show a negative inotropic response to nifedipine when, at the same time, a cardiovascular reflex stimulation of the sympathetic nervous system takes place. Such a sympathetic stimulation may result from a decrease in blood pressure following peripheral vasodilation by nifedipine. Obviously, nifedipine does not abolish the sympathetic self-defence mechanism against a critical reduction in cardiac output or against a dangerous fall in arterial blood pressure. Therefore, on the heart *in situ* of an intact animal, the negative inotropic effects of nifedipine are self-controlled and self-limited or even compensated as long as the sympathetic system can react (baroreceptor system).

5. Reduction of Myocardial Oxygen Requirement by Ca-Antagonistic Compounds

As mentioned previously Ca-ions regulate quantitatively the amount of ATP that is utilized by the contractile system for the production of mechanical tension. As a result, the oxygen requirement of the active myocardium is also highly "Ca-sensitive", since the intensity of ATP consumption strictly determines the rates of glycolysis and respiration. Therefore, as can be seen from the data in Fig. 7, obtained from a rabbit's papillary muscle, the correlation between isometric tension and the additional consumption of oxygen due to mechanical activity is strictly linear when the Ca concentration is varied from 0 to 8 mM/l. Similarly the Ca-antagonistic compounds are also capable of producing the same proportional change of isometric peak tension and extra consumption of oxygen when they are applied in different doses. Therefore, cardiac oxygen consumption is always decreased by nifedipine to the same extent that the Ca-dependent splitting of ATP declines and contractile force diminishes.

As shown in Fig. 8 with 10–20 µg/l nifedipine, a 50% reduction in the oxygen requirement and isometric tension of a rabbit papillary muscle could be obtained. With a higher dose (0.1 mg) of nifedipine, both tension and oxygen consumption dropped nearly to resting level since the influence of the persisting electrical activity of the myocardial fibers on the rate of respiration is insignificant. Nevertheless, an appropriate extra dose of $CaCl_2$ restored mechanical activity and oxygen consumption to normal (as represented by the black dot) even when previously, the contractile system had been completely paralyzed.

6. Therapeutic Aspects

As to the therapeutic significance of these findings, the oxygen-saving effect of the Ca-antagonistic compounds is of practical use in patients with a hyperkinetic heart function or in cases of angina pectoris and of other forms of coronary disease. Here a certain restriction of the cardiac activity metabolism may be helpful in order to reestablish a suitable balance between a reduced coronary oxygen supply and the actual cardiac oxygen requirement. In this respect the Ca-antagonistic drugs exert the same beneficial influence on patients with angina pectoris as the adrenergic β-receptor blocking agents do. But more importantly, the Ca-antagonistic compounds have the therapeutic advantage that, apart from lowering the myocardial oxygen requirement, they also produce coronary vasodilation. Furthermore, the Ca-antagonistic compounds decrease the load on the heart because, by additional vasodilator action on the peripheral resistance vessels, they also reduce the arterial blood pressure.

So, in summation, I should like to emphasize that the improvement of the cardiac energy balance by nifedipine is rather complex. The contributing factors are as follows:

a) a reduction of the myocardial oxygen demand,
b) an increase in coronary oxygen supply,
c) a facilitation of heart work at a reduced level of arterial blood pressure.

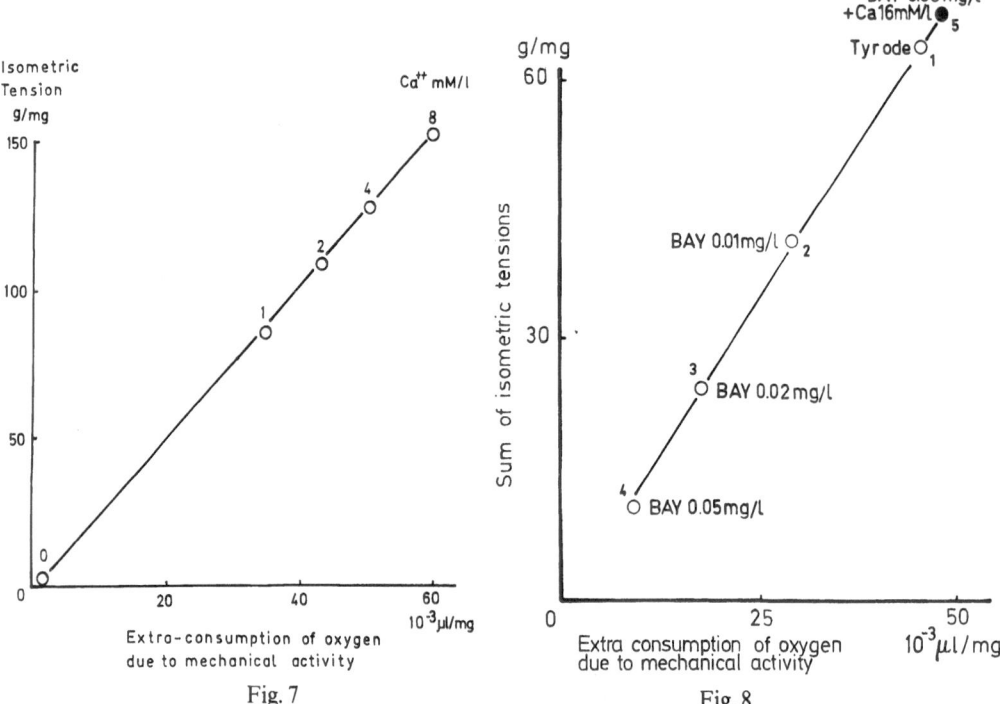

Fig. 7. Variation of extracellular Ca: Linear correlation between isometric tension and the additional consumption of oxygen due to mechanical activity (exceeding the oxygen uptake at rest) of a rabbit papillary muscle in Tyrode solution of different Ca concentrations (0, 1, 2, 4, and 8 mM/l). The muscle (1.6 mg wet weight) was incubated at rest in the different media each time for 20 min and then stimulated for 3.5 min at a frequency of 60/sec. Measurements of the rates of oxygen consumption (with a platinum electrode) and of mechanical tension (with a mechano-electronic displacement transducer) were made throughout the experiment. The graph shows the sum of the isometric peak tensions produced during each stimulation period plotted against the corresponding additional consumptions of oxygen (BYON and FLECKENSTEIN [7])

Fig. 8. Nifedipine (BAY a 1040): Linear reduction of isometric tension and extra-consumption of oxygen due to activity under the influence of increasing doses of the drug. Neutralization by additional Ca (1 = Tyrode solution without drug; 2 = Tyrode + 0.01 mg/l; 3 = Tyrode + 0.02 mg/l; 4 = Tyrode + 0.05 mg/l; 5 = Tyrode + 0.05 mg nifedipine/l + excess Ca (16 mM/l). Rabbit papillary muscle; wet weight 0.8 mg; stimulation period 3.0 min; frequency 60/min; temperature 30° C; methods as in Fig. 7 (BYON and FLECKENSTEIN [7])

The relaxing effects on the coronary and peripheral smooth muscle cells are also caused by a block of excitation-contraction coupling. In the following paper of Dr. FLECKENSTEIN-GRÜN, the vascular effects of the Ca-antagonistic compounds are discussed in more detail.

Abstract

Nifedipine produces coronary vasodilation and simultaneously lowers the oxygen requirement of the beating heart. As to the molecular mechanism of action, nifedipine restricts the transmembrane Ca influx during excitation so that excitation-contraction coupling in both cardiac and vascular smooth muscle fibers is affected. Biochemically, in reducing the Ca supply to the contractile system, nifedipine interfers with the activation of the Ca-dependent myofibrillar ATPase by which phosphate-bond energy is transformed into mechanical work. Thus, in the heart, the production of mechanical tension and activity oxygen consumption decreases, while the tone of vascular smooth muscle fibers, particularly in the coronary arteries, is also diminished. This improves the cardiac energy balance, as can be seen from a rise in the myocardial high-energy phosphate content, and augments the tolerance of the heart to hypoxia. In contrast to the pronounced influences of nifedipine on the mechanical parameters, the height and the shape of single fiber action potentials of ventricular tissue as well as resting potential, excitability and impulse conduction remain practically unchanged. The fundamental action of nifedipine on cardiac tissues and smooth muscle preparations resembles that of other Ca-antagonistic inhibitors of excitation-contraction coupling such as verapamil, D 600 or—to a lesser extent—prenylamine.

In the intact animal the negative inotropic effects of nifedipine are much less pronounced than on isolated myocardium. This is probably due to a reflex activation of the sympathetic system when, under the influence of nifedipine, the peripheral vascular resistance is reduced. Therefore, generally, following administration of reasonable doses of nifedipine, coronary and peripheral vasodilation predominates in the intact animal while cardiac contractility appears much less affected.

References

1. BYON, K. Y., FLECKENSTEIN, A.: Parallele Beeinflussung von isometrischer Spannungsentwicklung und O_2-Verbrauch isolierter Papillarmuskeln unter dem Einfluß von Ca^{++}-Ionen, Adrenalin, Isoproterenol und organischen Ca^{++}-Antagonisten (Iproveratril, D 600, Prenylamin). Pflügers Arch. ges. Physiol. **312**, R 8/9 (1969).
2. FLECKENSTEIN, A.: Specific inhibitors and promoters of calcium action in the excitation-contraction coupling of heart muscle and their role in the prevention or production of myocardial lesions. In: HARRIS, P., OPIE, L. (Eds.): "Calcium and the Heart", pp. 135–188. London-New York: Academic Press 1971.
3. FLECKENSTEIN, A.: Neuere Ergebnisse zur Physiologie, Pharmakologie und Pathologie der elektromechanischen Koppelungsprozesse im Warmblütermyokard. In: KEIDEL, W.D., PLATTIG, K.-H. (Hrsg.): Vorträge der Erlanger Physiologentagung 1970, S. 13–52. Berlin-Heidelberg-New York: Springer-Verlag 1971.
4. FLECKENSTEIN, A.: Drug-induced changes in cardiac energy. In: The Myocardium. Adv. Cardiol. V. 12, pp. 183–197. Basel: Karger 1974.
5. FLECKENSTEIN, A., TRITTHART, H., DÖRING, H.J., BYON, K.Y.: BAY a 1040 — ein hochaktiver Ca^{++}-antagonistischer Inhibitor der elektro-mechanischen Koppelungsprozesse im Warmblüter-Myokard. Arzneim. Forsch. (Drug Res.) **22**, 22–33 (1972).
6. KAMMERMEIER, H., DÖRING, H.J.: Eine neue Methode zur fortlaufenden, direktschreibenden Registrierung des Mechanogramms sowie der Dilatation am freigelegten Herzen im Tierexperiment. Wegmessung mit tastlosen induktiven Aufnehmern. Pflügers Arch. ges. Physiol. **273**, 311–314 (1961).
7. KOHLHARDT, M., BAUER, B., KRAUSE, H., FLECKENSTEIN, A.: New selective inhibitors of the transmembrane Ca conductivity in mammalian myocardial fibers. Studies with the voltage-clamp-technique. Experientia **28**, 288–289 (1972).
8. KOHLHARDT, M., BAUER, B., KRAUSE, H., FLECKENSTEIN, A.: Differentiation of the transmembrane Na and Ca channels in mammalian cardiac fibers by the use of specific inhibitors. Pflügers Arch. ges. Physiol. **335**, 309–322 (1972).

Ca-Dependent Changes in Coronary Smooth Muscle Tone and the Action of Ca-Antagonistic Compounds with Special Reference to Adalat

G. FLECKENSTEIN-GRÜN and A. FLECKENSTEIN

Physiological Institute, University of Freiburg, Fed. Rep. Germany

One of the most important facts in vascular smooth muscle physiology is that contractility of all types of vessels depends entirely on Ca ions. Therefore, contractile vascular smooth muscle tone is abolished and vasodilation produced by withdrawal of Ca ions from the environment. This can be achieved by chelation of Ca with a high dose of EDTA (ethylene diamine tetraacetic acid) or, in isolated vascular smooth muscle preparations, by administration of a Ca-free Ringer or Tyrode solution.

1. Relaxation of Potassium-Contractured Coronary Strips by Ca Withdrawal or Ca-Antagonistic Compounds

Figure 1 shows an experiment in which a spiral strip of a great coronary artery of a pig was first depolarized by increasing the potassium concentration of the surrounding fluid up to 43 mM/l. It is well known that the potassium contracture

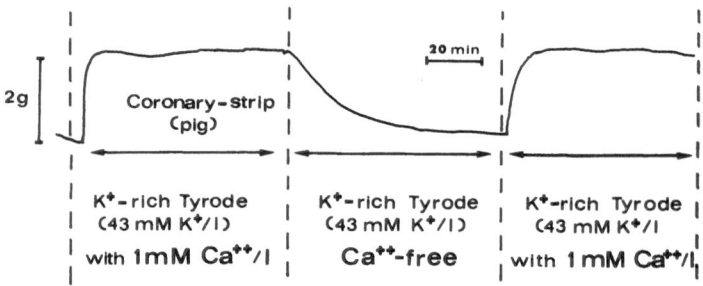

Fig. 1. Relaxation of a potassium-depolarized coronary strip by Ca withdrawal in a Ca-free K-rich Tyrode solution. Recovery of tone upon return to the Ca-containing medium. Fresh spiral strip (wet weight 10 mg) dissected from a great epicardial coronary artery of an adult pig. Before administration of the K-rich solutions, the coronary strip was kept in a Tyrode solution with a normal K content (concentrations in mM/l: NaCl 155; KCl 4; NaHCO$_3$ 11.9; CaCl$_2$ 1.0; NaH$_2$PO$_4$ 0.48; glucose 5.6) for a period of 60 min under a load of 2.0 g. Throughout the experiment a gas mixture of 97% O$_2$ and 3% CO$_2$ was used for oxygenation of the bath at a constant temperature of 35° C and at a pH of 7.4. Isometric tension was continuously recorded with the use of a mechano-electronic transducer

produced by this procedure is mediated by an increased Ca influx through the potassium-depolarized smooth muscle cell membrane. Therefore, it is not surprising that relaxation occurred when—as shown in the middle part of the picture— the coronary strip was transferred into a Ca-free solution—despite the fact that the high depolarizing potassium concentration remained unchanged. Obviously, excitation-contraction coupling is abolished in the absence of Ca. However, as can be seen on the right of Fig. 1, the contractile tone was completely restored after return to the Ca-containing medium.

As we found several years ago, the coronary vasodilator effects of verapamil, D 600, prenylamine, nifedipine and other musculotropic smooth muscle relaxants clearly depend on their ability to interfere with the Ca action in excitation-contraction coupling (see the comprehensive report of GRÜN and FLECKEN-STEIN [2]).

Figure 2 demonstrates, as an example, the complete loss of tone of 3 potassium-depolarized coronary strips upon addition of prenylamine, verapamil or nifedipine. In coronary smooth muscle, one molecule of these compounds is capable of blocking the effect of several thousand Ca ions in excitation-contrac-

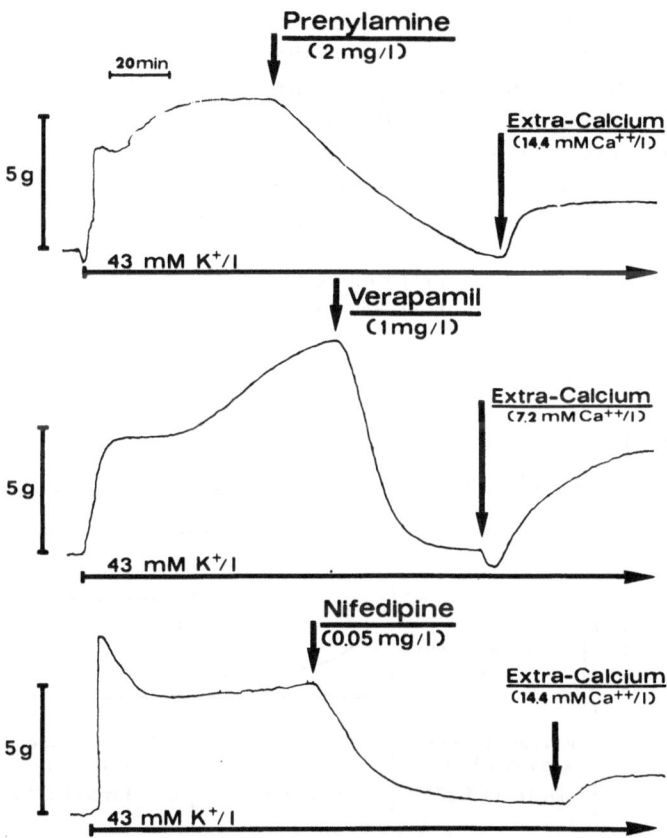

Fig. 2. Relaxation of potassium-depolarized coronary strips by Ca-antagonistic inhibitors of excitation-contraction coupling. Restitution of contractile tension by additional Ca. Principal procedure in these and the following experiments as in Fig. 1

tion coupling. It is to be assumed that these Ca-antagonistic compounds reduce the Ca influx through the depolarized smooth muscle cell membrane in a similar way as in heart muscle. So, even in the presence of a normal extracellular Ca concentration, less Ca is available to the contractile system. Only by increasing the extracellular Ca concentration above normal can the reduction in transmembrane Ca inflow be partially compensated.

2. Peculiarities of Ca-Antagonistic Coronary Smooth Muscle Relaxation Produced by Vasodilators of the Nitrite Group

It is very interesting in this connection that nitroglycerin and other coronary vasodilators of the nitrite group also interfere with the Ca-dependent processes of excitation-contraction coupling in smooth muscle, despite the fact that these drugs have no corresponding action on myocardial fibers (see Grün and Fleckenstein [2]; Weder and Grün [5]). However, the kinetics of the coronary effects of the nitrites proved to be very different when compared with the coronary vasodilators of the verapamil-nifedipine-type. For instance, the nitroglycerin-induced coronary relaxation is very rapid and reaches its maximum within a few minutes, as can be seen from Fig. 3. On the other hand, the coronary smooth muscle relaxation produced by simple Ca withdrawal or by nifedipine, D 600 or verapamil is considerably slower. But the rapid nitroglycerin-induced coronary relaxation always remains incomplete, even if the drug concentration is considerably increased. Apart from this, the nitroglycerin-induced relaxation is transient, so that the coronary tone tends to recover spontaneously even in the presence of

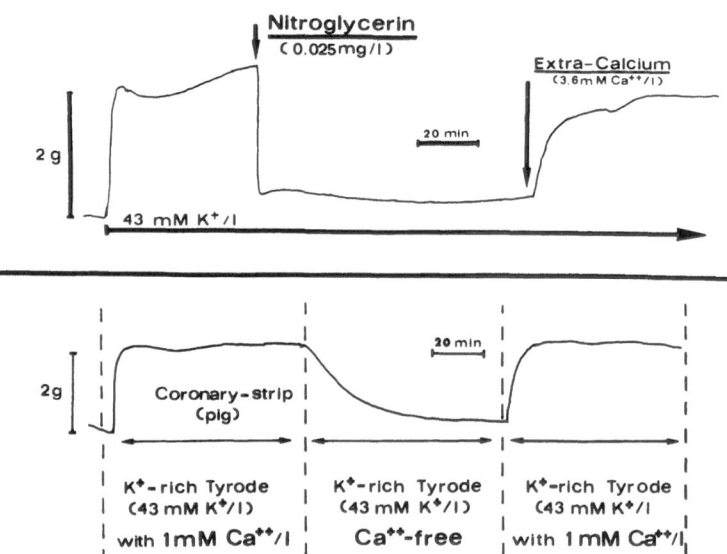

Fig. 3. Extremely rapid relaxation of a potassium-depolarized pig coronary strip produced by the Ca-antagonistic action of nitroglycerin. Comparison with the slower relaxation following simple Ca withdrawal

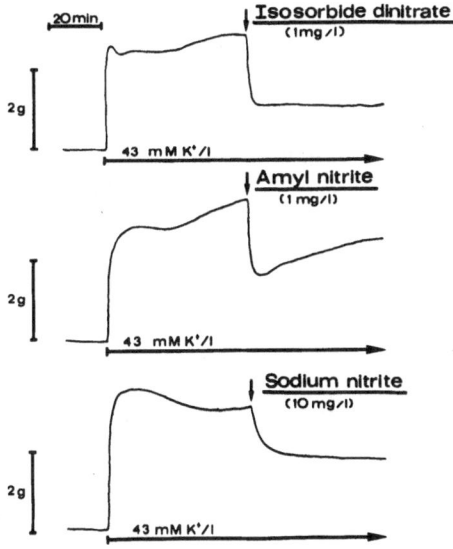

Fig. 4. Rapid but incomplete relaxation of potassium-depolarized pig coronary strips by the Ca-antagonistic action of other drugs of the nitrite group

an elevated drug level. Isosorbide dinitrate and sodium nitrite act like nitroglycerin, in that they also produce a rapid but incomplete relaxation of potassium-depolarized coronary strips (see Fig. 4). Again the drug action is spontaneously reversible, particularly in the case of amylnitrite.

In contrast, the coronary relaxation following administration of verapamil, D 600, prenylamine or nifedipine, proceeds more slowly and persists for many hours at a dose-dependent maximum. Only the drugs of the verapamil-nifedipine-type can abolish the coronary vascular tone completely and permanently. The peculiarities of coronary relaxation induced by the Ca-antagonistic actions of nitroglycerin and other nitrites are compiled in Table 1. Obviously both our experimental findings on isolated preparations and clinical observations confirm the general opinion that, due to their rapid action, the nitrites are very useful drugs in the therapy of an acute anginal attack. But for the basic long-term treatment of coronary disease the Ca-antagonists of the verapamil-nifedipine-type seem to be of greater value since these drugs produce long-lasting coronary vasodilation and exhibit prophylactic antianginal potencies.

Table 1. Particularities of coronary relaxation induced by the Ca-antagonistic action of nitroglycerin and other nitrites

---

1. *Rapid onset of relaxation* within 1 minute even at very low drug concentrations.
2. *Incomplete relaxation* (20—40% nitrite-resistant residual contractures in potassium-depolarized coronary strips even at high drug concentrations).
3. *Spontaneous recovery of coronary tone* even in the presence of increasing drug concentrations (particularly in the case of amyl nitrite).
4. *Easy reversibility of drug action* by extra Ca or by alkaline Tris-buffered Tyrode solution.

---

3. Coronary Vasodilators Lacking Ca-Antagonistic Properties— Site of Action and Questionable Efficacy in Coronary Disease

We have also examined the effects produced by some other coronary vasodilators such as adenosine, theophylline, dipyridamole (Persantine), chromonar (carbocromene, Intensain) and caffeine on isolated coronary strips. But none of these compounds interferes with Ca-dependent excitation-contraction coupling, even in very large doses, whereas a fraction of a milligram of nifedipine per liter produces full relaxation (see Fig. 5). Adenosine, dipyridamole, chromonar and theophylline preferably dilate the small coronary resistance vessels in the ventricular wall, but,

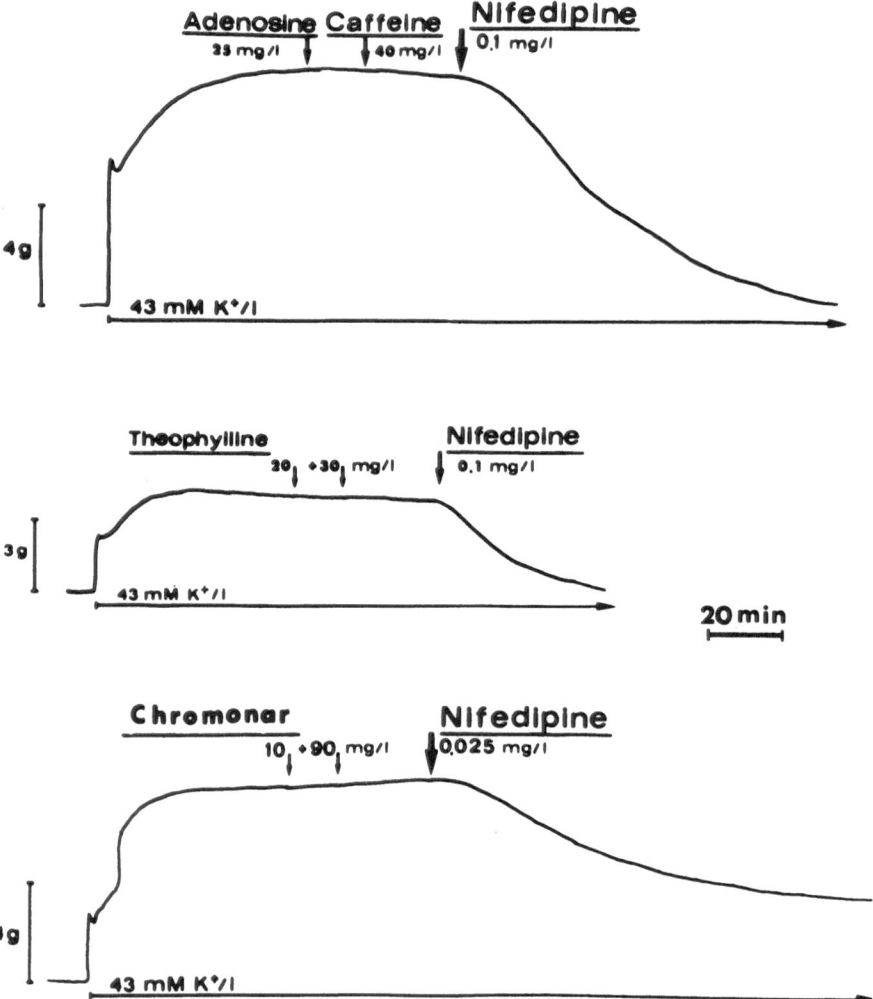

Fig. 5. Inability of 25 mg/l adenosine, 50 mg/l caffeine, 50 mg/l theophylline and 100 mg/l chromonar (carbocromene, Intensain) to interfere with excitation-contraction coupling in 3 potassium-depolarized pig coronary strips. Complete uncoupling by only 0.1 mg/l nifedipine

practically, do not diminish the Ca-dependent vascular tone of the large myocardial coronary arteries where most of the arteriosclerotic intima processes (approx. 95%) found in patients with coronary disease are localized. Therefore, the efficacy of these compounds in augmenting the blood flow through a diseased big coronary artery is questionable. In contrast, the Ca-antagonistic drugs such as nifedipine, verapamil, prenylamine, papaverine, and the nitrites are capable of relaxing the smooth musculature of the great epicardial coronary vessels. This fact is made particularly obvious by our present observations on coronary strips, which originated exclusively from arteries of large diameter. Because the big extramural coronary arteries are not closely exposed to the physiological vasodilator effects of a hypoxic accumulation of hydrogen ions in the myocardium, vasodilation by pharmacological means, particularly, with Ca-antagonistic drugs, seems to be a most reasonable method to use in the therapy of coronary disease as long as the sclerotic vessels remain responsive.

4. Ca-Synergistic Augmentation of Coronary Smooth Muscle Tone by Cardiac Glycosides.—Neutralization of the Vascular Glycoside Effects by Ca-Antagonistic Compounds

The last chapter of this paper deals with another interesting problem, namely the interaction of cardiac glycosides and Ca-antagonistic coronary vasodilators of the verapamil-nifedipine type. It is commonly known among clinicians that cardiac glycosides are not always well tolerated by patients with coronary disease. Some patients with coronary sclerosis may respond to the glycoside treatment with more frequent anginal attacks or with signs of cardiac ischemia in the electrocardiogram. Therefore, many drug combinations were introduced into therapy, in which cardiac glycosides were joined with coronary vasodilators, to avoid such complications.

One reason for the sometimes unpleasant side effects of cardiac glycosides in patients with coronary disease seems to be an increase in myocardial oxygen demand resulting from the glycoside-induced augmentation of stroke work. But apart from this the possible role of direct glycoside action on coronary smooth muscle cells should not be overlooked. Indeed, coronary vascular tone may be increased under the influence of digitalis or strophanthin. This increase in coronary smooth muscle tone is obviously due to a Ca-synergistic glycoside action. Therefore, it is not surprising that the Ca-antagonistic vasodilators of the verapamil-nifedipine type are able, even in very low doses, to suppress the vasoconstrictor action of the cardiac glycosides, as we have recently published [1, 3, 4]. As illustrated in Fig. 5, 6, and 7, cardiac glycosides such as ouabain, digoxin, lanatoside C, proscillaridin A, digitoxin and k-strophanthin produce considerable contractures of the coronary strips at a dose as low as 0.5 mg/l. But this vasoconstrictor effect is readily neutralized by addition of verapamil or nifedipine to the glycoside-containing medium. In the case of a simultaneous administration of the Ca-antagonistic compounds and the glycoside, no increase in tone occurs. Prenylamine and papaverine also possess Ca-antagonistic properties and produce relaxation of glycoside-contractured coronary strips. But when compared with nife-

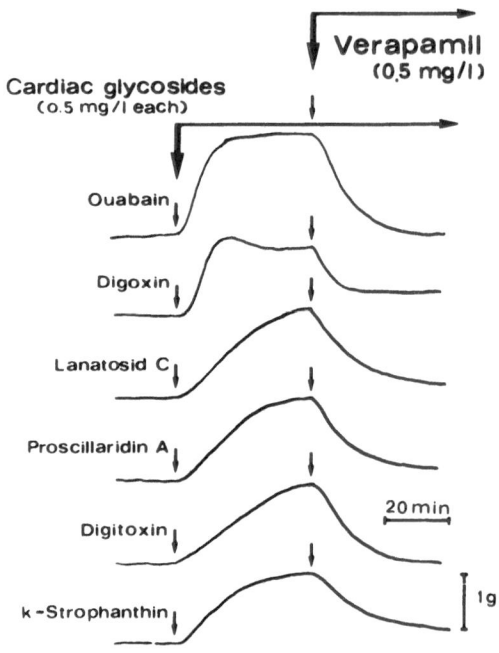

Fig. 6. Neutralization of the coronary vasoconstrictor effect of a number of cardiac glycosides by the Ca-antagonistic action of verapamil

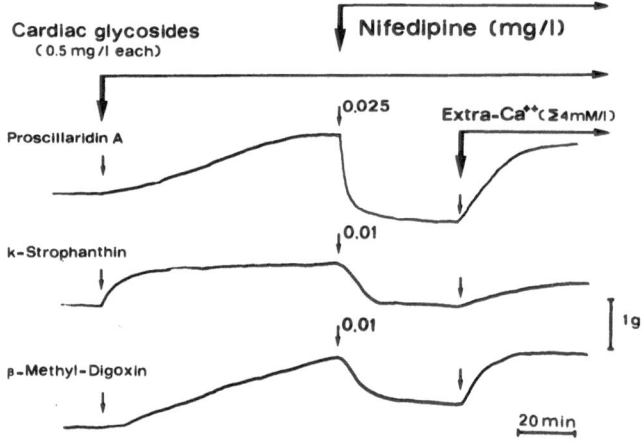

Fig. 7. Neutralization of the coronary vasoconstrictor effects of cardiac glycosides by the Ca-antagonistic action of nifedipine in a dosage range of 10–25 µg/l

dipine or verapamil, their coronary relaxant potencies are weaker. Figure 8 shows the relaxing effects of 2 mg/l prenylamine and 10 mg/l papaverine.

In contrast to the Ca-antagonistic compounds, other coronary vasodilators, which do not significantly interfere with excitation-contraction coupling, are practically unable to prevent or abolish the glycoside-induced coronary contractures. This applies, for instance, to chromonar (Intensain). As can be seen from

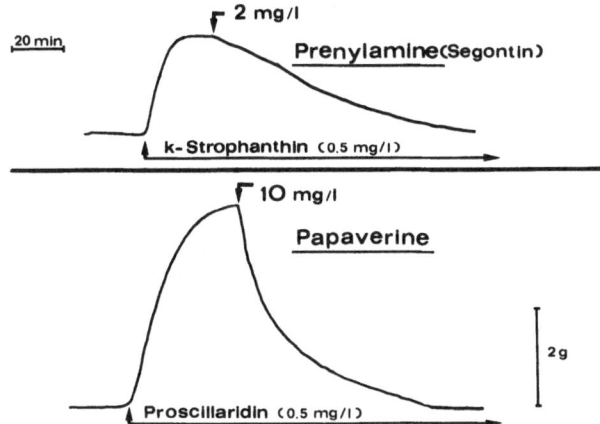

Fig. 8. Neutralization of the vasoconstrictor effect of cardiac glycosides on coronary smooth muscle by the Ca-antagonistic action of prenylamine (Segontin) and papaverine

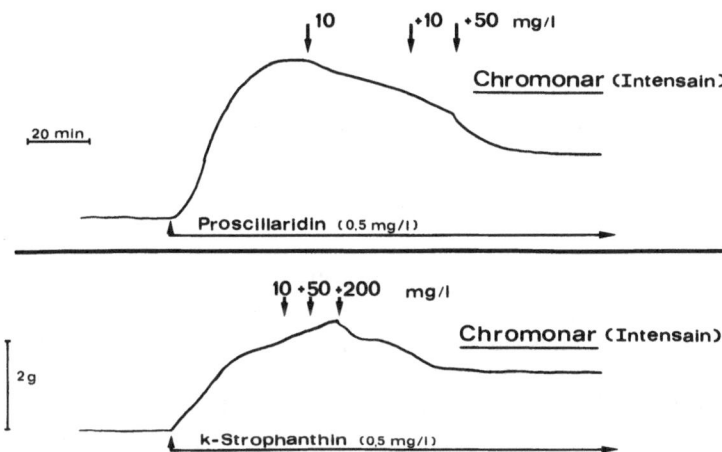

Fig. 9. Weak inhibition of glycoside-induced contractures of coronary strips by excessively large doses (70–260 mg/l) of chromonar (Intensain)

Fig. 9, even with 260 mg/l of Intensain, no complete inhibition of the glycoside-induced contractures of coronary strips could be obtained. Adenosine and dipyridamole (Persantine) also proved to be very weak, since doses as high as 60 mg/l were needed to produce relaxation (see Fig. 10). Theobromine and caffeine are totally inefficient. One must conclude from these results that it is of questionable value to choose dipyridamole, chromonar, theophylline or theobromine for drug combinations with cardiac glycosides. Glycoside-induced coronary vasoconstriction can be prevented only with the Ca-antagonistic vasodilators to a sufficient extent.

It should be noted that the Ca-antagonistic compounds neutralize the glycoside-induced coronary vasoconstriction in a dosage range that is too low to diminish the inotropic glycoside action on the myocardium. Or, in other words:

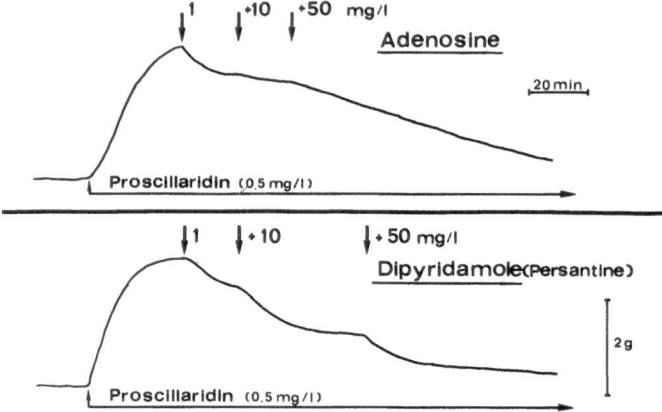

Fig. 10. Attenuation by adenosine or dipyridamole (Persantine) of glycoside-induced contractures of coronary strips

In a suitable drug combination of a cardiac glycoside and a Ca-antagonistic compound, the desired positive-inotropic glycoside effect on the myocardium can retain its full potency, whereas the unpleasant coronary vasoconstriction is eliminated. The clinical significance of these results is obvious.

Abstract

The tone of vascular smooth muscle as well as autoregulation depends quantitatively on the presence of Ca ions, which are required for the activation of myofibrillar ATPase. Thus vasoconstriction occurs if the extracellular Ca concentration rises, whereas vasodilation is produced by Ca deficiency. The present report deals with observations obtained from more than 1000 spiral strips from big epicardial coronary arteries of pig and cattle. A pharmacological way of interfering with the basic action of Ca on vascular smooth muscle tone has been opened by the recent discovery of the extremely potent Ca-antagonistic properties of some drugs such as verapamil, D 600 (a methoxy-derivative of verapamil) and nifedipine. These compounds obviously block the transmembrane Ca supply to the contractile system, so that a "musculotropic" relaxation is produced even by very low drug concentrations. The coronary smooth muscle cells seem to be particularly susceptible to these agents. The well-known coronary dilation produced by nitroglycerin and other compounds of the nitrite group is also due to an interference with Ca at certain membrane sites. By increasing the extracellular Ca concentration, the coronary vascular tone quickly recovers. Other coronary vasodilators such as adenosine, dipyridamole (Persantine), chromonar (carbocromene, Intensain), theophylline etc. do not possess Ca-antagonistic properties; these substances preferably dilate the small coronary resistance vessels, but, practically, do not relax the smooth musculature of the major epicardial arteries, which are primarily affected in patients with angina and other forms of coronary disease. Thus the therapeutic value of the latter drugs is questionable. Cardiac glycosides, on the other hand, even increase the smooth muscle tone of the big epicardial coronary arteries due to their well-known Ca-synergistic action. Nevertheless this unpleasant glycoside-induced coronary contracture, which may promote anginal attacks, can be easily prevented by Ca-antagonistic agents. In contrast, the foregoing coronary vasodilators that lack Ca-antagonistic properties are more or less unable to neutralize glycoside-induced coronary vasoconstriction.

References

1. FLECKENSTEIN, A., BYON, K. Y.: Prevention by Ca-antagonistic compounds (verapamil, D 600) of coronary smooth muscle contractures due to treatment with cardiac glycosides. Naunyn-Schmiedeberg's Arch. Pharmacol. (Suppl.) **282**, R 20 (1974).
2. GRÜN, G., FLECKENSTEIN, A.: Die elektro-mechanische Entkoppelung der glatten Gefäß-muskulatur als Grundprinzip der Coronardilatation durch 4-(2'-Nitrophenyl)-2,6-dime-thyl-1,4-dihydropyridin-3,5-dicarbonsäure-dimenthylester (BAY a 1040, Nifedipine). Arzneim. Forsch. (Drug Res.) **22**, 334–344 (1972).
3. GRÜN, G., FLECKENSTEIN, A., WEDER, U.: Changes in coronary smooth muscle tone produced by Ca, cardiac glycosides and Ca-antagonistic compounds (verapamil, D 600, prenyl-amine ect.). Pflügers Arch. ges. Physiol. (Suppl.) **347**, R 1 (1974).
4. GRÜN, G., WEDER, U.: Augmentation of coronary smooth muscle tone and sensitization to Ca by cardiac glycosides. Naunyn-Schmiedeberg's Arch. Pharmacol. (Suppl.) **282**, R 28 (1974).
5. WEDER, U., GRÜN, G.: Ca^{++}-antagonistische elektro-mechanische Entkoppelung der glatten Gefäßmuskulatur als Wirkungsprinzip vasodilatatorischer Nitroverbindungen. Naunyn-Schmiedeberg's Arch. Pharmacol. (Suppl.) **277**, R 88 (1973).

Discussion Remarks

to contributions FLECKENSTEIN and FLECKENSTEIN-GRÜN

KRAUPP: We studied the effect of ouabain on coronary resistance on the dog heart *in situ* after an intracoronary injection and we used the same doses in coronary arterial blood as GRÜN. We actually got an increase in coronary resistance of about 20–30%. However, this concentration was extremely toxic and cardiac rhythm disturbances occurred, but at this high dosage the reactive hyperemic response was uninfluenced. The concentrations used in these experiments were in the range of 0.5–1 µg/ml and since the clinical effective concentration of cardiac glycosides are about 0.5–1 ng/ml, it seems questionable whether this effect of cardiac glycoside in coronary resistance plays a significant role in clinical glycoside therapy.

FLECKENSTEIN: Cardiac glycosides have two effects on coronary circulation:

1. A direct coronary vasoconstrictor effect due to calciumsynergistic augmentation of coronary smooth muscle tone.

2. An indirect coronary vasodilator effect due to the positive inotropic action on the myocardium. These two effects neutralize each other under normal conditions in a healthy dog. I think if you had carried out your experiments on arteriosclerotic dogs, then the results of the experiments would be perhaps quite different. Another question is the dose. We have carried out dose-response curves for coronary strips and for isolated papillary muscles of the same animal (rabbit), and

if we compare the glycoside action on isolated papillary muscle and on an isolated strip of a bigger branch of the coronary artery of the same animal, we find that the coronary strip is always more sensitive to glycosides than the isolated papillary muscle. We cannot influence myocardial contractility without influencing the coronary smooth muscle cells too.

As to the effective doses of cardiac glycosides on rabbit coronary strips, there is an increase in tone and height of phasic responses to electric stimuli with 3 ng/ml k-strophanthin. This dose is totally inefficient on papillary muscles.

TAIRA: Dr. FLECKENSTEIN, is it your opinion that the primary action of nifedipine is the depressive action on the myocardium instead of the dilating action on the coronary vasculature? If one uses the blood perfused papillary muscle preparation and nifedipine in a dose which almost doubles the blood flow through the artery which supplies the papillary muscle preparation, it does not affect the contractility force. So, in my opinion, the primary action of nifedipine, which underlies its antianginal efficacy, is a vasodilative but nondepressant action on the myocardium.

FLECKENSTEIN: We fully agree with you. The extramural coronary arteries, according to our experiments, are more sensitive to nifedipine than the ventricular myocardium. In the unanesthetized animal nifedipine produces primarily vasodilation and if the dose is not too high no appreciable inhibition of myocardial contractility takes place.

LOCHNER: What is the present stage of knowledge on the specificity of those drugs regarding special organs? Is there any idea of the basic mechanism of such a possible specificity?

FLECKENSTEIN: Nifedipine is the strongest and probably the most specific calcium-antagonistic drug. Nevertheless, D 600, a methoxy derivative of verapamil, has similar potency. Perhaps nifedipine exerts a more pronounced vasodilator effect on the limbs so that the reflex activation of the sympathetic system is more obvious. But the basic calciumantagonistic action is the same. Verapamil is somewhat weaker than nifedipine but this can be compensated for by increasing the dose. Perhaps there are differences in the intestinal absorption rates. Prenylamine, apart from its calcium-antagonistic action and a reserpine-like influence on catecholamine stores, exerts sodium-antagonistic side effects. The consequence is that the excitatory processes (action potential, ectopic automaticity, impulse conduction, etc.) of the ventricular myocardium are somewhat more affected by prenylamine than by nifedipine.

Myocardial Oxygen Consumption under the Influence of Nifedipine (Adalat) in the Anesthetized Dog

W. VATER

Pharma Research Center, Bayer AG, Wuppertal 1, Fed. Rep. Germany

FLECKENSTEIN et al. [3] demonstrated that nifedipine decreases the contractility and oxygen consumption of the isolated papillary muscle of guinea pig. These results were confirmed by RAFF et al. [5], who demonstrated negative inotropic effects and a decreasing action on the oxygen consumption of nifedipine in the isolated Langendorff-guinea pig heart preparation.

Negative inotropic effects of nifedipine and diminished cardiac oxygen consumption did not occur in intact superficially anesthetized dogs as shown by MAXWELL and RENCIS [4] as well as by RAFF et al. [5].

This lack of correspondence between the effects of nifedipine in isolated organs and in the intact animal is probably due to the ability of the intact organism to counteract the direct cardiac muscle effects of the drug through circulatory reflexes.

In order to abolish compensatory reactions, dogs were deeply anesthetized with cyclobarbital. The influence of nifedipine on cardiac oxygen consumption was assessed by different methods:

In a first series of experiments, the tension-time-index—an indirect measure of cardiac oxygen demand—was estimated in intact dogs.

In a second series of experiments, direct measurements of left ventricular oxygen consumption were performed in open-chest dogs.

Materials and Methods

Experimental animals were dogs weighing between 18–20 kg, anesthetized with cyclobarbital, 80 mg/kg intraperitoneally.

a) The tension-time-index was calculated from left ventricular ejection time, the mean systolic pressure and heart rate. The ejection time was assessed phonocardiographically as the interval between the first and the second heart sound.

b) The dogs were artificially respirated using a tracheal catheter and a Starling pump.

The chest was opened and the heart exposed. The preparation of the heart is demonstrated in Fig. 1.

Coronary flow was monitored from the intraventricular ramus of the left coronary artery using a Statham SP 2202 magnetic flowmeter and a flow probe of 1.5 mm in diameter.

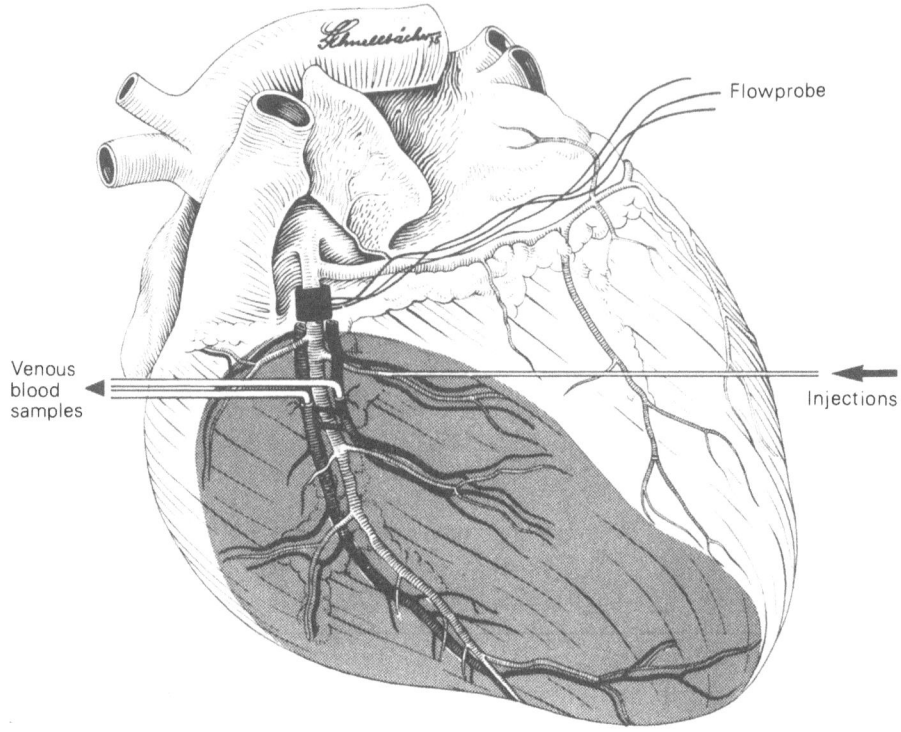

Fig. 1. Demonstration of the dog heart preparation

By inserting cannulas in the concomitant veins, blood samples were withdrawn. The oxygen tension, the carbon dioxide tension and the pH were determined by a blood gas analyzer (Instrumentation Laboratories 313). The oxygen content of the blood—given in percent volume—was calculated using the oxygen binding curve for dog blood according to BARTHELS and HARMS [7]. The oxygen consumption was calculated by multiplying the coronary flow by the arteriovenous oxygen difference.

At the end of each trial, a 3% Evans blue solution according to ECKENHOFF et al. [2] was injected into the intraventricular ramus of the left coronary artery until the dye stuff was visible in the concomitant veins. The stained part of the heart muscle, which is approximately equal to the area perfused by the intraventricular ramus, was excised and weighed immediately.

Results and Discussion

As indicated in Fig. 2, intravenous injections of nifedipine in the dose range between 1 to 10 µg/kg diminish the tension-time-index dose dependently, the maximum effect being −31% with the 10 µg/kg dose.

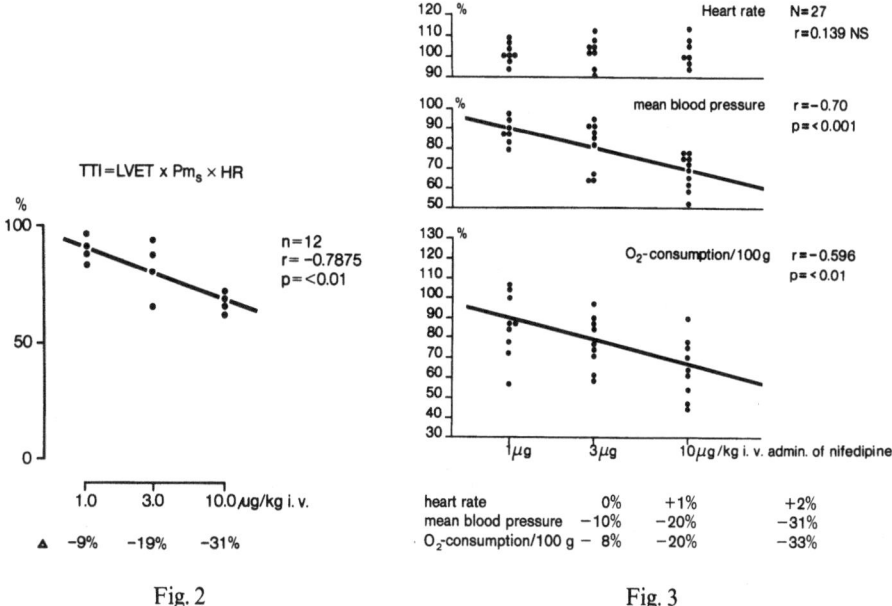

Fig. 2   Fig. 3

Fig. 2. Tension time index after nifedipine in anesthetized intact dog

Fig. 3. Influence of intravenous administration of nifedipine on heart rate, mean blood pressure and O_2-consumption of the anesthetized dog

Although assessed by an indirect method, these results favor a diminishing effect of nifedipine on cardiac oxygen consumption in the deeply anesthetized intact animal.

As shown in Fig. 3, nifedipine injected intravenously in doses from 1 to 10 µg/kg exerts no effect on the heart rate. Mean blood pressure decreases up to − 31% after the 10 µg/kg dose. Oxygen consumption of the measured area of the myocardium also decreases dose dependently.

Since in these experiments nifedipine was administered systemically, influences of extracardial hemodynamic effects on cardiac oxygen consumption cannot be excluded. Therefore the question remains open as to whether the decrease in oxygen consumption of the heart after intravenous nifedipine is a result of a direct action of the drug on the heart muscle itself or it is achieved indirectly, e.g. by reduction of the afterload.

In order to exclude extracardial actions of nifedipine, experiments with intracoronary administration were carried out. Under the conditions of intracoronary administration our experimental set-up permits assessment of regional pharmacogenic effects on contractility and oxygen consumption without major effects on contractility of the heart as a whole.

Figure 4 indicates that oxygen consumption of the perfused part of the heart muscle drops dose dependently after intracoronary administration of 0.3–3 µg/kg. Although with this route of administration a considerable decrease in oxygen consumption was achieved, there were no changes in mean blood pressure and heart rate.

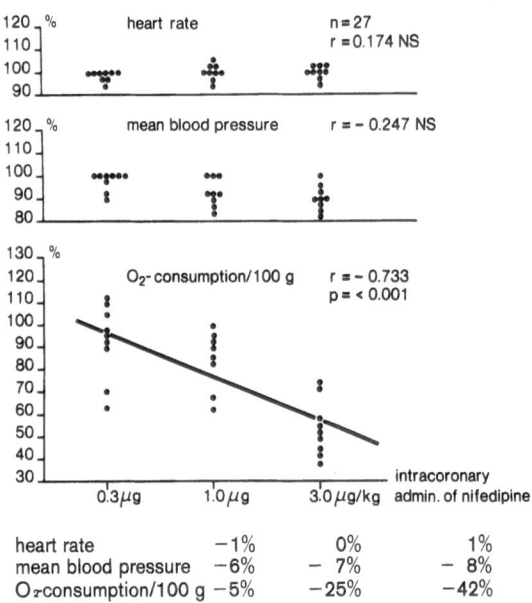

Fig. 4. Influence of intracoronary administration of nifedipine on heart rate, mean blood
pressure and O_2-consumption of the anesthetized dog

Since in these experiments nifedipine does not influence the blood pressure
and heart rate, it can be concluded that the compound does diminish the oxygen
consumption of the heart by acting directly on the heart muscle.

Preliminary experiments on the influence of nifedipine on contractility of the
perfused part of the heart muscle showed that decrease in oxygen consumption
seems to be correlated with a decrease in contractility.

The results demonstrated show and confirm that nifedipine decreases contractility and oxygen consumption not only in isolated organs but under certain
conditions also in the intact organism.

Abstract

In anesthetized artificially respirated open chest dogs coronary flow was
measured in the left coronary artery using magnetic flowmeters. Blood samples
were withdrawn from the concomitant veins and oxygen tension was determined
using a blood gas analyzer. Blood pressure and heart rate were monitored from
the femoral artery.

Myocardial oxygen consumption was calculated from coronary blood flow
and arterio-venous difference of oxygen content of the left coronary artery and
the concomitant vein. The size of the studied myocardial region was established
by staining with Evans blue and weighing the stained tissue. Nifedipine reduced
the oxygen consumption of the myocardium as well as the mean blood pressure
dose dependently (1–10 µg/kg) when given i.v.

With intracoronary application, myocardial oxygen consumption also decreased dose dependently (0.3–3 µg/kg i.c.). With this route of administration blood pressure and heart rate remained unchanged.

The results suggest that the decreased myocardial oxygen consumption caused by nifedipine is not only due to peripheral hemodynamic effects but probably is the consequence of a direct action of nifedipine on the myocardium.

References

1. BARTHELS, H., HARMS, H.: Sauerstoffdissoziationskurven des Blutes von Säugetieren. Pflüg. Arch. Bd. **268**, 334–365 (1959).
2. ECKENHOFF, J. E., HAFKENSCHIEL, J. H., LANDMESSER, C. M.: The coronary circulation in the dog. Amer. J. Physiol. **148**, Nr. 3, 582 (1947).
3. FLECKENSTEIN, A., TRITTHART, H., DOERING, H.-J., BYON, K. Y.: BAY a 1040 — ein hochaktiver Ca^{++}-antagonistischer Inhibitor der elektro-mechanischen Koppelungsprozesse im Warmblütermyokard. Arzneim.-Forsch. (Drug Res.) **22**, 22–33 (1972).
4. MAXWELL, G. M., RENCIS, V.: The effects of a new coronary vasodilatator (BAY a 1040, nifedipine) on the coronary and systemic hemodynamics in the anesthetized dog. Aust. J. Exp. Biol. Med. Sci. **51**, 117–120 (1973).
5. RAFF, K. H., KOSCHE, F., LOCHNER, W.: Untersuchungen mit Nifedipin, einer coronargefäßerweiternden Substanz mit schneller sublingualer Wirkung. Arzneim.-Forsch. (Drug Res.) **22**, 33–39 (1972).

Discussion Remarks

STRAUER: As has been shown in your slides, the oxygen consumption decreased under nifedipine. Heart rate and systolic pressure were kept constant. Was the decrease in oxygen consumption primarily due to a change in coronary blood flow, to a change of arterial-coronary venous oxygen difference, or was it due to a change of both?

VATER: I assume both. The decrease in myocardial oxygen consumption depends primarily on a decrease in contractility, as has been confirmed in several cases with the help of a strain-gauge screwed into the myocardium.

STRAUER: It seems to be generally accepted that nifedipine exerts an increase in coronary blood flow. With increments in coronary blood flow, however, the arterialcoronary venous oxygen difference would be expected to decrease more than the increase of coronary blood flow in order to result in a decrease of the overall oxygen consumption of the myocardium.

VATER: This is understandably not excluded. Therefore, we measured oxygen consumption in constant flow. We could establish the dose-dependent oxygen consumption reduction in the same dose area as I have just shown.

Hemodynamic Effects of Adalat in the Unanesthetized Dog

H. KIRCHHEIM and R. GROSS

I. Physiologisches Institut der Universität Heidelberg, Fed. Rep. Germany

The effect of a drug on the cardiovascular system is determined not only by its principal mechanism of action on vascular smooth muscle and the myocardium, but also by the secondary activation of several control mechanisms. The vasodilator action of a Ca-antagonistic compound such as Adalat will necessarily induce reflex baroreceptor activation. According to the recent literature, supramedullary regions in the central nervous system are involved in the baroreceptor reflex pathways (KORNER [1]). These connections are known to be more susceptible to the action of an anesthetic, however, than the medulla oblongata itself (PEISS and MANNING [2]). In addition the neurons in the medullary reticular formation of an anesthetized animal—due to varying degrees of preparative trauma—receive a viscero-somatic afferent input not present under more physiological conditions.

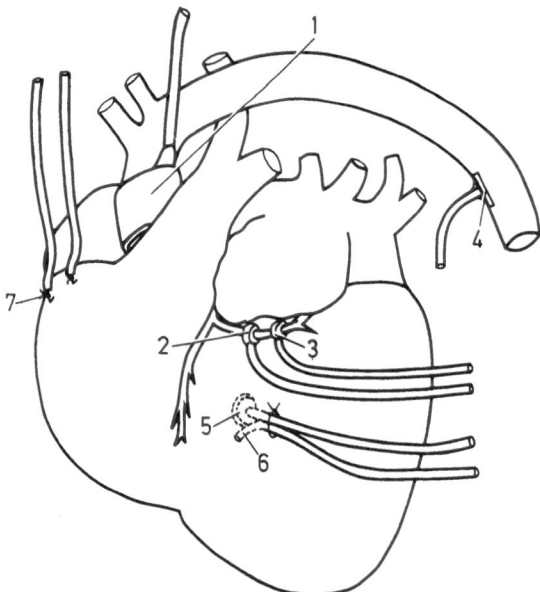

Fig. 1. Diagram of the instrumentation applied to the animal. *1*: Aortic flow probe, *2*: Coronary flow probe, *3*: Coronary occlusive cuff, *4*: Miniature pressure transducer (Konigsberg, P-19), *5*: Miniature pressure transducer (Konigsberg, P-21), *6*: Teflon catheter, *7*: Pacing electrodes

This poorly controlled "non-specific" input, which usually has a generalized activating effect on sympathetic efferents, may lead to alterations in the set point and gain of the baroreceptor reflex (KORNER [1]). In order to facilitate the application of results obtained from animals to man, the experiment in the trained conscious dog seems of great advantage (RUSHMER et al. [3]). We therefore studied the effects of Adalat on the coronary and systemic hemodynamics in the conscious dog.

Trained foxhounds of 23 kg body weight were used. Figure 1 contains a schematic diagram of the instrumentation applied to the animal. Electromagnetic flow probes were implanted around the ascending aorta and left circumflex coronary artery. A small pneumatic cuff downstream from the coronary flow probe was used to determine the zero-flow reference. Miniature pressure transducers (Konigsberg Instruments, type P-19 and P-21) had been implanted into the aortic arch and the left ventricle. A Teflon catheter was used to measure ventricular pressure at the same site in order to check the zero-reference when some drift of the solid-state pressure transducers occurred. Pacing electrodes approximately 2 cm apart were sutured to the base of the right ventricle close to the right atrium.

Figure 2 shows characteristic flow- and pressure signals that were recorded in the resting trained dog after full recovery from implantation surgery (usually not before the 14th postoperative day). At the left a control record is shown followed by registrations obtained 5, 15, 25, and 45 min after the sublingual application of 10 mg (0.43 mg/kg body weight) Adalat. Depicted are 1. left ventricular enddiastolic pressure, 2. aortic flow, 3. its first derivative with respect to time (maximum acceleration of blood in the ascending aorta), 4. left ventricular pressure, 5. its first derivative with respect to time *(dp/dt)*, 6. aortic pressure and 7. left circumflex coronary flow. The records demonstrate an increase of enddiastolic pressure, heart rate and coronary flow but only a small reduction in aortic pressure. At the

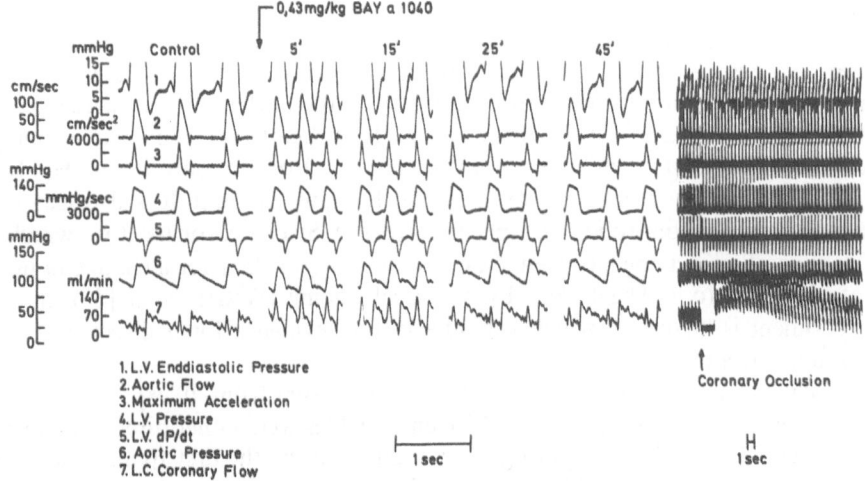

Fig. 2. Original record showing the effect of 0.43 mg/kg Adalat on characteristic flow- and pressure signals

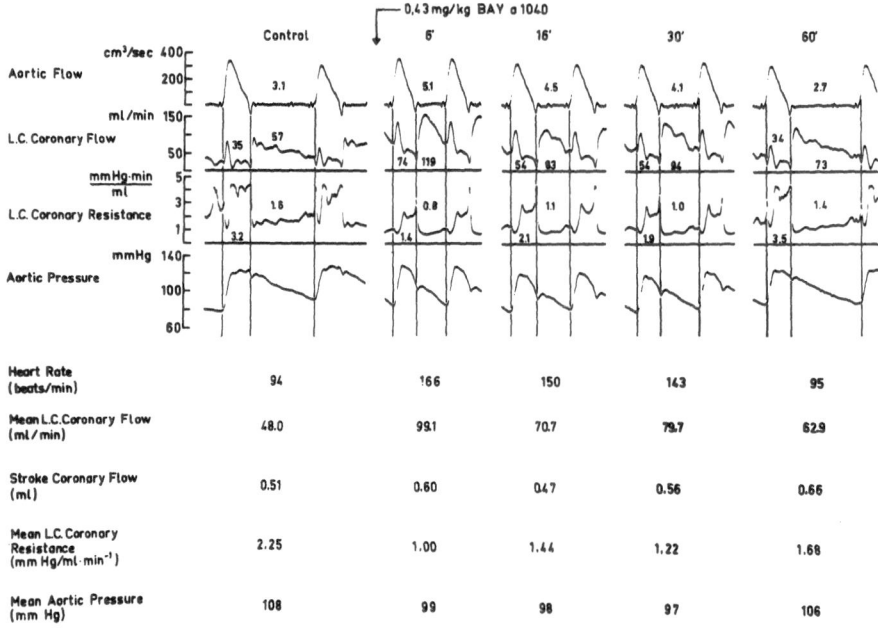

Fig. 3. Original record showing the effect of 0.43 mg/kg Adalat on phasic coronary blood flow and resistance

right of Fig. 2 the coronary artery was occluded in order to check the zero-flow reference; a reactive hyperemia was present after an occlusion of approximately 2 sec duration.

In Fig. 3 the changes in coronary flow and resistance are represented in more detail. In the original record, aortic flow, left circumflex coronary flow, instantaneously calculated coronary resistance (obtained by analog division) and aortic pressure are depicted. In addition several calculated variables are indicated below. The numbers in the coronary flow and resistance curves represent systolic and diastolic means evaluated by planimetry, while in the aortic flow record the numbers indicate cardiac output in 1/min. Both heart rate and cardiac output increase considerably while mean aortic pressure drops by only 10 mm Hg. Systolic and diastolic coronary flow increase by the same amount. It is also seen that systolic as well as diastolic resistance is decreased. Stroke coronary flow, which in the unanesthetized dog has been shown to decrease by 25% for a change of heart rate from 90 to 160 beats/min by electrical pacing (WHITE et al. [5]), in this experiment is increased, which provides further evidence for a direct coronary vascular effect of Adalat.

Figures 4 and 5 show means and standard errors from 10 experiments performed in one and the same dog. Thirteen variables were either directly recorded or evaluated by analog computing every minute during the first 10 min and every 2 min thereafter; the variables are plotted versus time in minutes. A statistically significant difference from control is indicated by the crosses on the reference lines. The initial transient increases of heart rate, aortic pressure, stroke work, $dp/$

dt and left ventricular peak pressure are part of a startle reaction accompanied by licking and chewing due to the crushing of the drug-capsule under the dogs tongue. From the changes in total peripheral resistance (Fig. 4) it is clearly seen that the effect of the drug started about 2 min after sublingual application and lasted for roughly 1 h. Total peripheral resistance decreased by 45% (5th to 10th minutes) and induced a reflex rise of heart rate and cardiac output that was 65% and 61% of that in the control, respectively. The maximum decrease in aortic mean pressure was 11%. Between the 5th and 10th minutes coronary flow was elevated by 91% of that of the control while mean coronary resistance was 56% below control. It should be noted that there was no significant change in stroke volume, although heart rate rose by 62 beats/min. This suggests that a reflex sympathetic inotropic effect was already present, since a similar rise in heart rate induced by electrical pacing would decrease stroke volume in the dog by at least 20% of control (STONE and BISHOP [4]).

Variables that allow more conclusions regarding left ventricular contractility after the application of Adalat are shown in Fig. 5. The data demonstrate a small but statistically significant increase in maximum acceleration (+9%), peak aortic flow velocity (+8%) and left ventricular maximal dp/dt (+13%). While the changes in left ventricular peak pressure are small (+3%), left ventricular end-diastolic pressure rises significantly by 37% of control. During the first 30 min after drug application, when enddiastolic pressure is elevated, left ventricular stroke work is not changed significantly; this indicates a shift of the "ventricular function curve" (stroke work versus enddiastolic pressure) to the right and suggests a primary negative inotropic effect of Adalat on the ventricular myocardium.

From the data presented it seems reasonable to conclude that the primary vasodilator action of Adalat, as evidenced by the remarkable decrease in total peripheral resistance, is probably counterregulated by the activation of the arterial baroreceptors; with the dose used in our experiments this results in almost complete control of arterial mean pressure. Although the data presented so far make it highly probable that the constancy of stroke volume and stroke work is due to a positive inotropism mediated by reflex sympathetic activation, they do not provide direct evidence in favor of this hypothesis. Furthermore the effects of the reflex tachycardia on the metabolic demands of the myocardium possibly could account for a significant fraction of the total observed increase in coronary blood flow. In order to approach these problems, further experiments were performed.

Figure 6 demonstrates the effects of Adalat at a constant heart rate. The control record at the left shows 1. aortic flow, 2. cardiac output, 3. aortic pressure, 4. mean left circumflex coronary flow, 5. left ventricular dp/dt and 6. left ventricular pressure. The heart was electrically paced at a rate that was usually observed after the application of Adalat, i.e. at 150 beats/min. Pacing itself reduced peak velocity and stroke volume (the latter variable is not directly indicated in Fig. 6) while it increased cardiac output. Aortic mean pressure rose by 20 mm Hg, coronary mean flow increased by 15 ml/min, dp/dt was slightly decreased whereas left ventricular peak pressure was slightly increased. The application of Adalat at a paced rate of 150 beats/min caused a rise in aortic peak flow, stroke

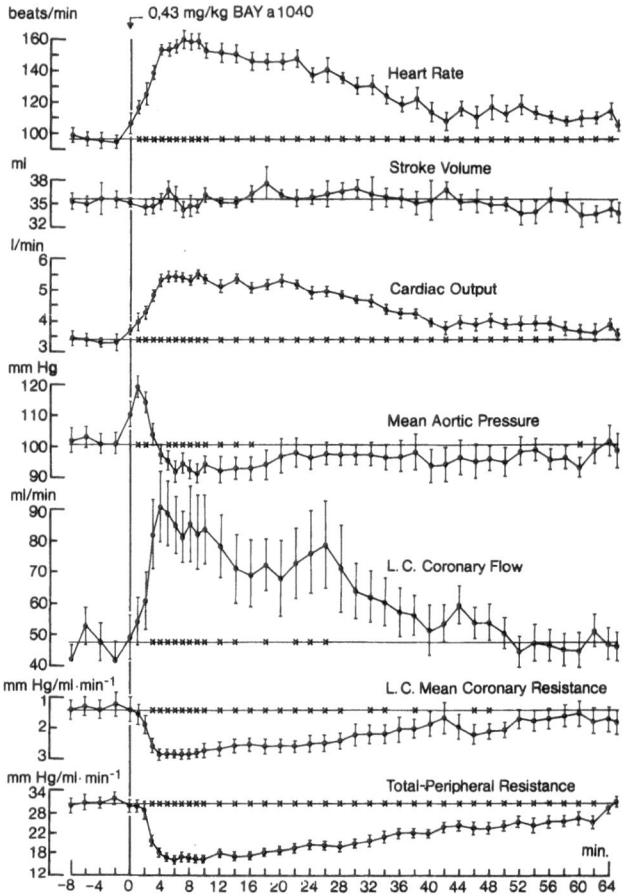

Figs. 4 and 5. Effect of 0.43 mg/kg Adalat on thirteen hemodynamic variables. Depicted are means and standard errors from 10 experiments in one dog

volume, cardiac output and coronary mean flow while mean aortic blood pressure decreased by roughly 20 mm Hg. Left ventricular maximal dp/dt is increased 4 and 14 min after the administration of Adalat while the changes in peak ventricular pressure are small. The oscillations seen in this record are caused by overriding normal excitations from the sinus node.

In order to obtain stronger effects on total peripheral resistance and thus possibly to induce more prominent reflex sympathetic activation, in the experiment shown in Fig. 7 the dose of Adalat was doubled. The control at the left shows 1. aortic mean pressure, 2. cardiac output, 3. left ventricular dp/dt, 4. left ventricular pressure, 5. heart rate, 6. left ventricular enddiastolic pressure and 7. instantaneously calculated left ventricular stroke work. Changes similar to those shown previously were observed after Adalat. With this dose, however, mean aortic pressure dropped by 20 mm Hg, and there was a marked decrease in stroke work accompanied by a small decrease in left ventricular enddiastolic

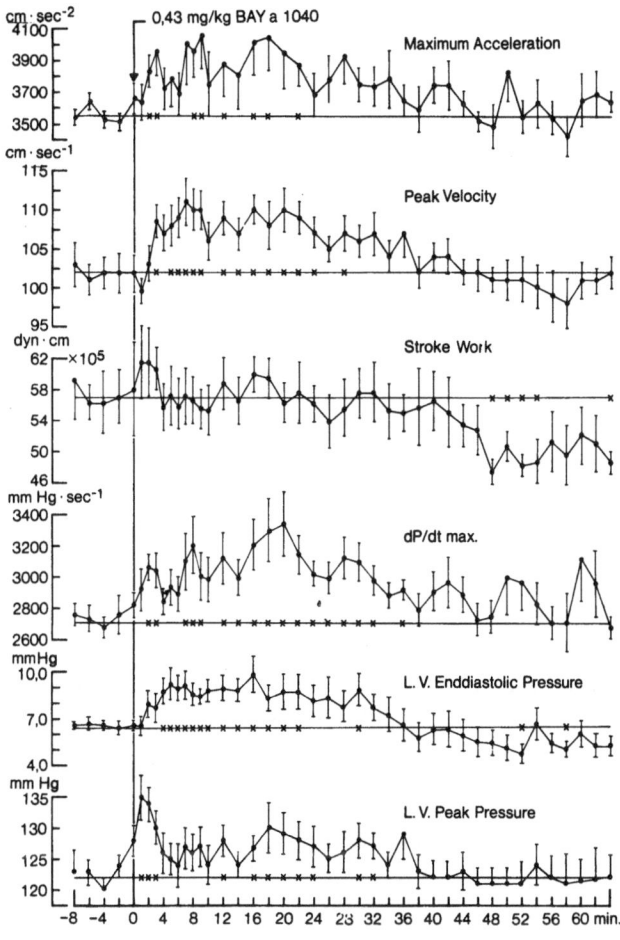

Fig. 5

pressure. Although heart rate rose by as much as 86 beats/min, stroke volume was only slightly reduced (−6%). At the 12th minute following the application of Adalat, 0.5 mg/kg propranolol was given. The β-blockade induced a prominent decrease in stroke volume (−23%), cardiac output (−26%), dp/dt and stroke work. Aortic mean pressure was left practically unchanged, while left ventricular enddiastolic pressure increased. It is interesting to note that heart rate dropped by only 6 beats/min following β-blockade. This experiment demonstrates that a probably reflex mediated sympathetic β-adrenergic stimulus to the myocardium is responsible for the constancy of stroke volume, despite the remarkable tachycardia. The decrease of stroke work in view of an increased enddiastolic pressure following propranolol (17th minute, Fig. 7) indicates that the primary negative inotropic effect of Adalat is unmasked when the reflex sympathetic activation is eliminated by β-blockade. The small decrease of heart rate (5 beats/min) following β-blockade suggests that the greater part of the tachycardia is mediated by reflex vagal inhibition.

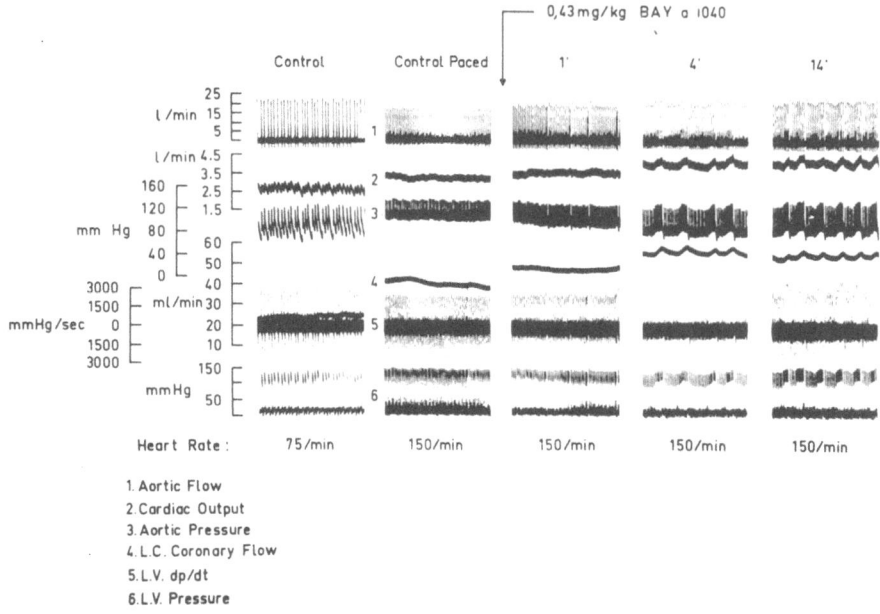

Fig. 6. Hemodynamic effect of 0.43 mg/kg Adalat at a constant heart rate of 150 beats/min (electrical pacing)

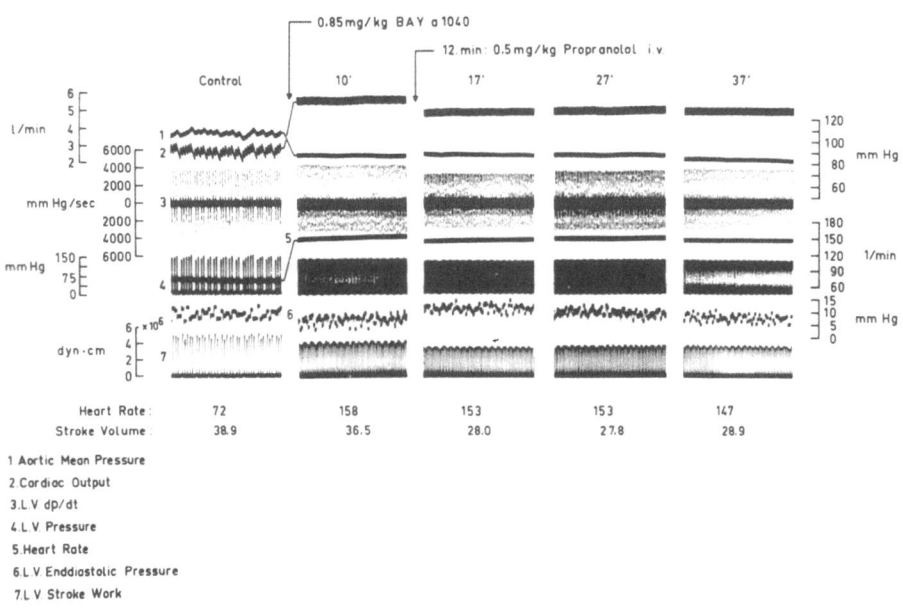

Fig. 7. Hemodynamic effect of 0.85 mg/kg Adalat and the influence of β-adrenergic blockade thereupon (original record)

In summary, we should like to conclude that Adalat in the unanesthetized dog has a powerful vasodilator action in the peripheral and coronary vasculature. After a sublingual dose of 10 mg (0.43 mg/kg) the decrease of total peripheral resistance is compensated by a reflex heart rate dependent rise in cardiac output, probably elicited by the arterial baroreceptors; this results in an almost complete regulation of aortic mean blood pressure. The tachycardia is caused predominantly by reflex vagal inhibition. The primary negative inotropic effect of Adalat on the heart is almost completely countered by reflex sympathetic β-adrenergic stimulation of the myocardium.

Abstract

The hemodynamic effects of Adalat were studied in resting unanesthetized foxhounds after full recovery from implantation surgery. Electromagnetic flow probes had been implanted around the ascending aorta and left circumflex coronary artery, and miniature pressure transducers had been inserted into the left ventricle and aortic arch. The dogs had been further instrumented with a Teflon catheter in the left ventricle, pacing electrodes on the base of the right ventricle, a pneumatic cuff around the left circumflex coronary artery downstream of the flow probe, and a second pneumatic cuff around the descending aorta.

Two minutes after sublingual application of 10 mg (0.43 mg/kg) Adalat the first hemodynamic effects were observed. The effects were most pronounced between 5 and 30 minutes and lasted for one hour, approximately. A remarkable decrease of total peripheral resistance (-45%) induced a reflex rise of heart rate ($+66\%$) which caused an increase of cardiac output by 61%; this resulted in a decrease of aortic mean blood pressure by only 11%. A decrease of mean coronary resistance by 56% caused mean coronary flow to rise by 91%. The vasodilator action of Adalat was furthermore shown by a decrease of coronary diastolic resistance (-50%). Although heart rate rose by 62 beats/min stroke volume was not changed significantly. Corresponding to the increase of heart rate left ventricular mean power rose by 62%. Left ventricular stroke work was not changed significantly, whereas left ventricular enddiastolic pressure increased by 37%. Peak flow velocity and maximum acceleration in the ascending aorta were elevated by 8% and 9%, respectively; left ventricular dp/dt_{max} was increased by 13%.

During the maximum of the drug effect total peripheral resistance was raised by compressing the descending aorta; this caused heart rate and cardiac output to decrease again and demonstrated the reflex nature of the tachycardia. Administration of Adalat after β-adrenergic blockage (0.5 mg/kg propranolol) showed that this tachycardia is in greater part due to vagal inhibition.

When the effect of heart rate on the metabolic demands of the myocardium was eleminated by electrical pacing at 150 beats/min, the application of Adalat caused no significant changes in left ventricular mean power and stroke work but still a decrease of coronary resistance by 20%. Left ventricular dp/dt_{max} under these experimental conditions increased by 8%.

It is concluded that Adalat in the unanesthetized dog has a powerful vasodilator action both in the peripheral and coronary vasculature. The increased enddiastolic pressure at an unchanged stroke work suggests a negative inotropic effect of the drug. Since dp/dt_{max} still demonstrated a small rise in the paced heart its increase can probably be attributed only in part to the rise of heart rate and suggests a slight reflex sympathetic stimulation of the heart.

References

1. KORNER, P. I.: Integrative neural cardiovascular control. Physiol. Rev. **51**, 312–367 (1971).
2. PEISS, C. N., MANNING, J. W.: Effects of sodium-pentobarbital on electrical and reflex activation of the cardiovascular system. Circ. Res. **14**, 228–235 (1964).
3. RUSHMER, R. F., VAN CITTERS, R. L., FRANKLIN, D.: Some axioms, popular notions, and misconceptions regarding cardiovascular control. Circulation **27**, 118–141 (1963).
4. STONE, H. L., BISHOP, U. S.: Ventricular output in conscious dogs following acute vagal blockade. J. appl. Physiol. **24**, 782–786 (1968).
5. WHITE, S., PATRICK, T., HIGGINS, C. B., VATNER, S. F., FRANKLIN, D., BRAUNWALD, E.: Effects of altering ventricular rate on blood flow distribution in conscious dogs. Amer. J. Physiol. **221**, 1402–1407 (1971).

Discussion Remarks

LYDTIN: We have had similar sympathetic activation following the nifedipine administration in the human. We repeated our studies following the administration of atropine in order to rule out that vagal withdrawal contributes to these response patterns. Following atropine we saw increased resting heart rates. There the inverse relationship between the resting heart rate and the increases in heart rate following nifedipine was the same with and without atropine. In the human vagal withdrawal does not seem to contribute to the sympathetically mediated increases in heart rate.

My second comment concerns the administration of propranolol. Propranolol is a beta blocking agent which acts also in the periphery. You gave about 20 mg propranolol which should cause strong β-adrenergic inhibition in the periphery. This could antagonize your nifedipine effect in the periphery. When we used practolol, which is a more selective drug as far as the heart is concerned, we were able to decrease the increases in heart rate induced by nifedipine. Whereas vagal withdrawal does not contribute to the response patterns following nifedipine, β-adrenergic drive takes part in it.

KIRCHHEIM: We usually use 0.2–0.5 mg/kg atropine to block the parasympathetic effects on the heart. LEON et al. [Am. Heart J. **80**, 729–739 (1970)] found, after 2 mg of atropine in man, heart rates of 120–130 beats/min. This rate is very close to the heart rate in the transplanted human heart; so it seems that following vagal blockade heart rate in man is probably about 120–130 beats/min. Another finding of LEON et al. was that after inducing mean blood pressure reductions by 30 mm Hg with amylnitrite, beta blockade only partly reduced the resulting reflex tachycardia; that is, 80% of the heart rate increase was due to vagal inhibition.

On the other hand there is a difference between dog and man as shown in a recent study by SCHER et al. [Fed. Amer. Soc. Exp. Biol. **31**, 1219 (1972)]. They found that predominantly primates react with a sympathetic response; the dog is primarily a vagal responder whereas man—lying in between—reacts more closely to the dog than to primates.

We also have used another beta blocker with less peripheral effects, namely MJ 1999 (Sotalol) and also observed little effect on heart rate.

KRONEBERG: Did you control whether the propranolol dose was able to inhibit other heart rate increases elicited by sympathetic, nonisoprenaline induced β-stimulation?

KIRCHHEIM: There are studies in the unanesthetized dog that provide evidence that the doses used are sufficient to eliminate the effects of sympathetic stimulation to the heart [BERGAMASCHI et al., Amer. Heart J. **86**, 216–226 (1973)].

KRONEBERG: It is very difficult in the conscious dog to inhibit heart rate increase with propranolol per se, so it might be that this is more a technical and a pharmacologic problem, that it seems the drug has properties like atropine.

We have investigated all pharmacologic properties and none have been comparable to atropine. This should be emphasized.

KIRCHHEIM: I think the main difference is actually that in the anesthetized dog a baroreceptor reflex response is observed which is not seen in the conscious animal. If you reduce blood pressure in the conscious dog the reflex increase in heart rate is predominantly mediated by vagal inhibition. So I think the regulation is entirely different in the two preparations.

LOCHNER: Could you define under what conditions or with which doses in your experiments you see a decrease of the preload, that is, the end-diastolic intraventricular pressure, either of the right or of the left ventricle?

KIRCHHEIM: For a total dose of 10 mg—this is 0.45 mg/kg sublingually—we found an increase in end-diastolic pressure by 37% of control. When we doubled this dose we found a slight decrease in end-diastolic pressure (Fig. 7). I would suggest that under the influence of the higher dose there are stronger sympathetic reflex influences and the primary negative inotropic effect of the drug is compensated by reflex sympathetic activation. However, we do not have enough experiments with the higher dose; in most of our experiments we used the small dose and we observed this increase in end-diastolic pressure.

Investigations on the Development of Collaterals, Coronary Flow, Tachyphylaxis and Steal Phenomenon in Dogs after Application of Adalat

J. Schmier, K. van Ackern, U. B. Brückner, B. Hakimi, W. Heger, and J. Simo

Abteilung für experimentelle Chirurgie, Universität Heidelberg, Fed. Rep. Germany

As long as there is no causal therapy of coronary disease, treatment of coronary insufficiency can only be symptomatic and prophylactic. Animal experiments by Vater et al. [4] demonstrated that nifedipine causes a rapid, long-lasting increase of coronary blood flow.

Loos and Kaltenbach [3] reported a long-lasting antianginous effect in patients. There is an improved ST segment in the ECG with an increased capacity for physical activity. These findings are in line with results from double-blind studies published by Kimura et al. [2] and Hayase et al. [1] and other studies.

Long-term therapy, however, is possible only in cases in which no tachyphylaxis occurs. Furthermore it is important to know whether nifedipine induces coronary collaterals. In order to investigate these questions, long-term studies were performed on dogs under standardized experimental conditions.

Eleven mongrel dogs [with a mean body weight of 28.7 kg] were fed 30 mg/day of nifedipine for 39 days. The experiments were performed under light aneste-

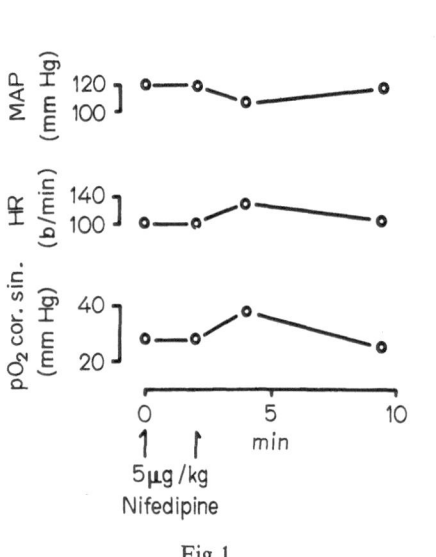

Fig. 1

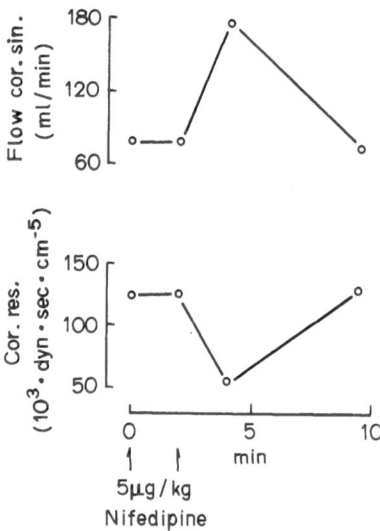

Fig. 2

Table 1. Chronic application

$n = 11$	Before		After		Control group
	Control period	$5\ \mu g \cdot kg^{-1}$ Nifedipine i.v.	Control period	$5\ \mu g \cdot kg^{-1}$ Nifedipine i.v.	
Coron. sin. flow ml · min⁻¹	77.1 ± 16.4	171.6 ± 58.0	76.9 ± 9.5	192.8 ± 52.9	84.0 ± 13.0
Art. press mm Hg	120 ± 14.8	108 ± 10.7	121 ± 15.8	105 ± 12.2	109 ± 24.0
Coron. art. resist. dyn · sec · cm⁻⁵	125 836 ± 29 373	54 559 ± 16 353	120 598 ± 19 865	45 038 ± 17 130	159 478 ± 21 344
Heart rate b · min⁻¹	100 ± 27.0	131 ± 28.0	91 ± 15.8	147 ± 34.3	127 ± 33.0
pO₂ coron. sin. mm Hg	28.0 ± 5.0	38.0 ± 5.2	24.6 ± 6.3	38.5 ± 6.0	24.2 ± 3.3

sia with 15 mg/kg of Nembutal before and after chronic administration of the coronary agent. In the *closed chest state*, coronary blood flow was monitored with an electromagnetic flow probe, which is advanced into the coronary sinus via the jugular vein.

Coronary sinus flow and arterial pressure, measured in the femoral artery with a Statham strain-gauge transducer, were continuously recorded. Heart rate was counted from the ECG. Arterial and coronary sinus pO_2, pCO_2, and pH were measured at constant time intervals. Anticoagulation was induced with 1 mg/kg of heparin. After a control period 5 µg/kg of nifedipine were injected over a 2-minute period.

Figure 1 shows the averages of acute changes of hemodynamic parameters before chronic feeding of nifedipine. From top to bottom: arterial pressure, heart rate and coronary sinus pO_2. The double arrows indicate intravenous injection of nifedipine. There is a slight decrease in arterial pressure to 108 mm Hg. Heart rate increases 30%. Coronary sinus pO_2 rises from 28 to 38 mm Hg.

Figure 2 shows coronary sinus flow and coronary resistance. During injection of nifedipine, coronary sinus flow increases from a control value of 77 ml/min and reaches a maximum of 172 ml/min after 2 min, which is an increase of 123%. Coronary resistance is diminished by 57%. After 10 min, coronary sinus flow reaches the control level.

In a second experiment, after 39 days of chronic feeding of 30 mg/day of nifedipine, the same parameters were recorded during acute injection of 5 µg/kg of nifedipine. In Table 1 the average changes during acute injection of the coronary agent before and after chronic feeding are compared.

Control values from 11 non-pretreated dogs are compared with controls of the pretreated dogs before and after chronic administration of the drug. For example coronary sinus flow is 77 millimeters per minute before and after chronic application of the drug. When compared to a control group there is practically no difference.

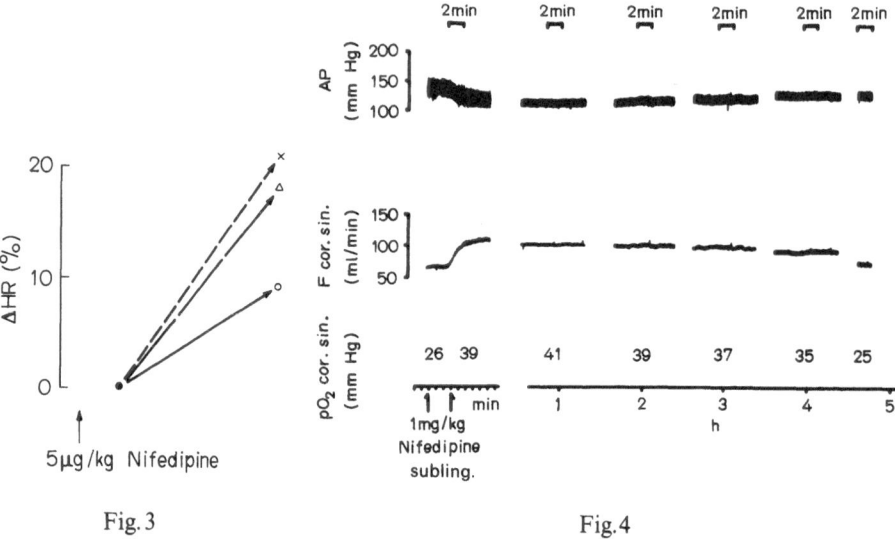

Fig. 3   Fig. 4

Also, changes in coronary resistance and pO_2 as well as in heart rate and arterial pressure are nearly identical before and after chronic administration of the drug.

Chronic therapy with nifedipine does not change the hemodynamic control state. Moreover no signs of tachyphylaxis were observed. Acute injection of the coronary dilator results in identical hemodynamic changes regardless of whether the drug has been chronically fed to the dogs.

In another 7 dogs, the influence of 5 mg of propranolol on the increase in heart rate after i.v. injection of 5 µg/kg of nifedipine was studied. The results are shown in Fig. 3.

Injection of nifedipine alone caused a 20%, increase in heart rate. Propranolol diminished the heart rate by no more than 2%. However, if 5 mg of propranolol were injected before the application of nifedipine, heart rate rose only 9%. This reduced increase in heart rate is statistically significant ($p < 0.05$).

Clinical application requires the rapid and good intestinal absorption of a coronary agent. This is the case with nifedipine, which is absorbed by the mucous membranes of the whole *gastro-intestinal* tract. Figure 4 demonstrates a typical example of an original recording of sinus flow and arterial pressure in an anesthetized dog after sublingual administration of 1 mg/kg of nifedipine. Coincident with a slight decrease in arterial pressure, coronary blood flow increases to a maximum of 120 ml/min after 3 min. After 5 h and 40 min coronary flow has returned to control level. The numbers in the lower part of the figure represent coronary sinus pO_2.

Two different methods are used to determine whether i.v. injection of Adalat increases myocardial blood flow exclusively in well perfused healthy myocardium in comparison to low perfused areas of the heart muscle.

In Fig. 5 blood flow in the circumflex coronary artery and in the left anterior descending coronary artery is measured with electromagnetic flow probes.

Table 2

	Control	Clamp before	5 µg after
M. Ao. Pr. mm Hg	105	100	103
Flow left. ant. desc. ml · min⁻¹	35	18	24
Flow cor. circ. art. ml · min⁻¹	57	49	84

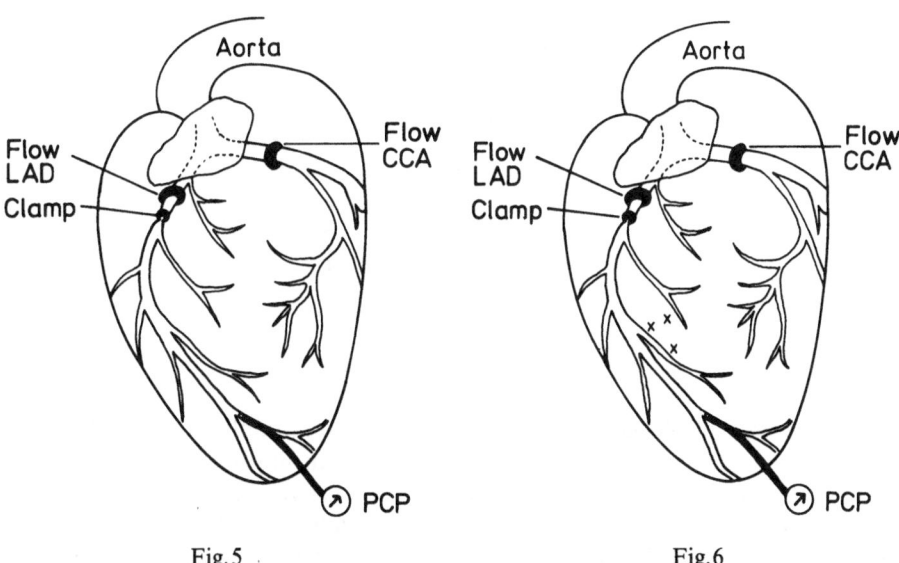

Fig. 5   Fig. 6

Table 3. ^{133}Xenon-Clearance

	Control	Clamp before	5 µg after
ml · min⁻¹ · 100 g⁻¹	98	40	59

As shown in Table 2 flow in the LAD (left anterior descending coronary artery) is initially reduced to 50% by a constrictor. Mean aortic pressure is kept as constant as possible. After injection of 5 µg·kg⁻¹ of Adalat the flow behind the constrictor rises by 30%, although the lumen of the coronary artery is narrowed by about 85%. The flow in the circumflex coronary artery increases by more than 70% ($p<0.01$). The flow resistance is decreased in the constricted LAD by 20% and in the unaffected CCA by 40%. Furthermore myocardial blood flow is determined by the ^{133}xenon clearence (Fig. 6).

After constriction of the LAD myocardial blood flow measured in the area supplied by the LAD decreases from 98 ml/100 g·min to 40 ml/100 g·min (Table 3). Intravenous injection of 5 µg·kg⁻¹ of Adalat results in an increase of myocardial blood flow to 59 ml/100 g · min.

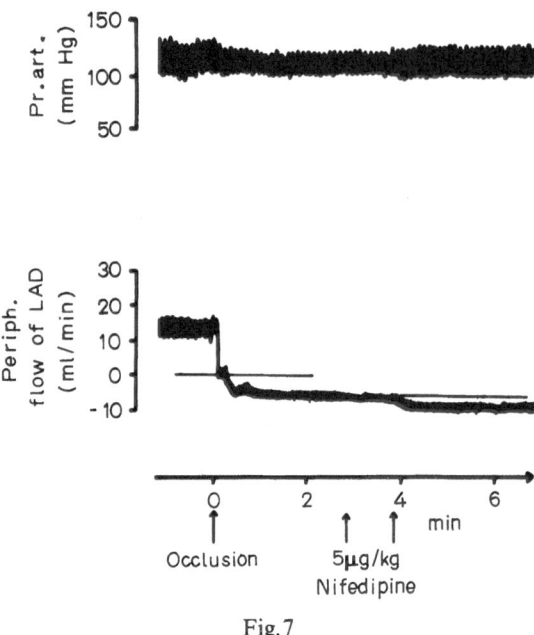

Fig. 7

The increase of blood flow in the poststenotic area implies that Adalat does not produce a steal phenomenon. With regard to an improved tolerance of an acute occlusion, it should be known, whether the active coronary agent induces the development of a collateral circulation. Determination of the functional significance of the collateral circulation posed a difficult problem. We attempted to study the functional and morphologic aspects of this question in the following way: in 10 chronically pretreated dogs, the anterior descending branch of the left coronary artery was acutely ligated 1 cm distal to its origin. Coronary flow was monitored in the distal segment of the occluded coronary artery. Figure 7 shows the results of a typical experiment. Before coronary ligation coronary flow amounted to 13 ml/min at this peripheral location. After occlusion of the vessel, the *direction of flow was reversed* and a retrograde flow of 5 ml/min was observed. After intravenous injection of 5 μg/kg of Adalat retrograde flow increased to 9 ml/ min in the ischemic region.

In nearly all cases, flow was reversed in the occluded coronary artery with the exception of one animal, which had large collaterals distal to the ligature but proximal to the flow probe.

Seven out of 14 pretreated dogs, i.e. 50%, survived a high ligation of the LAD. Only 8% of the controls with equal age and weight survived the same procedure. The increase in survival rate after pretreatment with 30 mg/day of Adalat is statistically significant ($p < 0.02$), even taking into consideration that the deaths of three pretreated animals were from causes other than cardiac.

The coronary arteries were perfused post-mortem with a synthetic resin at physiological pressures. The myocardium was macerated with KOH (potassium hydroxide). The interarterial collaterals of the corrosion casts were counted microscopically and their smallest diameter was measured. In 11 hearts of the pre-

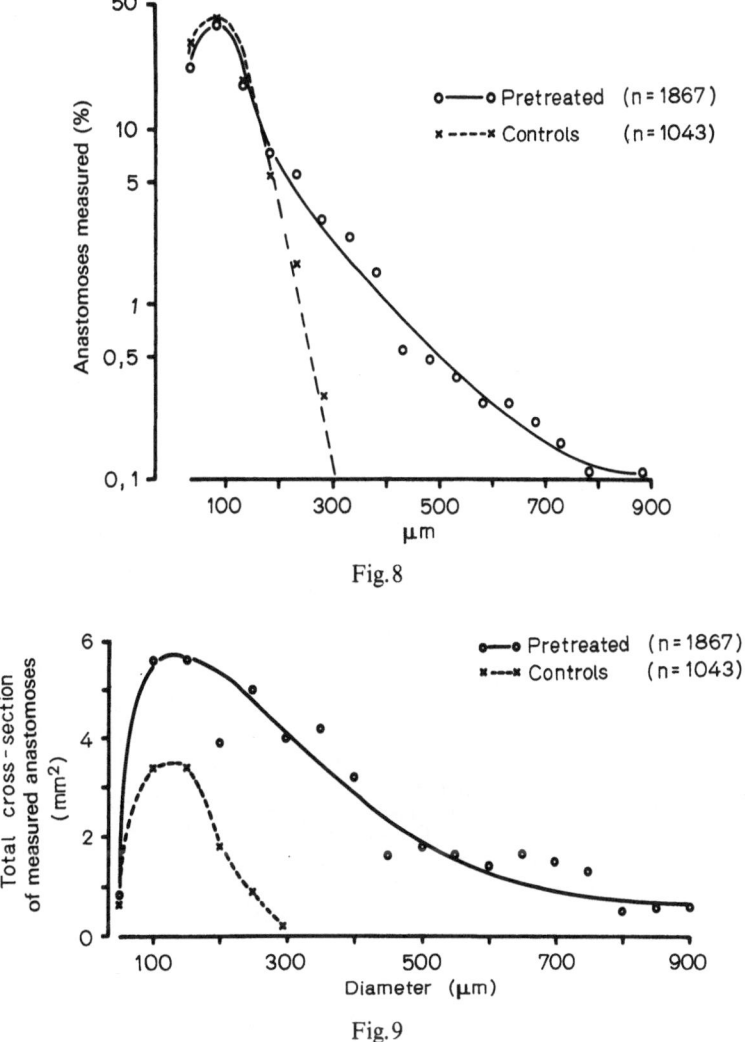

Fig. 8

Fig. 9

treated dogs, a total of 1867 mainly superficially located collaterals were counted. Their smallest diameter was 50 μm. Seven control hearts had a total of 1043 collaterals. On Fig. 8 the collaterals of pretreated and non-pretreated dogs are compared. The collateral diameter in μm is plotted on the abscissa versus the percentage of measured anastomoses on the ordinate. Most of the collaterals of the non-pretreated animals are about 100 μm in diameter. The largest are 300 μm.

Collateral diameters of the hearts of pretreated dogs were significantly larger. In more than 6%, the diameter at its narrowest segment exceeded 300 μm and went as high as 1 mm.

The difference between the collaterals of controls and pretreated animals becomes even more evident when the cross section is calculated in either group, as shown in Fig. 9. In the pretreated dogs the overall cross section of anastomoses is about 4 times as large as that in the controls.

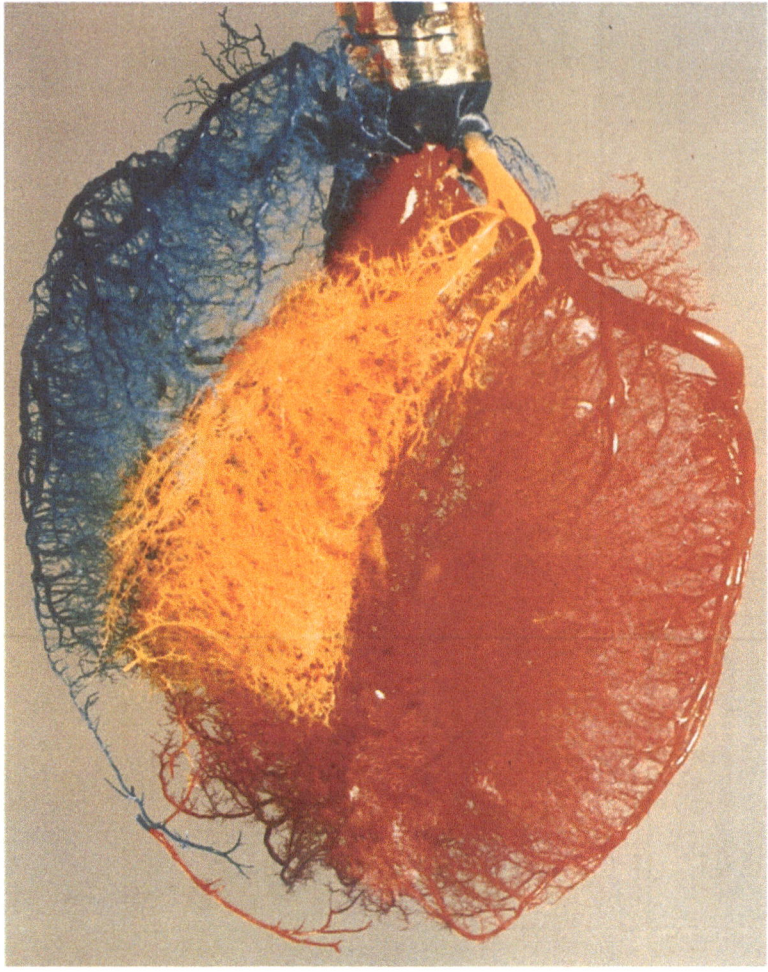

Fig. 10

As the vascular resistance is reciprocal to the fourth power of the radius, the total resistance of the collaterals is significantly smaller in the hearts of pretreated dogs than in control hearts.

After high ligation of the LAD in control animals, the infarct area can generally not be filled with resin via anastomotic channels. This is demonstrated in Fig. 10. Distal to the coronary occlusion, a large portion of the vasculature is not filled.

After identical coronary ligation in the pretreated animals there is complete retrograde filling of the vasculature in the infarct areas demonstrated in Fig. 11.

In conclusion the experiments demonstrate that chronic treatment with Adalat does not cause tachyphylaxis. The substance is a long-acting drug which is absorbed by the mucous membranes. When administered over the chronic in dogs, it induces a protective collateral circulation.

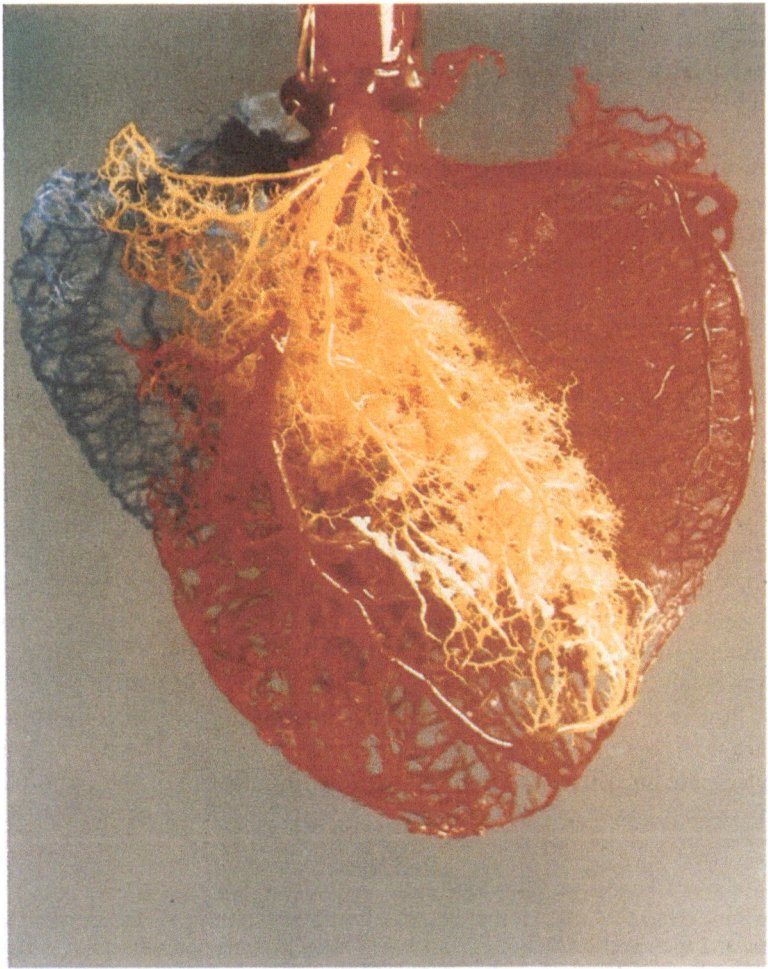

Fig. 11

Abstract

Physiological adaption to coronary vasodilators (CD) is a phenomenon which excludes their use in chronic therapy. In experiments, the action of nifedipine (BAY a 1040) was studied before and after chronic p.o. administration. Two groups were studied. One received no treatment ($n = 11$) and the experimental group ($n = 11$) was administred 30 mg/day of nifedipine for 39 days. Before and after the chronic treatment period the dogs were anesthetized and 5 µg/kg of nifedipine was injected i.v. In the closed chest preparation the following parameters were monitored: coronary sinus flow (electromagnetic probe), arterial pressure, heart rate, arterial and coronary sinus pO_2, pCO_2 and pH.

After the chronic administration of nifedipine the control values of all monitored parameters had not changed. Furthermore, the effects of intravenous injection of nifedipine were the same before and after chronic p.o. treatment. Long-term feeding with nifedipine does not result in tachyphylaxis.

Sublingual administration of 1 mg/kg resulted in a peak increase of coronary flow of more than 100%. This flow increase lasted up to 5 h. Similar results were observed in unanesthetized dogs.

Post-mortem corrosion casts of coronary arteries were made. In chronically pretreated dogs the coronary collaterals were significantly larger in diameter than in nonpretreated dogs. In the pretreated group the left anterior descending coronary artery (LAD) was completely filled distal to its occlusion due retrograde flow.

In 10 chronically pretreated animals blood flow was monitored in the peripheral LAD. After coronary occlusion the direction of flow was reversed. A small retrograde flow was observed. After a slow i.v. injection of 5 µg/kg of nifedipine the retrograde flow increased in the ischemic region. This occurs always when there is no or only a minor decrease in arterial blood pressure.

In 11 pretreated dogs the LAD was ligated close to its origin. Seven animals (63.6%) survived the coronary ligation. The lower coronary mortality after pretreatment with nifedipine is statistically significant (< 0.05).

With 8 measurements the influence of nifedipine on coronary blood flow to a hypo-perfused myocardial region was studied. Flow in the left anterior descending coronary artery was mechanically reduced by 50%. When steady state was reached, $5 \, \mu g \cdot kg^{-1}$ of nifedipine were slowly injected.

The flow resistance in the area of reduced perfusion decreased by 20%; thus coronary flow rose by 31%. The heart rate was unchanged. There is no evidence that nifedipine affects only the normal myocardium but not the hypo-perfused heart tissue.

References

1. HAYASE,S., HIRAKAWA,S., HOSOKAWA,S., MORI,N., KANYAMA,S., IWASA,M.: Hemodynamic and therapeutic effect of BAY a 1040 on the patients with ischemic heart disease. Arzneim.-Forsch. (Drug Res.) **22**, 370–372 (1972).
2. KIMURA,F., MABUCHI,G., KIKUCHI,H.: The clinical effect of 4-(2'-nitrophenyl)-2,6-dimethyl-3,5-dicarbomethoxy-1,4-dihydropyridine(BAY a 1040) on angina pectoris evaluated by sequential analysis. Arzneim.-Forsch. (Drug Res.) **22**, 365–367 (1972).
3. LOOS,A., KALTENBACH,M.: Die Wirkung von Nifedipine (BAY a 1040) auf das Belastungs-Elektrokardiogramm von Angina-pectoris-Kranken. Arzneim.-Forsch. (Drug Res.) **22**, 358–365 (1972).
4. VATER,W., KRONEBERG,G., HOFFMEISTER,F., KALLER,H., MENG,K., OBERDORF,A., PULS,W., SCHLOSSMANN,K., STOEPEL,K.: Zur Pharmakologie von 4-(2'-Nitrophenyl)-2,6-dimethyl-1,4-dihydropyridin-3,5-dicarbonsäuredimethylester (Nifedipine, BAY a 1040). Arzneim.-Forsch. (Drug Res.) **22**, 1–14 (1972).

The Effect of Adalat on the Mechanical and Electrical Activity of Isolated Rat Cardiac Muscle, with Special Reference to Calcium Antagonism of the Compound

K. LANDMARK and H. REFSUM

Institute of Pharmacology, University of Oslo, and Medical Departement B, Rikshospitalet, Oslo, Norway

Introduction

Adalat has been classified as a calcium antagonistic inhibitor of the electrome-chanical coupling process (FLECKENSTEIN et al. [5]). In isolated heart prepara-tions, the compound depresses contractile force and reduces the spontaneous frequency (HASHIMOTO et al. [9]). The drug also causes a dilation of the coronary vessels (VATER et al. [17]; HASHIMOTO et al. [9]; KOSCHE et al. [11]), and when given intra-arterially into the AV node artery, AV conduction was depressed (HASHIMOTO et al. [9]). In the ventricular myocardium of the rabbit and guinea pig, FLECKENSTEIN et al. [5] found that the height and the shape of the single fiber action potential as well as resting potential, excitability and impulse conduction remained practically constant. *In vivo*, the QRS complex was not altered by Adalat (VATER et al. [17]).

The present study was performed in order to investigate the effects of the drug in isolated rat cardiac muscle, with special reference to the calcium antagonistic activity of the compound.

Methods

Isolated Rat Atria

Female, albino rats (about 200 g) were used. The hearts were excised under ether anesthesia, and the atria were quickly removed by dissection and suspended in a water-jacketed organ bath containing a Ringer solution kept at 32° C. The calcium concentration, $(Ca^{++})_0$, of the solution was either 2.0, 5.0 or 8.0 meq/l. The solution also contained glucose, 1.8 mg/ml, and it was bubbled with 95% O_2 and 5% CO_2; pH was 7.4. A preload of 400 mg was put on the preparations and contractile force was recorded isometrically with a Grass force-displacement transducer connected to a Grass polygraph. The stimulation and recording tech-niques, the measurements of the excitability and refractory period as well as the methods used in studying single action potentials derived from rat atrial muscle, have been described before (LANDMARK [12, 13]).

Isolated Rat Hearts

The isolated rat hearts were perfused in a perfusion set-up, and the Ringer solution was continuously recirculated by a peristaltic pump. Cannulation of the aorta was performed with the hearts submerged in ice-cold saline; they were then transferred to a heart chamber. Systolic pressure, atrial rate and coronary flow were recorded, and ECG tracings were obtained by attaching recording electrodes to the aortic cannula and to the cannula draining the chamber in which the hearts were mounted. The temperature of the Ringer solution was kept at 32° C, and $(Ca^{++})_0$ was either 2.0 or 5.0 meq/l. The solution contained glucose and was bubbled with O_2 and CO_2 as described previously.

Calcium-induced ventricular tachyarrhythmias of isolated rat hearts were obtained by a method described by GRUMBACH et al. [8] with some minor modifications. The potassium concentration of the Ringer solution was low (1.325 meq/l) and ventricular tachyarrhythmias were induced by increasing $(Ca^{++})_0$ from 2.0 to 8.0 meq/l.

Calculations

In isolated rat atria, control experiments were performed after a 30 min period of equilibration before Adalat was added. Test experiments were then performed after 10 min. In the isolated rat hearts, continuous recordings of the effect of the drug were made after a 20 min period of equilibration. In order to compare the results, the values obtained at the end of the equilibration period were in some experiments called 100% and used as reference.

Results

Adalat caused a dose-dependent decrease in the frequency of contractions (Fig. 1). The sinus node discharge was higher at 5.0 than at 2.0 meq/l of calcium, and the negative chronotropic effect of the drug was stronger at the lower calcium level (Fig. 2). The drug increased the sinus node recovery time (Fig. 3). In electrically stimulated left atria, Adalat caused a progressive decline in contractile force (Fig. 4). In isolated rat hearts, the systolic aortic pressure was almost the same at the two calcium levels tested. The product of the systolic pressure and the frequency (work index, LOEB [14]) is considered to be a valid expression of the myocardial work. Hence, work index was lower at 2.0 than at 5.0 meq/l of calcium, and the reduction in mechanical performance induced by Adalat 100 µg/l was more pronounced at the lower $(Ca^{++})_0$ (Fig. 5).

The resting membrane potential derived from isolated rat atria stimulated at a frequency of 180 per min remained unchanged at varying calcium levels. The maximum rate of rise of the action potential (dv/dt) and the overshoot, however, increased with an increase in $(Ca^{++})_0$. Adalat 100 µg/l reduced the dv/dt ratio, an effect which was pronounced at low, but negligible at high $(Ca^{++})_0$ (Fig. 6). Increasing $(Ca^{++})_0$ decreased the time for 50 and 90% repolarization. Adalat caused a shortening of the action potential duration, but this action was negligible at higher Ca-levels (Fig. 6).

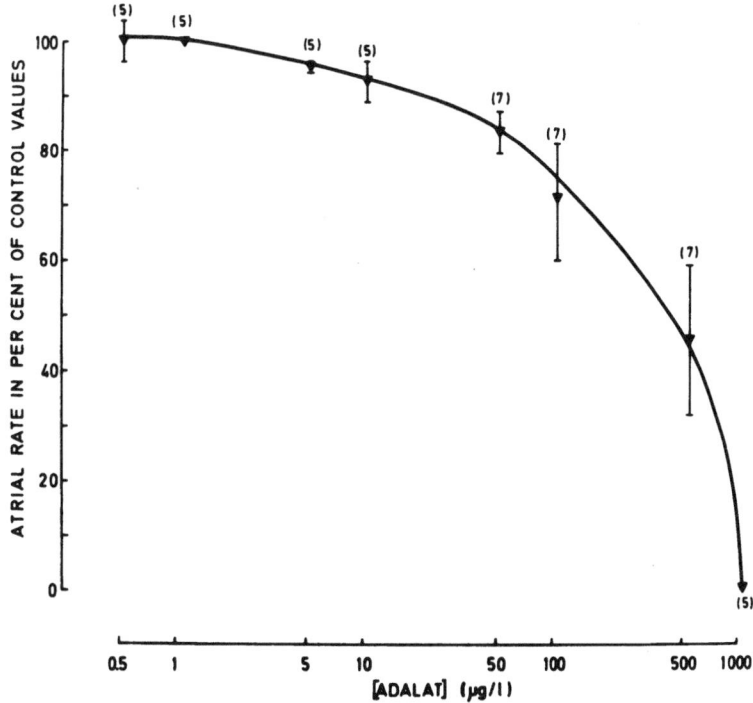

Fig. 1. Changes in atrial rate after addition of Adalat. The values (mean value ± S.E.M.) are calculated as a percentage of the rates measured after an initial equilibration period of 30 min (in brackets, number of experiments)

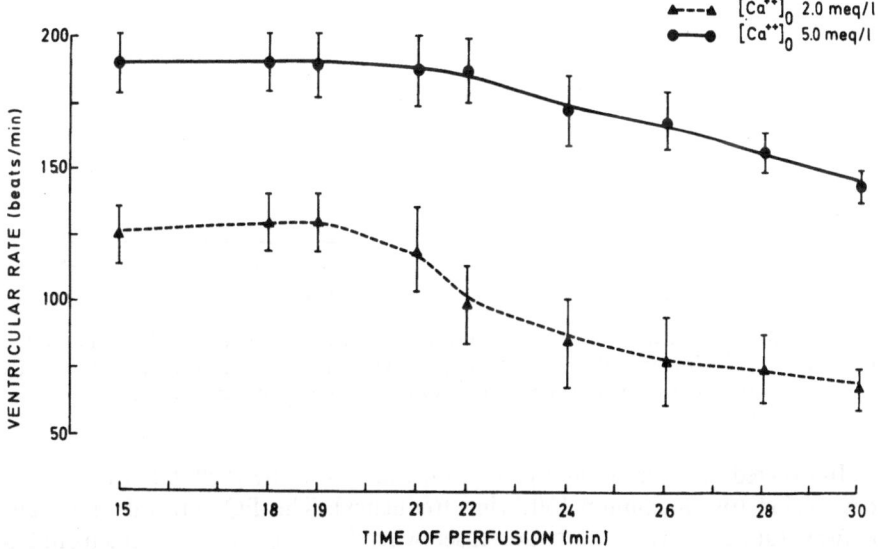

Fig. 2. The ventricular rate in the presence of 2.0 and 5.0 meq/l of Ca^{++}, and the effect of Adalat 100 µg/l after an initial equilibration period of 20 min. Mean value ± S.E.M. of 6 hearts in each group

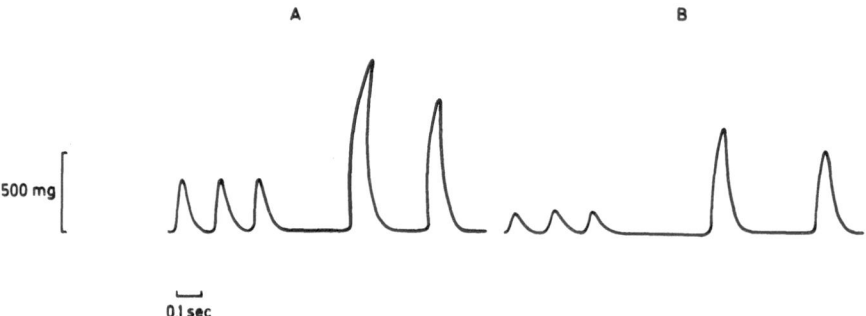

Fig. 3 A and B. The sinus node recovery time in the absence (A) and the presence of Adalat
100 µg/l (B)

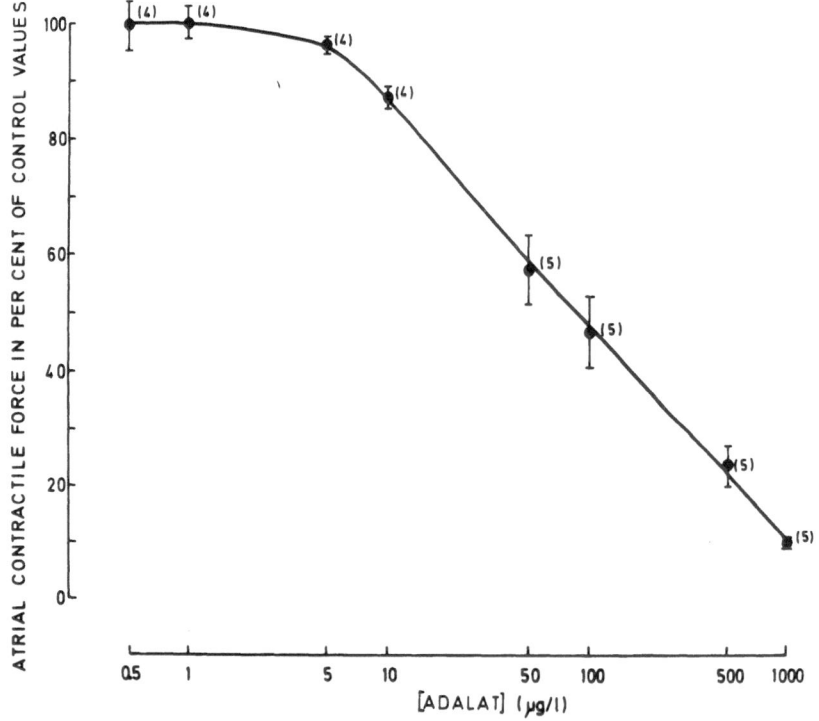

Fig. 4. Changes in contractile force of stimulated left rat atria caused by Adalat. The values
(mean value ± S.E.M.) are calculated as a percentage of the values measured after an initial
equilibration period of 30 min (in brackets, number of experiments)

In isolated rat atria, Adalat caused no changes in the excitability and refractory period (the maximum following frequency). The PQ interval of isolated perfused rat hearts was slightly decreased when $(Ca^{++})_0$ was increased from 2.0–5.0 meq/l. Adalat 100 µg/l increased AV conduction time, the effect being more pronounced at 2.0 than at 5.0 meq/l of calcium, and in these experiments AV blocks of varying degrees appeared (Fig. 7). The R wave voltage of the ECG was

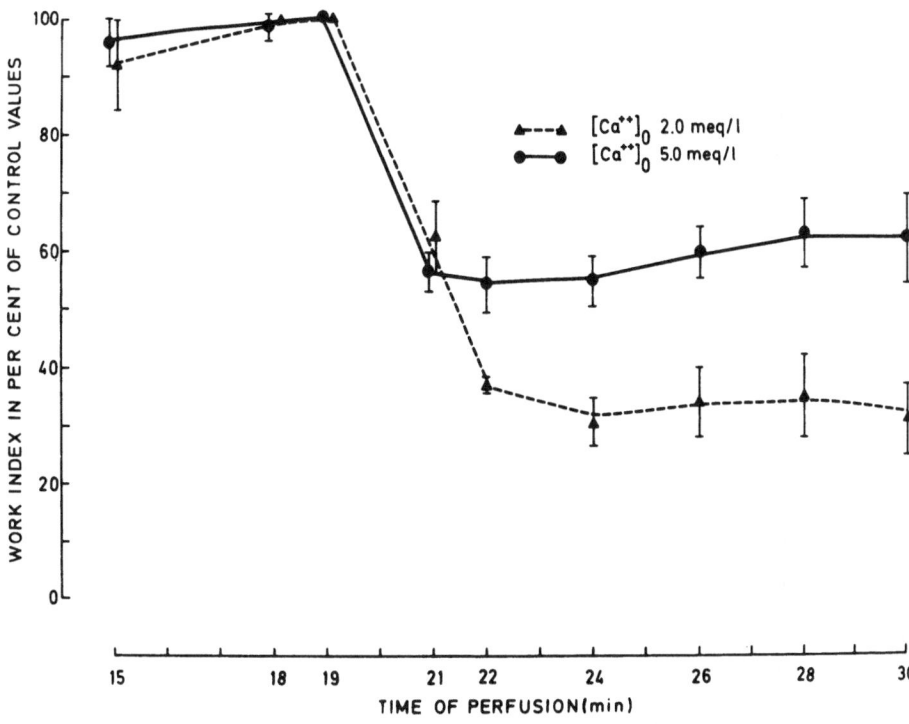

Fig. 5. Work index in the presence of 2.0 and 5.0 meq/l of Ca^{++}, and the effect of Adalat 100 μg/l after an initial equilibration period of 20 min. The values (mean value ± S.E.M.) are calculated as a percentage of the values measured at the end of the equilibration period. 6 hearts in each group

3.2±0.3 mV and 1.7±0.3 mV at the end of the equilibration period in the presence of 5.0 and 2.0 meq/l of calcium, respectively (6 hearts in each group). Adalat 100 μg/l reduced R wave voltage—the percentage reduction was approximately 25 and 35 in the presence of 5.0 and 2.0 meq/l of calcium, respectively.

Adalat 100 μg/l caused a small and transient increase in coronary flow (Fig. 8).

Ventricular tachyarrhythmias were observed in 7 out of 7 hearts when $(Ca^{++})_0$ was increased. In three hearts ventricular fibrillation occured; in the four remaining hearts, ventricular extrasystoles were found (Fig. 9). In 8 out of 8 hearts, pretreatment with Adalat 100 μg/l completely protected the preparations against calcium-induced ventricular arrhythmias.

Discussion

It has been suggested that the generation of action potentials in the sinus and AV node depend on a slow ionic current carried by Ca^{++} or Ca^{++}/Na^{+} ions (VASSORT et al. [16]; ZIPES and MENDEZ [21]; ZIPES and FISCHER [22]). In addition, ARONSON and CRANEFIELD [1] found that under certain circumstances, Ca^{++} can carry the current necessary for pacemaker activity in Purkinje fibers.

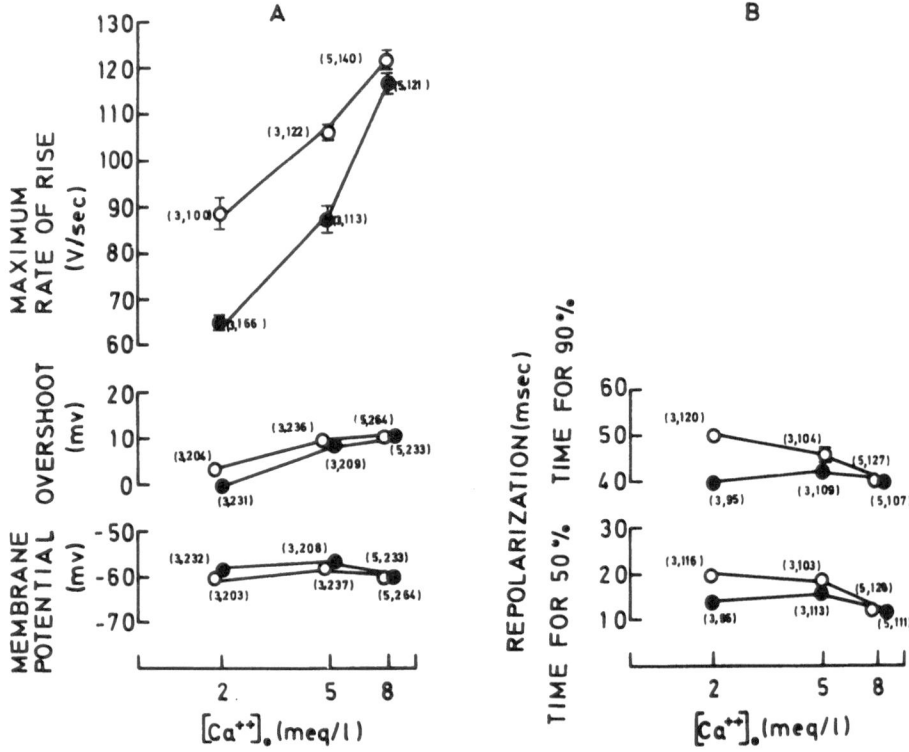

Fig. 6 A and B. The membrane potential, the overshoot and the maximum of rate of rise of the action potential (A), and the time for 50% and 90% repolarization (B) of isolated left rat atria in the presence of 2.0, 5.0, and 8.0 meq/l of Ca^{++}. Control values (○—○) and the effect of Adalat 100 µg/l (●—●). (In brackets, number of atria and penetrations, respectively)

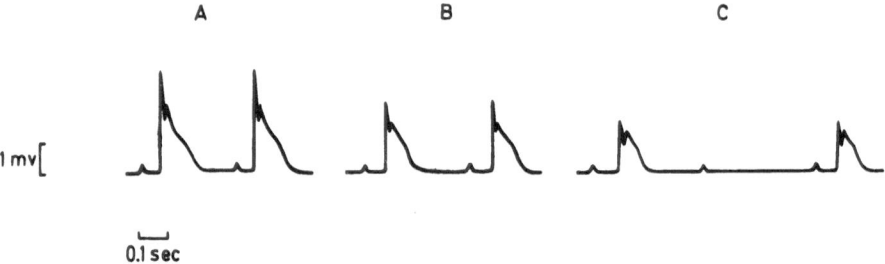

Fig. 7 A–C. ECG-tracings obtained from isolated rat hearts. (A) Control ECG (5.0 meq/l of Ca^{++}), (B) the effect of Adalat 100 µg/l in the presence of 5.0 meq/l of Ca^{++}, and (C) the effect of Adalat 100 µg/l in the presence of 2.0 meq/l of Ca^{++}

The results described above show that Adalat, which inhibits this slow current, depresses sinus node automaticity, increases the sinus node recovery time and impairs AV nodal conduction. The present study also confirms our previous observation that Ca^{++} ions contribute directly to the fast phase of the depolarization in the rat myocardium (LANDMARK and REFSUM, in preparation). The re-

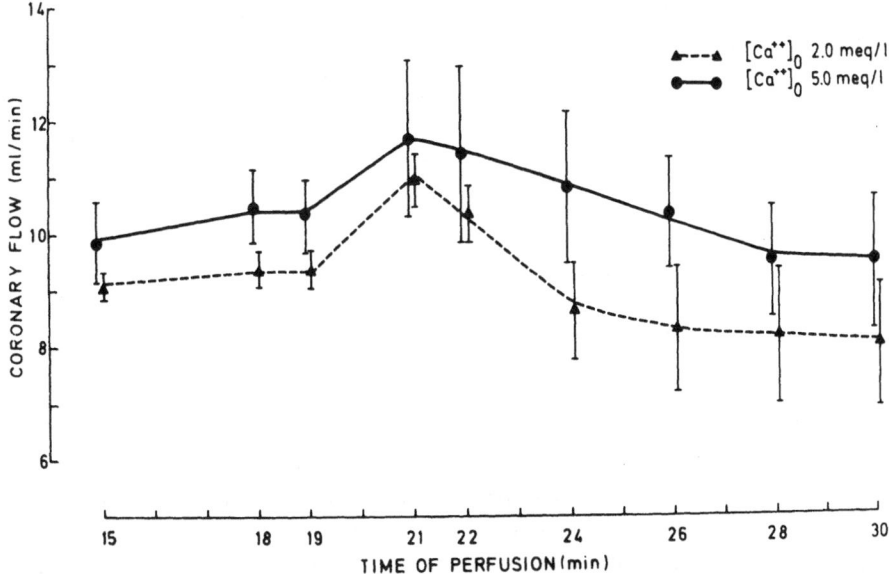

Fig. 8. Coronary flow in the presence of 2.0 and 5.0 meq/l of Ca^{++}, and the effect of Adalat 100 µg/l after an initial equilibration period of 20 min. Mean value ±S.E.M. of 6 hearts in each group

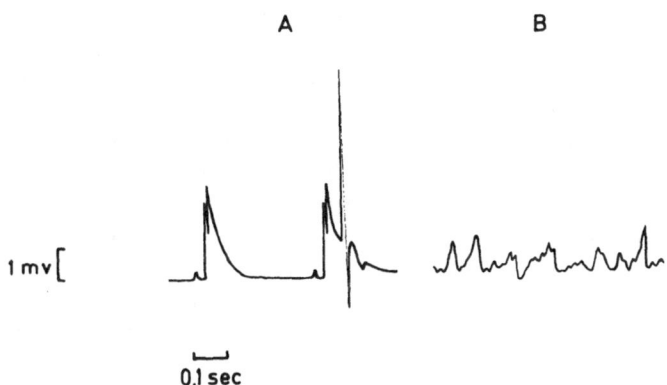

Fig. 9A and B. ECG-tracings of Ca^{++}-induced ventricular extrasystole (A) and ventricular fibrillation (B)

duced R wave voltage in the presence of low $(Ca^{++})_0$ and the Adalat-induced decrease in the R wave voltage are further evidences for this assumption. In the dog heart *in situ*, no effect of Adalat has been observed in the QRS complex (VATER *et al.* [17]). Increasing $(Ca^{++})_0$ decreased the time for 50 and 90% repolarization; this is in accordance with previous observations (CORABOEUF and VASSORT [3]). Adalat 100 µg/l caused a further shortening of the action potential duration, but this action was negligible at higher calcium levels.

Adalat did not exert any effect on the excitability of isolated rat atria. Determination of the maximum following frequency has been used as a test of the effective refractory period (VAUGHAN, WILLIAMS and SZEKERES [18]; LAND-MARK [12]). Although Adalat caused a shortening of the action potential duration, no alteration was observed in the maximum following frequency.

In the isolated rat left atrium, Adalat caused a progressive decline in contractile force, and in the isolated rat heart preparation, the reduction in mechanical performance was more pronounced at the lower calcium concentration. It has been supposed that the Adalat-induced decrease in the transmembrane Ca^{++} influx during excitation reduces contractile tension (FLECKENSTEIN et al. [5]).

In our experiments, Adalat caused only a small, transient increase in coronary flow. This finding is in contrast to previous observations in the isolated guinea-pig heart (KOSCHE et al. [11]), and species differences may account for this phenomenon.

All the Adalat effects described above were more pronounced at low than at high calcium levels.

Pretreatment with Adalat completely protected isolated hearts against Ca^{++}-induced ventricular tachyarrhythmias. The relevance of calcium currents in the origin of arrhythmias has been questioned. However, production of hypercalcemia in the intact animal (HOFF and NAHUM [10]; WINBURY and HEMMER [20]) or elevation of $(Ca^{++})_0$ in isolated perfused hearts (BEAULNES and LAVALLEE [2]) often causes cardiac irregularities, especially ventricular extrasystoles, and it has been suggested that an action on the ventricular conduction system is important. According to WEIDMANN [19], increased influx of Ca^{++} at membrane potentials in the range of -50 to -60 mV, could contribute to ectopic activity. TEMTE and DAVIS [15] assumed that Ca^{++}-induced changes in automaticity and conduction in Purkinje fibers may favour the development of ventricular arrhythmias. Reentry can occur in networks of Purkinje fibers that show slow conduction and unidirectional block within areas of low resting potential (CRANEFIELD et al. [4]). It has been assumed that conduction within these areas depends on a slow inward current carried by calcium ions (ARONSON and CRANEFIELD [1]), thus a drug which inhibits this current could probably suppress reentrant arrhythmias, originating either within the AV node (GOLDREYER and BIGGER [6]; GOLDREYER and DAMATO [7]) or within networks of Purkinje fibers (CRANEFIELD et al. [4]).

Our study confirms earlier observations that Adalat is a powerful calcium antagonist.

Abstract

In isolated rat cardiac muscle (atria- and retrogradely perfused hearts), Adalat caused a dose-dependent decrease in the spontaneous frequency of contraction as well as in the contractile force. These effects were more pronounced at low than at high concentrations of calcium $(Ca^{++})_0$ in the perfusion fluid. Adalat prolonged the PQ interval, and the effect on AV transmission characteristics was increased at low $(Ca^{++})_0$. A varying degree of AV block occurred in many experiments. Adalat reduced the R wave voltage in the ECG of isolated rat hearts. In isolated atria, the velocity (dv/dt) of the depolarization of the action potential increased with increasing $(Ca^{++})_0$. Adalat reduced the dv/dt ratio and caused a shortening of the action potential. These effects were small at high, but pronounced at low Ca^{++} levels. Pretreatment with Adalat completely protected the isolated hearts against Ca^{++}-induced ventricular arrhythmias. The drug produced a small and transitory increase in coronary flow.

The results presented in this investigation indicate that the Ca^{++} current contributes directly to the fast phase of depolarization in rat cardiac muscle. The study also confirms earlier observations that Adalat is a powerful Ca^{++} antagonist.

References

1. ARONSON, R. S., CRANEFIELD, P. F.: The electrical activity of canine cardiac Purkinje fibers in sodium-free, calcium-rich solutions. J. Gen. Physiol. **61**, 786 (1973).
2. BEAULNES, A., LAVALLEE, M.: Differential effects of some phenothiazine derivatives against calcium-induced ventricular arrhythmias in the isolated rabbit heart. Canad. J. Physiol. Pharmacol. **42**, 845 (1964).
3. CORABOEUF, E., VASSORT, G.: Effects of some inhibitors of ionic permeabilities on ventricular action potential and contraction of rat and guinea-pig hearts. J. Electrocardiology **1**, 19 (1968).
4. CRANEFIELD, P. F., ARONSON, R. S., WIT, A. L.: Effect of verapamil on the normal action potential and on a calcium-dependent slow response of canine cardiac Purkinje fibers. Circ. Res. **34**, 204 (1974).
5. FLECKENSTEIN, A., TRITTHART, H., DOERING, H.-J., BYON, K. Y.: BAY a 1040 — ein hochaktiver Ca^{++}-antagonistischer Inhibitor der elektro-mechanischen Koppelungsprozesse im Warmblüter-Myokard. Arzneim.-Forsch. (Drug Res.) **22**, 22 (1972).
6. GOLDREYER, B. N., BIGGER, J. T.: The site of re-entry in paroxysmal supraventricular tachycardia in man. Circulation **43**, 15 (1971).
7. GOLDREYER, B. N., DAMATO, A. N.: The essential role of atrioventricular conduction delay in the initiation of paroxysmal supraventricular tachycardia. Circulation **43**, 679 (1971).
8. GRUMBACH, L., HOWARD, J. W., MERRIL, W. I.: Factors related to the initiation of ventricular fibrillation in the isolated heart: Effect of calcium and potassium. Circ. Res. **2**, 452 (1954).
9. HASHIMOTO, K., TAIRA, N., CHIBA, S., HASHIMOTO, K., JR., ENDOH, M., KOKUBUN, M., KOKUBUN, H., IIJIMA, T., KIMURA, T., KUBOTA, K., OGURO, K.: Cardiohemodynamic effects of BAY a 1040 in the dog. Arzneim.-Forsch. (Drug Res.) **22**, 15 (1972).
10. HOFF, H. E., NAHUM, L. H.: An analysis of the cardiac irregularities produced by calcium, and their prevention by sodium amytal. J. Pharmacol. Exp. Therap. **60**, 425 (1937).
11. KOSCHE, F., RAFF, W. K., LOCHNER, W.: Zum Wirkungsmechanismus der Coronardilatation durch Nifedipine. Arzneim.-Forsch. (Drug Res.) **22**, 39 (1972).
12. LANDMARK, K.: The action of promazine and thioridazine in isolated rat atria. 1. Effects on automaticity, mechanical performance, refractoriness and excitability. Europ. J. Pharmacol. **16**, 1 (1971a).
13. LANDMARK, K.: Changes in rat atrial action potentials induced by promazine and thioridazine. Acta pharmacol. et toxicol. **30**, 465 (1971b).
14. LOEB, T.: Comparative evaluation of methods used for the measurements of the effect of drugs on cardiac muscle. M. Sc. Thesis, University of Sydney, 1965.
15. TEMTE, J. V., DAVIS, L. D.: Effect of calcium concentration on the transmembrane potentials of Purkinje fibers. Circ. Res. **20**, 32 (1967).
16. VASSORT, G., ROUGIER, O., GARNIER, D., SAUVIAT, M. P., CORABOEUF, E., GARGOUÏL, Y. M.: Effects of adrenaline on membrane inward current during the cardiac action potential. Pflügers Arch. **309**, 70 (1969).
17. VATER, W., KRONEBERG, G., HOFFMEISTER, F., KALLER, H., MENG, K., OBERDORF, A., PULS, W., SCHLOSSMANN, K., STOEPEL, K.: Zur Pharmakologie von 4-(2'-Nitrophenyl)-2,6-dimethyl-1,4-dihydropyridin-3,5-dicarbonsäuredimethylester (Nifedipine, BAY a 1040). Arzneim.-Forsch. (Drug Res.) **22**, 1 (1972).

18. VAUGHAN WILLIAMS, E. M., SZEKERES, L.: A comparison of tests for antifibrillatory action. Brit. J. Pharmacol. **17**, 424 (1961).
19. WEIDMANN, S.: Ionic basis of ectopic activity. International symposium on recent advances in cardiac arrhythmias, Amsterdam 1972.
20. WINBURY, M. M., HEMMER, M. L.: Influence of antiarrhythmic agents on calcium-induced cardiac arrhythmias in the rat. Circ. Res. **3**, 474 (1955).
21. ZIPES, D. P., MENDEZ, C.: Action of manganese ions and tetradotoxin on atrioventricular nodal transmembrane potentials in isolated rabbit hearts. Circ. Res. **32**, 447 (1973).
22. ZIPES, D. P., FISCHER, J. C.: Effects of agents which inhibit the slow channel on sinus node automaticity and atrioventricular conduction in the dog. Circ. Res. **34**, 184 (1974).

Discussion Remarks

HASHIMOTO: I would like to comment briefly on the species differences of responses in the A-V node. When hearts of rabbits, rats or guinea pigs are isolated and perfused with Ringer solution for arranging Langendorff's preparation, we never observe fibrillation immediately after recirculation. But human, dog, and cat hearts respond differently: Even when one can find a good circulatory condition, ventricular fibrillation must be observed in the initial stage of recirculation. Fibrillation continues 30 min to one hour, but suddenly it disappears and sinus rhythm takes place. So you can get different results in the A-V conduction time or in the antiarrhythmic effects, when you study the properties of your agent with hearts of different species.

LANDMARK: I agree that it might be species differences, of course, but I think that our paper showed that the drug influences the calcium current within the A-V node. In the intact animal or in the human there might be reflectory mechanisms that will modify or neutralize the effects.

TAIRA: Dr. LANDMARK, the problem is that nifidipine is about 30 times more potent in producing vasodilation and depression of the myocardium. But verapamil, nifedipine and other calcium-antagonists are almost equally potent in depressing A-V conduction.

FLECKENSTEIN: Our results obtained in the guinea pig A-V node agree completely with those of Dr. LANDMARK on rats: We were also unable to find a basic difference between the negative-dromotropic action of verapamil and nifedipine. But one must certainly allow for species differences in the responsiveness of the A-V node to calcium-antagonistic compounds, as well as for differences in the strenght of β-adrenergic reflex activation of the A-V node when the blood pressure decreases under the influence of such drugs.

Session III

Clinical Pharmacology

Chairmen: K. Hashimoto (Tokyo), R.J.Esper (Buenos Aires)

Hemodynamic Studies on Adalat in Healthy Volunteers and in Patients

H. Lydtin, G. Lohmöller, R. Lohmöller, H. Schmitz, and I. Walter

Medizinische Poliklinik der Universität, München, Fed. Rep. Germany

In the dog nifedipine (= Adalat) lowers the resting tone of the coronary resistance vessels and increases coronary blood flow, concomitant peripheral effects being small and inconsistent [2, 6, 7, 18, 21]. On the other hand, good evidence has been presented for a nitrite-like action of the drug on other vascular smooth muscle cells and for a Ca^{++}-antagonistic effect in the myocardium [4]. Our own work with nifedipine in man started with a study of both the peripheral hemodynamic and the cardiac effects of this drug that accompany the coronary action. We felt that any increase in cardiac work could partly mask the direct action on the coronary arteries, when coronary AV-oxygen difference is used as an indicator of coronary blood flow [12]. At the same time a peripheral action of nifedipine would help to explain the immediate increase in exercise tolerance observed by other investigators [9, 10, 11, 20], since according to modern pathophysiologic concepts such an effect cannot be produced by a dilatation of the coronary vessels.

We set out to study the hemodynamic effects of nifedipine in healthy human volunteers using indirect methods in order to insure true resting (basal) conditions. Our experiments were designed to examine the direction and time course of these effects as well as the contribution of the vagal and/or sympathetic system whether stimulated directly or indirectly by nifedipine. The purpose of the investigation was also to determine the presence and magnitude of interactions of nifedipine with β_1-receptor blockade [1, 3, 13, 16], with nitrites and digitalis. In patients with ischemic heart disease, the mode of action was investigated by exercise tests under control of pulmonary artery and venous capillary pressures (pcvp). In patients with cerebral lesions we investigated whether nifedipine changes regional cerebral blood flow and/or whether it causes steal effects.

Methods

All studies in volunteers (healthy medical students, age 20–30) were done under BMR-conditions in the supine position. Heart rate (HR), arterial blood pressure (semi-automatic cuff method), pre-ejection period (PEP), left ventricular ejection time (LVET) and peripheral blood flow (PBF) (plethysmography, mercury-in-rubber strain gauges) were monitored by standard techniques. Cardiac output (CO) was determined by the dye dilution method.

0.015 mg/kg body weight nifedipine were injected intravenously before and after an intravenous dose of 1.0 mg atropine. 0.0075 mg/kg and 0.015 mg/kg body weight nifedipine were
injected intravenously before and after intravenous doses of 20 and 80 mg practolol (Eral-
din = Dalzic), respectively. We also studied the hemodynamic response patterns following
20 mg and 40 mg given orally (sublingually) either in capsules or in aqueous solution as
compared to the intravenous efficacy of the drug. Nitroglycerin was tested before and after
sublingual nifedipine (20 mg).

Exercise studies in patients with angina on effort were done before and after sublingual
application of nifedipine on a bicycle ergometer in the recumbent position (30° elevated),
pulmonary capillary pressure ("pcvp") being monitored by means of a flow-directed Swan-
Ganz catheter. Before and immediately after the exercise periods peripheral blood flow was
measured plethysmographically. Statistical analysis of our data was performed using Wilcox-
on's matched-paired-signed-rank-test or Student's T-test (for detailed description of some of
the methods used and of part of our data see Refs. [15] and [17]).

Regional cerebral blood flow (rCBF) was measured by an isotope clearance method
(^{133}Xe) in patients with cerebral lesions before and after the inhalation of carbon dioxide and
before and after the intravenous injection of nifedipine. ^{133}Xe was injected with a saline bolus
into the cannulated internal carotid artery. The "initial slope index" was determined using
15 scintillation detectors placed extracranially on the diseased hemisphere. Mean arterial
pressure (P art.) was monitored by an electronic transducer. Arterial $PaCO_2$ was also determined. Heart rate (HR) was registered through standard electrocardiographic leads, peripheral blood flow (PBF) was measured by venous occlusion plethysmography. The mercury-
in-rubber strain gauge was placed on the calf, the occlusion cuff on the thigh. Either 0.0075 or
0.015 mg/kg body weight nifedipine were injected intravenously during three minutes. rCBF
was measured four times at 20 min intervals, i.e. under basal conditions, after 4 min of CO_2-
inhalation, after a second control period and after the injection of nifedipine. The other
parameters were followed at 2–5 min intervals.

Results

It is impossible to describe in detail all our data in a short communication.
Results presented were therefore selected in order to highlight points of practical
importance (see also Refs. [15] and [17]).

Immediately after the injection of nifedipine (BAY a 1040), systolic and diastolic pressures as well as PEP (QA is equivalent to PEP) decreased (Fig. 1). PBF
increased to 250% of the control level in the mean. HR increased by a mean of
25 beats/min. The maximal effect occurred 1–2 min after the end of the injection
of nifedipine. All parameters returned to their respective control levels with a
"half-life time" of 2–3 min.

Fig. 2 shows the effect of repetitive injections of 0.0075 mg/kg body weight on
blood pressure, heart rate and systolic time intervals. There is no evidence of
immediate tolerance or tachyphylaxis.

The hemodynamic effects of 0.0075 mg/kg body weight nifedipine administered intravenously before and after the administration of 1 mg atropine are
shown in Fig. 3.

Atropine causes a rise in HR which plateaus at about 90 beats/min. The
immediate effects of intravenous nifedipine are not changed by the vagal blockade, all changes starting from different baselines ($p < 0.01$). In all experiments we
found an inverse relationship between the increase in heart rate following nifedipine and the respective control (resting) values. This relation is not changed by
atropine.

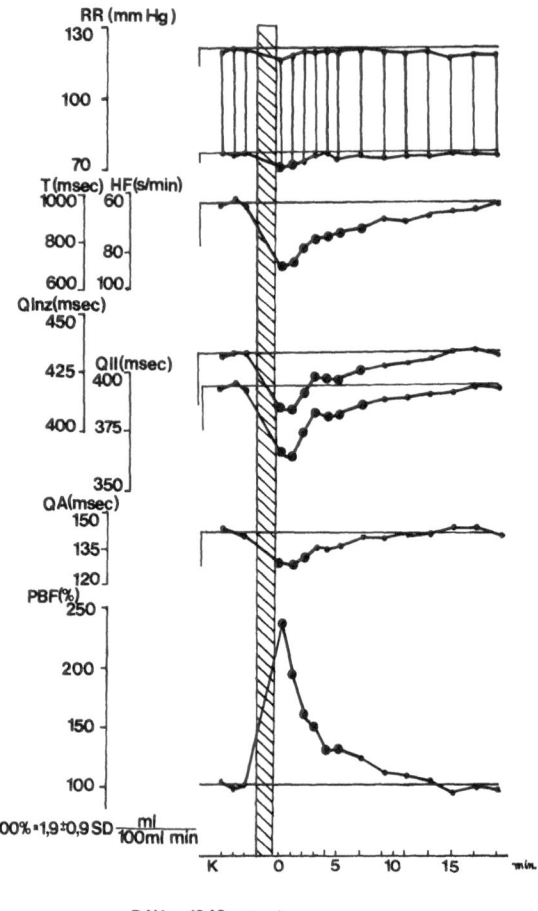

BAYa 1040 0,015mg/kg i.v.

Fig. 1. Arterial blood pressure (RR), heart rate (HF), systolic time intervals [QInz, QII, QA are the time intervals from the beginning of electrical activity in lead II of the electrocardiogram to the incisura of the carotid pulse (QInz), to the beginning of the second heart sound in the phonocardiogram (QII) and to the beginning of the upstroke of the carotid pulse (QA)] and peripheral blood flow (PBF) before and after 0.015mg/kg body weight nifedipine intravenously. The graph represents the mean values of 10 experiments in different volunteers. Time scale in minutes

Figure 4 shows changes in cardiac index (CI), heart rate (HR), stroke volume (SV), arterial mean pressure $\bar{P}_{art.}$ and calculated peripheral resistance $\bar{R}_{per.}$, peripheral blood flow (PBF), mean systolic ejection rate (MSER) and tension-time-index (TTI) in five experiments before, immediately and 7 min after the intravenous injection of nifedipine (0.0075 mg/kg body weight). There is a significant increase in cardiac output and heart rate with a clear drop in $\bar{R}_{per.}$. Left ventricular work index (LVWI), PBF and TTI also increase. Seven minutes later almost all parameters have nearly returned to their resting (basal) values.

Figure 5 shows the hemodynamic effects of intravenous nifedipine (0.0075 mg/ kg body weight) before and after the intravenous administration of practolol.

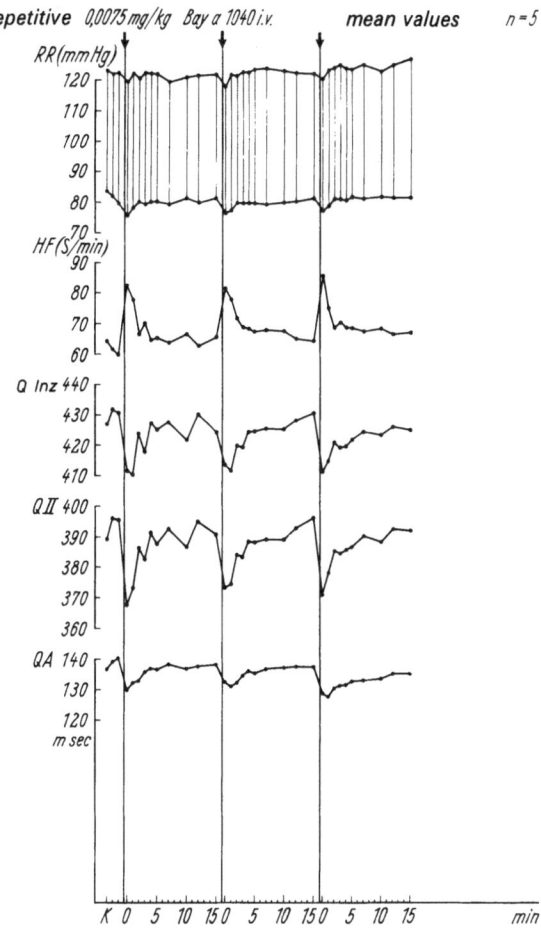

Fig. 2. Effect of repetitive intravenous injections of 0.0075 mg/kg nifedipine (BAY a 1040) in 5 experiments. RR: arterial pressure; HF: heart rate, QInz, QII, QA: see Fig. 1. For details see text

Whereas the effects of nifedipine on blood pressure and peripheral blood flow are not changed significantly by the β-blocking agent, the increase in heart rate and the shortening of the systolic time intervals are clearly ($p < 0.01$) diminished.

Figure 6 summarizes data from repetitive injections of nifedipine at different dosage levels in 5 subjects. Injections were made in randomized order. The data demonstrate a dose dependence of the hemodynamic activity of nifedipine, which is statistically significant ($p < 0.05$) between 0.0075 and 0.004 mg/kg body weight.

Following the series of experiments with intravenous injections of nifedipine, we studied the effect of its sublingual i.e. oral application in the same group of healthy volunteers thus facilitating paired comparisons of the individual dose response curves. Hemodynamic changes induced by oral nifedipine in general are much more variable as far as time course and absolute amount are concerned, the direction of the induced changes being the same following both methods of application.

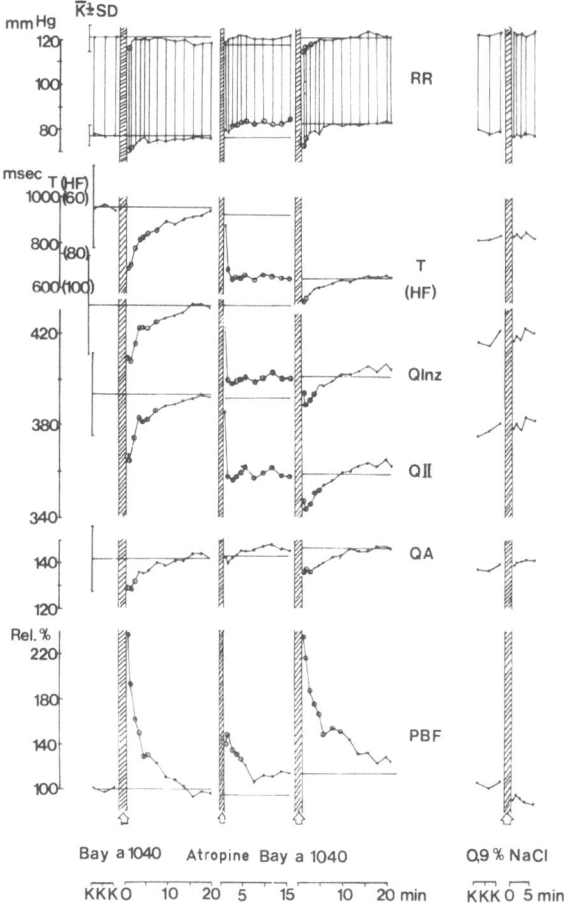

Fig. 3. Hemodynamic effects of nifedipine (BAY a 1040), atropine and placebo injections of saline. For explanation of symbols see Fig. 1, for details see text. Large dots indicate a statistical significance for differences versus respective control values, $p < 0.01$

In almost all experiments with oral administration of nifedipine, there is a distinctly phasic response pattern as observed after some of the intravenous injections of nifedipine. HR and PBF increase during the initial 30 min after administration of the capsules and reach a maximum between 10 and 40 min. Thereafter all measured parameters temporarily tend to return toward control levels followed by a second increase in HR, PBF and by a second shortening of systolic time intervals. In 4 out of 6 experiments with 20 mg and 40 mg nifedipine orally, PBF and HR did not reach a maximum during the 120 min-observation period following administration of the drug, i.e. they did not return to control values during this second phase of action. In additional experiments in which we extended the observation period to 180 min, PBF and HR were still distinctly above control values.

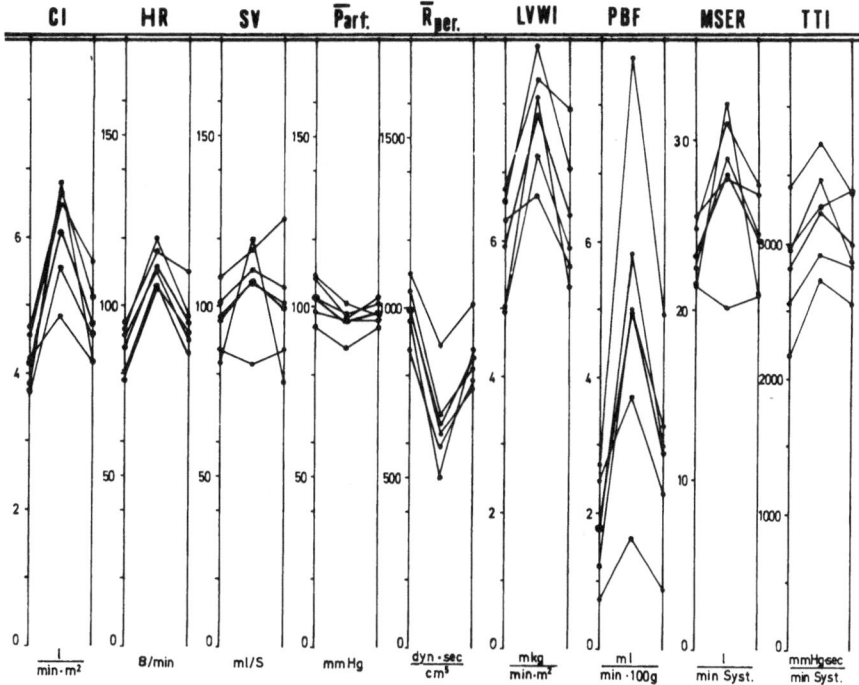

Fig. 4. Cardiac index (CI), heart rate (HR), stroke volume (SV), mean arterial pressure ($\overline{\text{P}}$ art.), calculated peripheral resistance ($\overline{\text{R}}$per.), left ventricular work index (LVWI), peripheral blood flow (PBF), mean systolic ejection rate (MSER) and tension-time-index (TTI) before, immediately and 7 min after the intravenous injection of 0.0075 mg/kg body weight nifedipine. For description and details see text

Because of the intraindividual variability of dose response curves following oral nifedipine, it is difficult to make an unbiassed comparison of intravenous and oral applications. If only the initial 15 min after administration are taken into account, we have to assume that only 1/40 of the amount brought into the mouth becomes active in the circulation during that time. If the total hemodynamic response is summed up during 120 min following oral nifedipine it can be compared with intravenous dose response curves of the same individual. If we neglect metabolism and excretion of the drug during the time, we then can speculate on the amount of nifedipine which is absorbed from the mouth and (since we allowed the volunteers to swallow after 10 min) from the intestine.

Depending on the parameter examined (HR, PBF or PEP), we found that between 10 and 40% must be absorbed by the oral and/or gastric mucosa.

Oral nifedipine causes no decrease in the effect of nitroglycerin on PBF and HR nor does nitroglycerin change the typical hemodynamic pattern following oral nifedipine. There is also no statistically significant change in systolic or diastolic blood pressure, a greater increase in HR following nitroglycerin after pretreatment with nifedipine suggests a higher degree of sympathetic activation.

After our studies on healthy volunteers we studied patients presenting symptoms of ischemic heart disease. In all cases in which exercise tolerance was in-

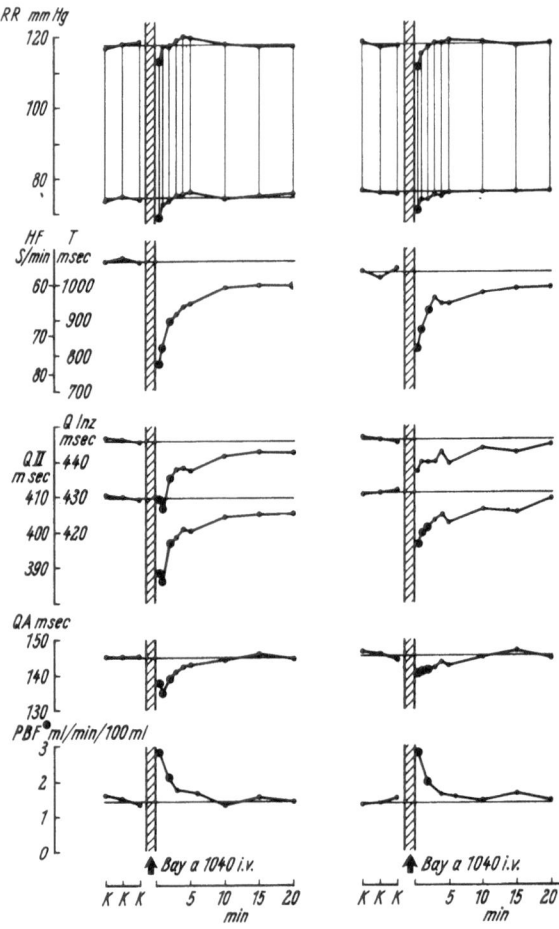

Fig. 5. Hemodynamic effects of 0.0075 mg nifedipine (BAY a 1040) administered intravenously before and after the intravenous injection of 20 and 80 mg practolol. For details see text

creased by nifedipine, systolic and diastolic blood pressure as well as "pcvp" was lowered as compared to the exercise levels in the control experiments. These data indicate that in patients with angina pectoris a peripheral effect of the drug is at least partly responsible for the increase in exercise tolerance observed by other investigators and by our group.

Thus far our own experience with nifedipine in open therapeutic trials on patients has been very favorable. Concomitant treatment with digitalis, nitrites and β-blocking agents was very well tolerated for periods of up to 18 months. If patients are put on placebo capsules in between, they immediately experience an increase in the number and severity of angina pectoris attacks. We did not observe any evidence that tolerance developed under prolonged application of nifedipine.

We did not observe any significant prolongation of the AV-interval due to nifedipine, either in our experiments on volunteers also taking practolol or in patients on practolol and digitalis. Since we have not yet measured AH-intervals, we cannot completely rule out an effect of nifedipine on conductance. Our data

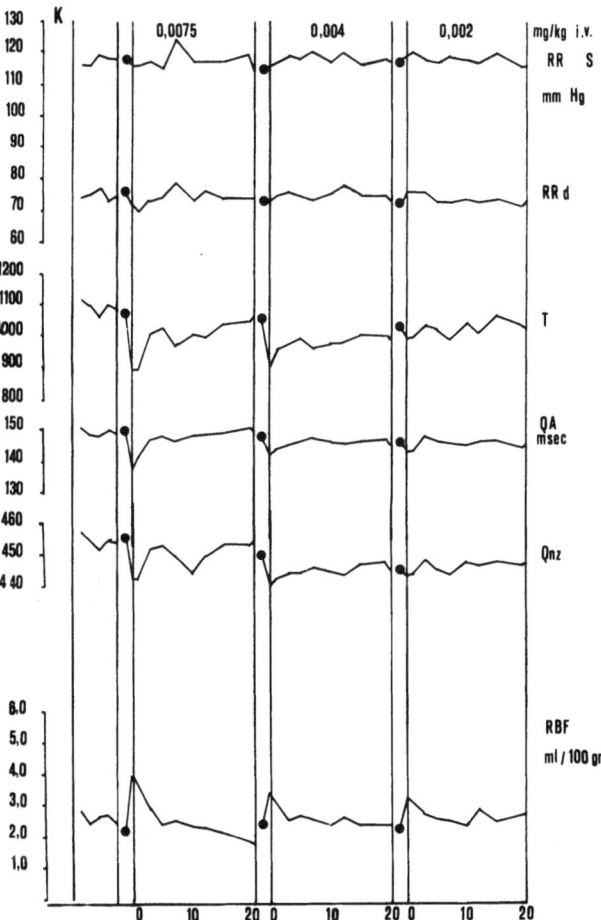

Fig. 6. Mean values of hemodynamic changes following different intravenous doses of nifedipine given in randomized order. For details see text

indicate however that this effect must be small and can only be of clinical importance if AV-conductance is severely damaged before the application of nifedipine.

Nifedipine is a strong vasodilator not only in the coronary vasculature. In individual patients with cerebral lesions nifedipine can increase cerebral blood flow to a limited extent when vessels react normally to an increase in arterial CO_2 tension [19]. However there is no marked dilatation of the cerebral arteries comparable to the marked peripheral response occurring at the same time. Autoregulatory adaptation of cerebral vascular resistance in response to changes in blood pressure apparently is not affected by nifedipine. From our data there is no evidence for steal effects caused by the drug. Larger series however are needed to confirm these results. Our data do not completely rule out the possibilities, that a completely normal cerebral circulation could have dissimilar response patterns and that there could be differences in the time response curves of the brain and of the peripheral arteries, i.e. that the cerebral effects occur distinctly later [14]. Possibly the cerebral resistance vessels react only when sufficient amounts of

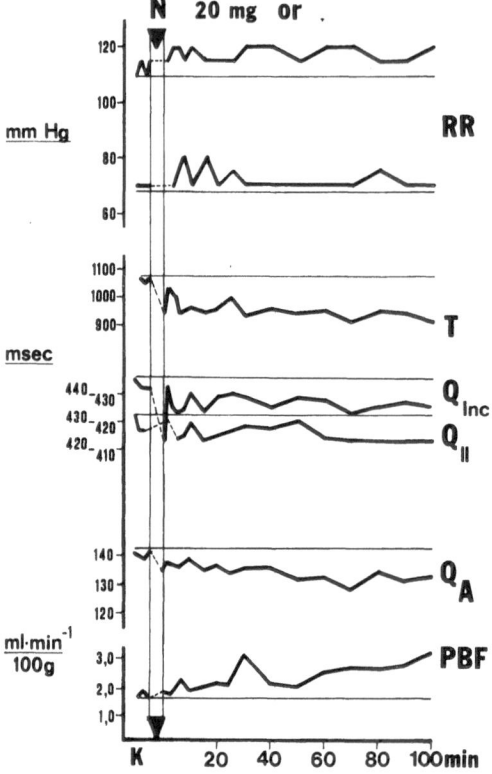

Fig. 7. Arterial blood pressure (RR), RR interval in the ECG (T), systolic time intervals (QInz, QII, and QA) and peripheral blood flow (PBF) after 20 mg nifedipine (N) administered sublingually. Time scale in minutes. For details see text

nifedipine have accumulated in the cerebral fluid following oral ingestion of the drug. Assuming a slow penetration of nifedipine into the cerebral fluid, the serum half-life times after intravenous administration would be to short for such an effect [8]. The time lag between the ingestion of the drug by the healthy volunteers and the occurrence of headache hints in that direction. So far our data speak against the hypothesis, that the use of this valuable drug in the treatment of angina pectoris could be limited by concomitant cerebral vascular disease.

Abstract

Nifedipine (BAY a 1040) was administered intravenously under BMR-conditions to healthy volunteers before and after atropine (1 mg i.v.) as well as before and after practolol (20 and 80 mg i.v.). Heart rate (HR), arterial blood pressure (BP), pre-ejection period (PEP), left ventricular ejection time (LVET) and peripheral blood flow (PBF) were monitored by standard techniques, cardiac output was measured by the dye dilution method. Following nifedipine, there was an increase of PBF by 250% which is 150% of the base line value, in HR of 25 beats/min. Systolic and diastolic pressures decreased, PEP was shortened by 13 msec.

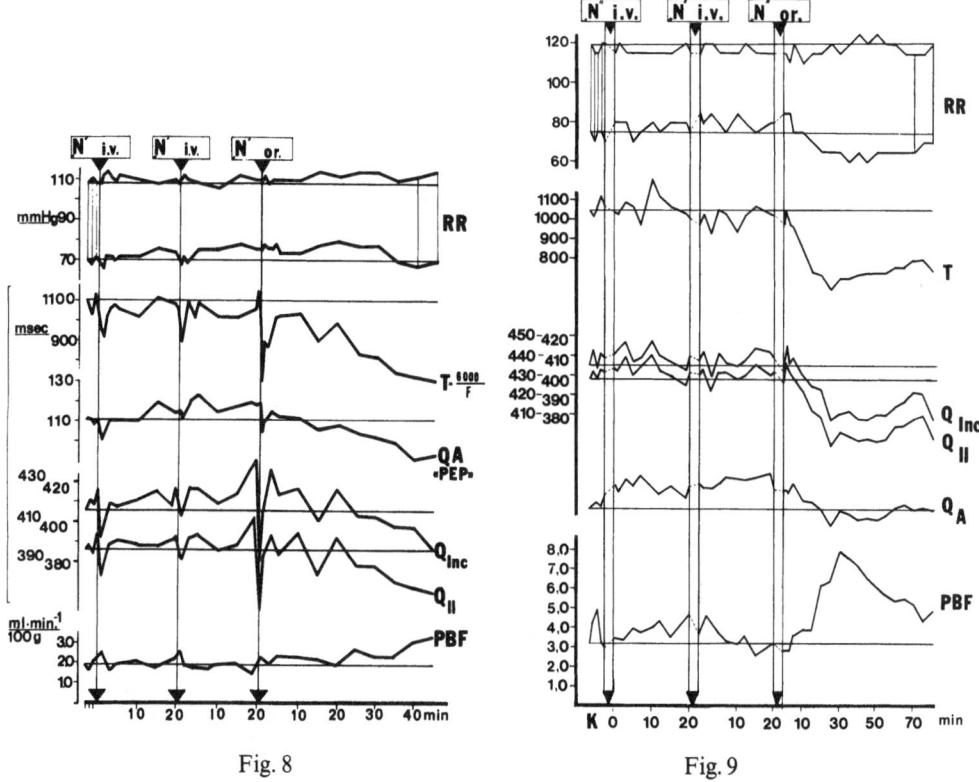

Fig. 8   Fig. 9

Fig. 8. Effect of 0.004 mg/kg i.v., 0.002 mg/kg i.v. and 40 mg = 0.53 mg/kg Nifedipine (N) administered sublingually on arterial blood pressure (RR), RR interval in the ECG (T), systolic time intervals (QA, Q II and QINz) and peripheral blood flow (PBF). Time scale in minutes. For details see text

Fig. 9. Effects of 0.002 mg/kg i.v., 0.004 mg/kg i.v. and of 40 mg = 0.56 mg/kg nifedipine (N) administered sublingually on arterial blood pressure (RR), RR interval in the ECG (T), systolic time intervals (QA, Q II and QInz) and peripheral blood flow (PBF). Time scale in minutes. Compare with Fig. 8 variability in response curves following oral application of nifedipine in healthy volunteers

Cardiac output increased after nifedipine from a mean of 8.3 l/min to 12 l/min. Changes of PEP indicated an increase in contractility, which can be explained at least in part by a β_1-stimulation of the heart, following a decrease of peripheral resistance. Whereas atropine did not change the hemodynamic action of nifedipine, cardioselective β_1-receptor blockage by practolol diminished significantly the positive chronotropic action of nifedipine, the increase of PBF induced by nifedipine remaining unchanged. After oral nifedipine, we found evidence for a sustained action of nifedipine for more than 180 min. Following oral nitroglycerin, similar response patterns were observed before and after nifedipine, nitroglycerin demonstrating much shorter action as compared to nifedipine.

In patients with coronary heart disease repetitive exercise tests were performed on a bicycle ergometer. Pulmonary capillar pressure was measured by means of a flow-directed Swan-Ganz catheter. There was clear evidence of an

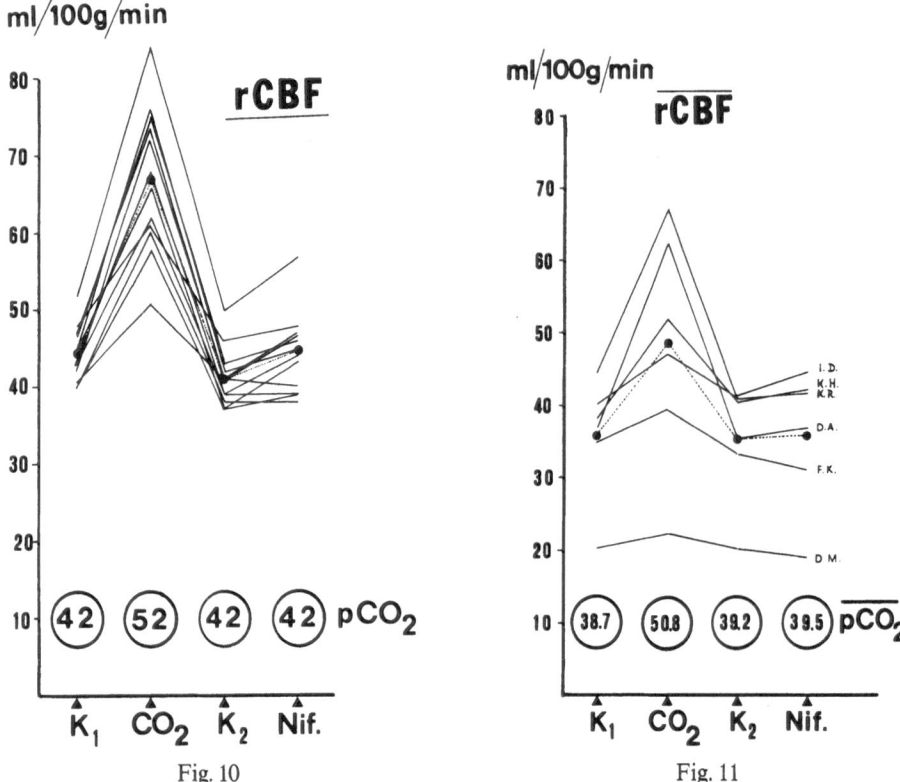

Fig. 10

Fig. 11

Fig. 10. Regional cerebral blood flow (rCBF) under basal conditions, under increased CO_2-tension after a second control period and following an intravenous injection of 0.015 mg/kg body weight nifedipine in one patient. Note small increase of rCBF in 9 out of 12 channels. PBF increased at the same time by 150%

Fig. 11. Mean changes in rCBF in 6 patients (and the mean thereof). Note tendency of rCBF to increase in patients with normal reaction to CO_2

increase in exercise tolerance following oral nifedipine paralleled by a decrease in pulmonary artery pressure. In conclusion, nifedipine offers a long acting nitrite action with significant protection against angina pectoris.

So far, we have not observed important adverse reactions in patients. The occurrence of headache and/or flush almost exclusively in the young healthy volunteers stimulated studies of regional and total cerebral blood flow by ^{133}Xe during diagnostic procedures in patients with cerebral lesions. In these studies cerebral blood flow did not change or increased much less than PBF immediately after the intravenous injection of nifedipine. However no true steal effect of the peripheral vasculature and/or of well-perfused cerebral regions compared to the regions with low flow could be observed.

References

1. BARRETT, A. M., CROWTHER, A., DUNLOP, D., SHANKS, R. G., SMITH, L. H.: Naunyn-Schmiedeberg's Arch. Pharmak exp. Path. **259**, 152–153 (1967/1968).
2. BOSSERT, F., VATER, W.: Naturwissenschaften **58**, 578 (1971).

3. DUNLOP, D., SHANKS, R. G.: Brit. J. Pharmacol. **32**, 201–218 (1968).
4. FLECKENSTEIN, A., TRITTHART, H., DÖRING, J., BYON, K. Y.: Arzneim.-Forsch. (Drug Res.) **22**, 22–33 (1972).
5. GUTMAN, J.: Herz/Kreisl. **3**, 365 (1971).
6. HASHIMOTO, K., TAIRA, N., CHIBA, S., HASHIMOTO, K., JR., ENDOH, M., KOKUBUN, M., KOKUBUN, H., LIJIMA, T., KIMURA, T., KUBOTA, K., OGURO, K.: Arzneim.-Forsch. (Drug Res.) **22**, 15–21 (1972).
7. HAYASA, S., HIRAKAWA, S., HOSOKAWA, S., MORI, N., KANAYAMA, S., IWASA, H.: Arzneim.-Forsch. (Drug Res.) **22**, 370–373 (1972).
8. HORSTER, F. A., DUHM, B., MAUL, W., MEDENWALD, H., PATZSCHKE, K., WEGNER, L. A.: Arzneim.-Forsch. (Drug Res.) **22**, 330–334 (1972).
9. KALTENBACH, M., BECKER, H. J., KOBER, G., LOOS, A.: Arzneim.-Forsch. (Drug Res.) **22**, 362–365 (1972).
10. KIMURA, E., MABUCHI, G., KIKUCHI, W.: Arzneim.-Forsch. (Drug Res.) **22**, 365–367 (1972).
11. KOBAYASHI, T., ITO, Y., TAWARA, I.: Arzneim.-Forsch. (Drug Res.) **22**, 380–389 (1972).
12. KOCHSIEK, K., NEUBAUR, J.: Arzneim.-Forsch. (Drug Res.) **22**, 353–358 (1972).
13. LANDS, A., ARNOLD, A., MCAULIFF, J. P., LUDUENA, F. P., BROWN, T. G., JR.: Nature (Lond.) **214**, 597–598 (1967).
14. LASSEN, N. A.: Circulat. Res. **34**, 749–760 (1974).
15. LOHMÖLLER, R., LYDTIN, H.: Int. J. clin. Pharmacol. **8**, 118–125 (1973).
16. LYDTIN, H.: Ergebn. inn. Med. Kinderheilk. **30**, 97–158 (1970).
17. LYDTIN, H., LOHMÖLLER, R.: Verh. dtsch. Ges. inn. Med. **78**, 1554–1559 (1972).
18. RAFF, W. K., KOSCHE, F., LOCHNER, W.: Arzneim.-Forsch. (Drug Res.) **22**, 33–39 (1972).
19. SCHMITZ, H., SCHIERL, W., BECK, I., LYDTIN, H.: World Congress of Cardiology Buenos Aires 1974.
20. SCHNEIDER, K. W., JESSE, R.: Arzneim.-Forsch. (Drug Res.) **22**, 373–377 (1972).
21. VATER, W., KRONEBERG, G., HOFFMEISTER, F., KALLER, H., MENG, K., OBERDORF, A., PULS, W., SCHLOSSMANN, K., STOEPEL, K.: Arzneim.-Forsch. (Drug Res.) **22**, 1–14 (1972).

Discussion Remarks

KIRCHHEIM: Dr. LYDTIN, after practolol you were not able to completely abolish the increase in heart rate. You commented that probably beta blockade was not complete. But I think your results could be easily interpreted in the same way as our results with the difference that the part played by the sympathetic system is probably a little more prominent in man as compared to the dog.

LYDTIN: I think we agree in principle. Practolol has a certain amount of intrinsic adrenergic activity per se, so that basal values with practolol would be different from those with propranolol. You have higher resting values with practolol than with propranolol under resting conditions. I do not see a change of getting "complete beta blockade" because these agents are competitive antagonists which induce only a parallel shift of your dose response curve—not a change in slope. And apparently the sympathetic drive, which is brought on as a reflex, is a very strong stimulus and can overcome part of the effect. The point made earlier in the discussion was that you did not get a change—no change at all—in your heart rate and this is what I am curious about.

If the vagal tone has any impact it should have more effect at low heart rates— at a rate of 60–70 where you know that the vagal tone is high.

Pharmacokinetics of Nifedipine-^{14}C in Man

F. A. HORSTER

2. Medizinische Klinik der Universität, Düsseldorf, Fed. Rep. Germany

The pharmacokinetic investigations were carried out at the 2nd University Clinic, Düsseldorf, and the results were determined in the Isotope Institute of Bayer, Wuppertal-Elberfeld, by Drs. Duhm, Maul, Medenwald, Patschke and Wegner.

Materials and Methods

Figure 1 shows the positions at which nifedipine was labelled with ^{14}C. This radioactive substance had already been tested by the Isotope Institute of Bayer in numerous animal experiments on rats and dogs.

Table 1 contains a description of the patients and doses; 20 patients were hospitalized, suffering from illnesses such as gastric ulcers, duodenal ulcers, pneumonia and unstable hypertension. None of the patients displayed a renal or liver insufficiency. Nine patients received no medication during the study; the others received digitalis preparations or antibiotics. Eight patients each received a capsule of 10 mg orally, 7 patients received a capsule of 10 mg sublingually and 5 patients 1 mg intravenously. The capsules were kept in aluminum foil and the injections were also protected from light.

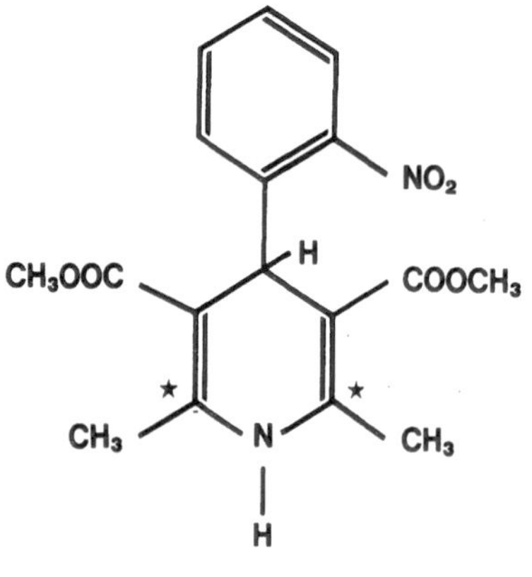

Nifedipine-^{14}C

Fig. 1

Table 1. Nifedipine-[14]C: Mode of administration

Administration	No. of Subjects	Dose mg/subject	mg/kg
Capsule, oral.	8	10	∼ 0.15
Capsule, subling.	7	10	∼ 0.15
Solution, i. v.	5	1	∼ 0.015

The fasted patients received a single dose in the morning. Thereafter blood was taken by venous puncture at regular intervals and urine quantitatively collected. The activity-content of the serum and urine samples was determined by liquid scintillation. In the following figures the values given are mean values. The variability was calculated as a standard deviation of the individual values.

Results

Figure 2 shows the course of concentration of the activity in the serum after sublingual or intravenous administration of the radioactive substance. The scale of the left ordinate is the dose ratio "P", which corresponds to the relation between the radioactivity per gram serum and the administered radioactivity per gram body weight.

This relative concentration permits the comparison of different doses of nifedipine, e.g. Fig. 3 contains a comparison of an i.v. dose of 15 µg/kg with a sublingual dose of 150 µg/kg. As early as 10 min after sublingual administration, the activity concentration is measurable in the serum.

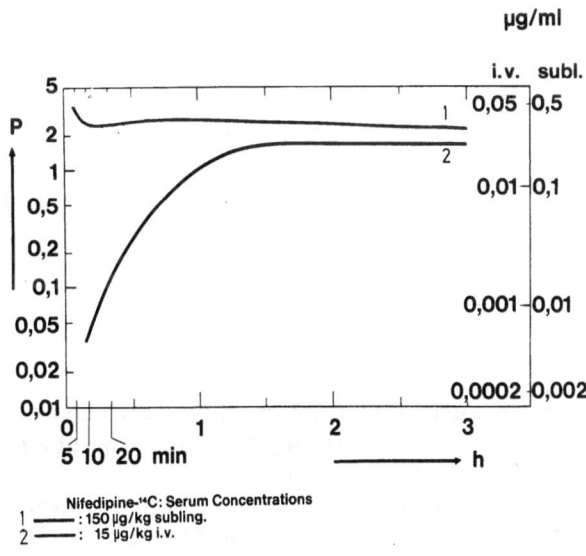

Nifedipine-[14]C: Serum Concentrations
1 ——— : 150 µg/kg subling.
2 ——— : 15 µg/kg i.v.

Fig. 2

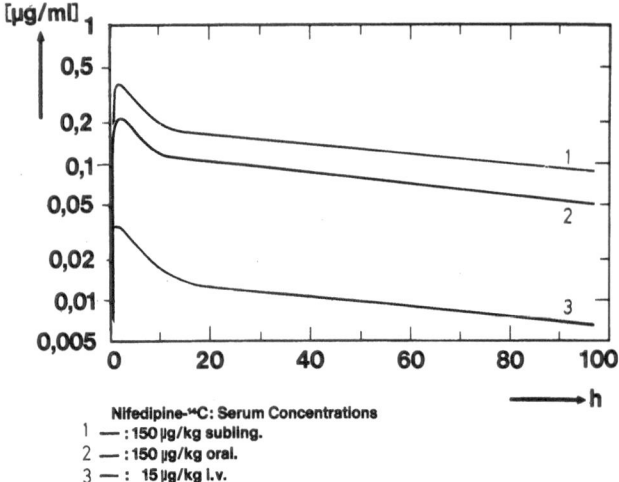

Nifedipine-¹⁴C: Serum Concentrations
1 — : 150 µg/kg subling.
2 — : 150 µg/kg oral.
3 — : 15 µg/kg i.v.

Fig. 3

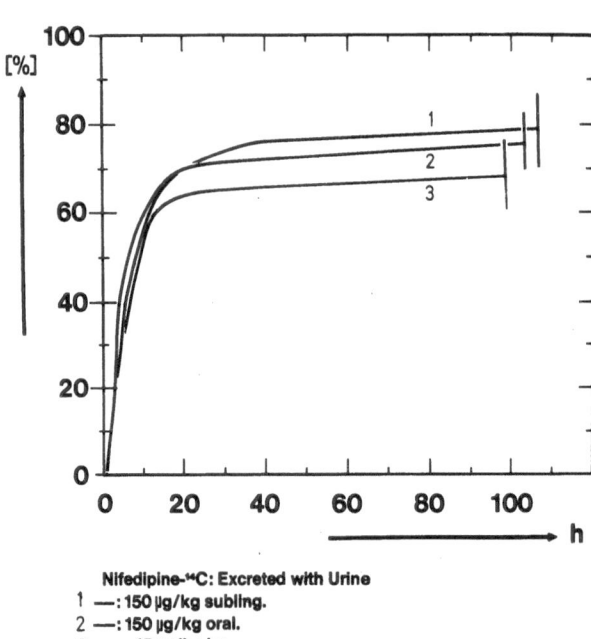

Nifedipine-¹⁴C: Excreted with Urine
1 — : 150 µg/kg subling.
2 — : 150 µg/kg oral.
3 — : 15 µg/kg i.v.

Fig. 4

Approximately 2 h after administration, the relative concentrations, either intravenous or sublingual, are statistically the same. The upward slope of the curve demonstrates the rate of absorption.

Figure 2 also shows that after i.v. administration, the serum concentration drops markedly within a few minutes, which could indicate a rapid distribution of the substance in the tissue.

Figure 3 is also concerned with serum concentrations; here the values given 100 h postadministration were taken into consideration. Equivalent concentrations based on nifedipine are on the ordinate. Because of the smaller doses the values obtained after i.v. administration are much smaller than after oral or sublingual administration. One can see that in the first 12 h the serum level drops rapidly and then decreases gradually. The slow decrease suggests that there is a marked protein binding of the radioactive substance in the serum. This figure raises the question of renal elimination of the substance, particularly the question: Is the rapid decrease of the serum concentration during the first 12 h in any way connected with the corresponding elimination of the substance via the urine.

Figure 4 gives a positive answer to this question: It clearly shows that the radioactivity is at first rapidly and then mainly eliminated via the urine. The scale of the ordinate shows the percentage of the total administered radioactive substance eliminated via the urine. One can see that independent of the application route, within 12 h, more than 50% and as much as 80% is eliminated via the urine. The rest of the radioactive substance, as preliminary studies showed, is eliminated via the feces.

Some words about biotransformation: Even in the first urine sample, i.e. 3 h postadministration, no unchanged nifedipine was detectable. This indicates a rapid and complete metabolization of the substance.

Abstract

Radioactive nifedipine was administered as a single dose sublingually, orally or intravenously.

More than 90% of the nifedipine was absorbed after oral or sublingual administration of a capsule of 10 mg.

Ten minutes after sublingual and 20 min after oral administration, ratioactivity was measured in the serum. In other words, the content of the sublingual capsule was absorbed more rapidly than that of the oral capsule. Maximal equivalent concentrations were achieved in the serum 1–2 h after enteral administration. These concentrations corresponded to the equivalent concentrations measured over the same period of time after intravenous administration.

After enteral and after intravenous administration, 70–80% of the activity was eliminated via the urine. Of this amount 90% had already been eliminated after 24 h.

Hemodynamic Studies on the New Coronary Therapeutic Drug Nifedipine (BAY a 1040)

P. F. Angelino, P. Tortore, and R. Algranati

Ospedale Civile S. Croce, Cuneo, Italy

Previous experimental investigations by several authors have shown that nifedipine has an antianginal action, due to the following mechanisms:
1. Relaxation of vascular smooth muscle, particularly in the coronary bed
2. Increase of total cardiac output due to increase of venous return
3. Slight negative inotropic effect on cardiac muscle [4–6, 8, 9].

The purpose of this paper is to demonstrate the pharmacological activity of nifedipine in humans, with regard to the following parameters:

Cardiac index, systolic index, pulmonary mean transit time, heart-to-brain mean circulation time, heart-to-femoral artery mean circulation time (Table 1).

These parameters have been evaluated using radioactive tracers before and after intravenous injection of 1 mg of nifedipine.

Table 1. Hemodynamics studies before and after i.v. acute administration 1 mg BAY a 1040

parameters
1. Cardiac Index
2. Systolic Index
3. Pulmonary mean transit time
4. Heart to brain mean circulation time
5. Heart to femoral artery mean circulation time

Methodology (Table 2)

Nifedipine (1 mg) was administered by slow intravenous injection (lasting 3 min), and hemodynamic parameters were measured before and after 5 min from the beginning of the injection.

Twenty subjects took part in the study, including 5 non-cardiac patients, 9 cardiac patients without clinical signs of heart failure and 6 patients with cardiac insufficiency.

Three sodium iodide scintillation detectors were collimated on the head (median frontal area), on precordium and on left groin to obtain a radiocardiographic curve (RCG) and to measure mean heart-to-brain and heart-to-femoral artery circulation times (Figs. 1, 2).

Table 2. Methodology

1. Radiocardiography acquired and processed by digital computer.
2. Isotopic measurement of pulmonary mean transit time.
3. Isotopic measurement of heart to brain and heart to femoral artery mean circulation time.

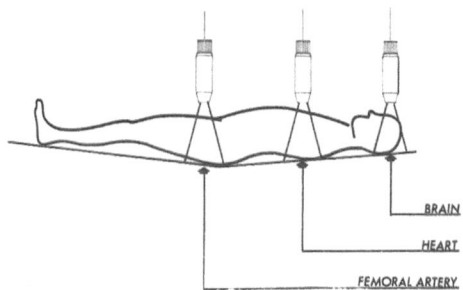

Fig. 1. Position of detectors for recording radiocardiogram, heart-to-brain and heart-to-femoral artery mean circulation times

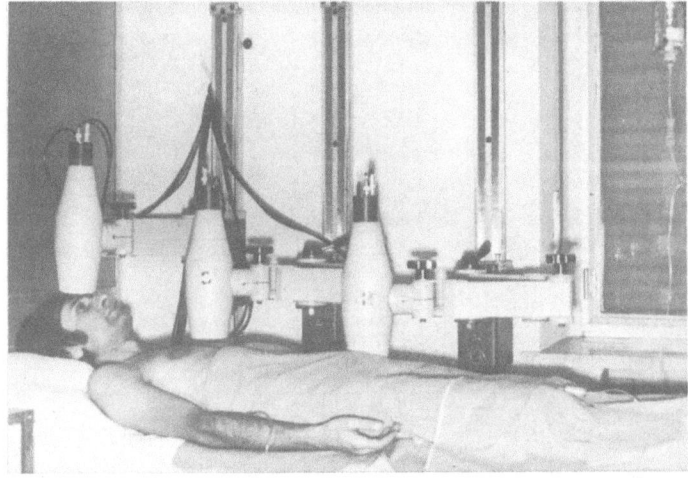

Fig. 2. Actual arrangement of detectors on patient studied in nuclear medicine department

Counts detected on each area were acquired directly by a computer (ND 812) working in a multichannel mode, stored in different memory groups, and displayed on oscilloscope as time-activity curves (Fig. 3).

In some patients suffering from acute coronary disease or cardiac infarction the radiocardiogram was recorded directly at the bed side and sent to computer by wire (Fig. 4).

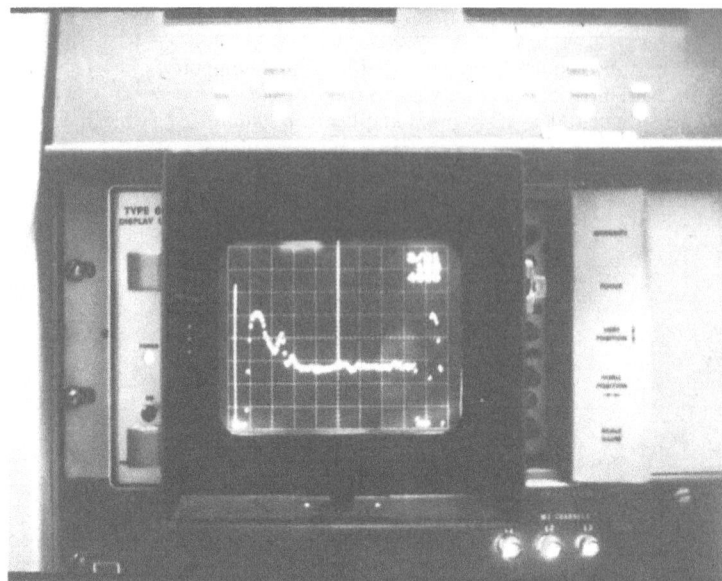

Fig. 3. Oscilloscope of the computer showing an activity-time curve

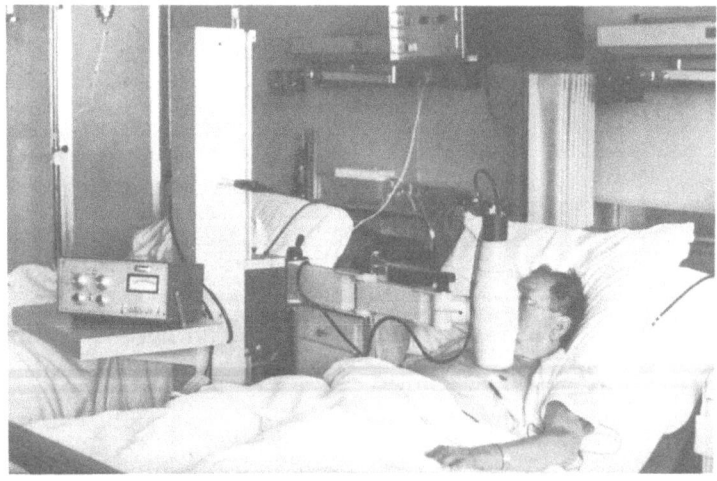

Fig. 4. Apparatus for recording radiocardiogram at bed side in coronary unit, connected by wire to computer

Indium (^{113}In), eluted from a tin-indium generator, was used as tracer; this radioisotope binds firmly to transferrin and therefore is very suitable as a tracer of circulatory space [10].

Indium was used in doses ranging from 600 to 1500 microcuries, included in a concentrated bolus not exceeding 0.4 ml volume.

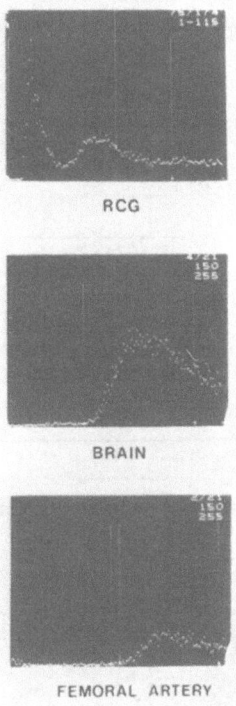

RCG

BRAIN

FEMORAL ARTERY

Fig. 5. Activity-time curve recorded simultaneously on precordium (radiocardiogram), on brain and on left femoral artery

Blood volume was measured beforehand by the dilution method, for each patient, using R.I.S.A. [125]I.

Indium was injected through an intracardiac catheter (Endocath) with the tip located in the right atrial cavity. Rapid injection was obtained by flushing with 10 ml of saline solution a short tracer bolus previously introduced into the catheter between two air bubbles.

Radiocardiographic curves, transit curves on head and femoral artery were immediately and simultaneously recorded (Fig. 5).

Ten minutes later, after complete mixing of tracer in the blood space, one minute recording of radioactivity at "equilibrium" was obtained from a detector collimated on the precordial area.

After the procedure was completed, recorded curves were tabulated and punched on paper tape and later processed by the same computer, using a conversational semi-automatic program written in ORCAL language.

Cardiac index, systolic index and pulmonary mean transit time were obtained from the radiocardiogram; heart-to-brain and heart-to-femoral artery mean circulation time were obtained simply by computing arithmetically the mean time elapsed between the left peak of the radiocardiogram and, respectively, the beginning of the ascending branch and the peak of curves detected on the brain and femoral artery.

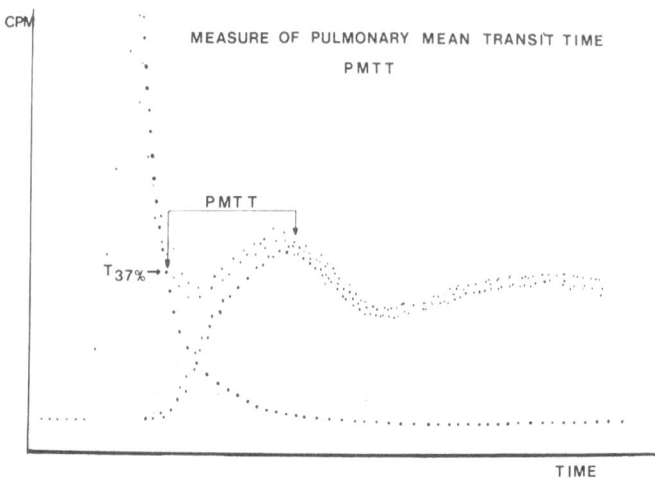

Fig. 6. Measure of pulmonary mean transit time

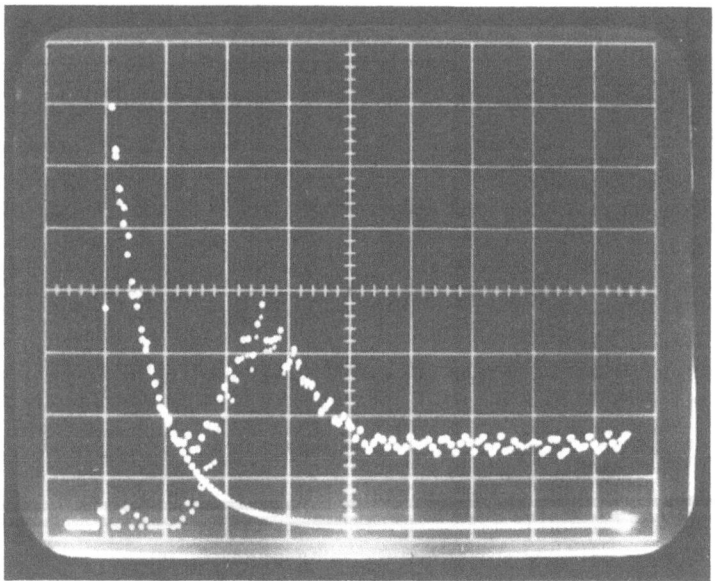

Fig. 7. Processing of radiocardiographic curve by computer. From original curve recorded on precordium, separate right curve and left curve are obtained

Computer processing of the radiocardiogram was done semi-automatically, leaving to the operator the choice of points corresponding to right or left peak of the radiocardiogram and the choice of the part of the curves to be fitted exponentially and extrapolated.

The program includes corrections for tracer decay (about 0.7% per minute) and background subtraction, which allows correct evaluation of hemodynamic parameters recorded by a second radiocardiogram carried out after injection of nifedipine.

Reproducibility of the measurements was previously tested in a patient not receiving pharmacological treatment after the first radiocardiogram.

Cardiac index was computed according to the following formula:

$$\frac{0.83 \times \text{counts at equilibrium recorded on precordium} \times \text{blood volume}}{\text{area under RCG curve} \times \text{skin area}}$$

Systolic index was computed by dividing cardiac index by heart rate.

Pulmonary mean transit time was obtained according to the method of GIUN-TINI *et al.* by measuring the time between the left peak of RCG and the point at which the exponential fitting the descending branch of the right curve of RCG reaches 37% of its peak value. This time is conveniently expressed in cardiac cycles [1–3, 7] (Fig. 6).

In order to obtain correct values for this parameter, the RCG curve is properly processed by computer, and time-activity curves corresponding to transit of the radioactivity bolus in the right and left heart are obtained separately (Fig. 7). Then, pulmonary mean transit time is computed as described previously.

Results and Comments

The study included twenty hospital patients (5 non-cardiac, 9 cardiac patients without cardiac failure and 6 cardiac patients with cardiac failure) (Fig. 8).

Parameters measured before and 5 min after i.v. administration of nifedipine were:

cardiac index, systolic index, pulmonary mean transit time, heart-to-brain and heart-to-femoral artery mean circulation time.

Evaluation was done at rest without sedation of patients, either in fasting subjects or a few hours after meals (Fig. 9).

Results of measurements were submitted to statistical analysis and tested for significance.

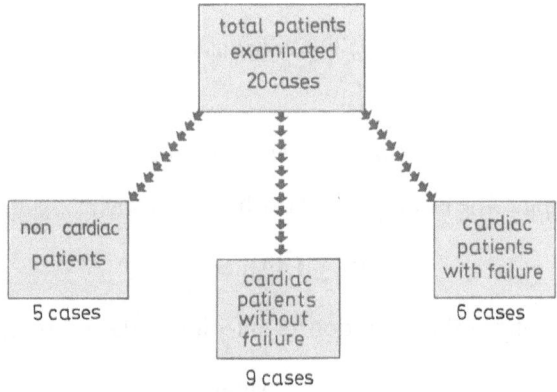

Fig. 8. Repartition of patients studied

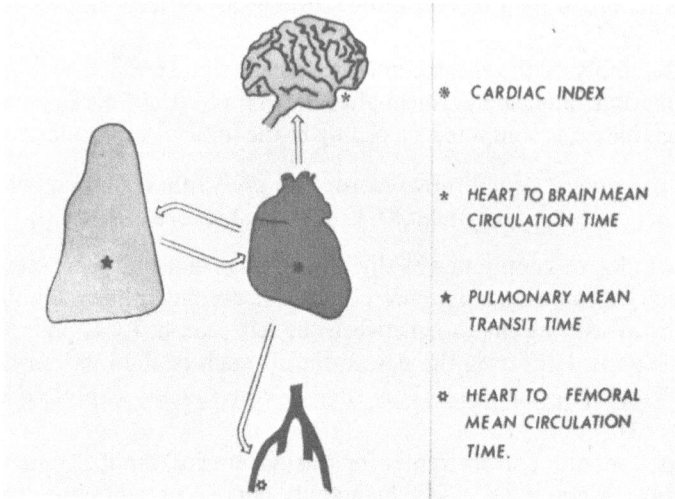

Fig. 9. Schematic drawing indicating parameters studied

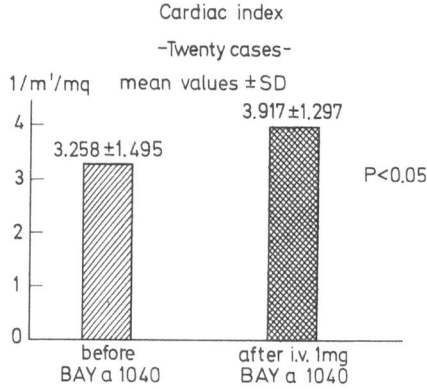

Fig. 10. Cardiac index

Cardiac Index (Fig. 10)

Before nifedipine, the mean value of cardiac index was:

$$3.258 \pm 1.49 \text{ liters}.$$

Five minutes after administration of nifedipine, the mean value of cardiac index was:

$$3.917 \pm 1.29 \text{ liters}.$$

The difference was statistically significant ($p < 0.05$).

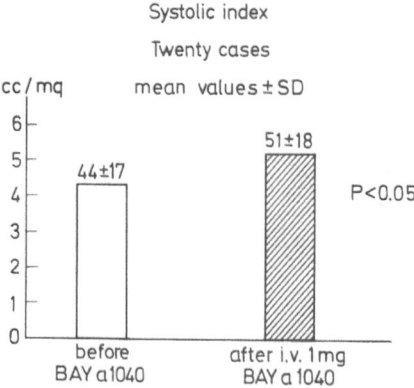

Fig. 11. Systolic index

Systolic Index (Fig. 11)

Before nifedipine, the mean value of systolic index was:

$$44.02 \pm 17 \text{ cc}.$$

Five minutes after administration of nifedipine, the mean value of systolic index was:

$$55.88 \pm 18 \text{ cc}.$$

The difference was statistically significant ($p < 0.05$).

Pulmonary mean transit time and heart-to-brain and heart-to-femoral artery mean circulation time were studied comparatively in order to assess possible differential activity of nifedipine in different vascular beds.

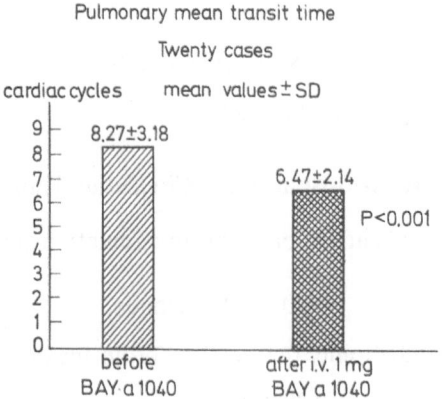

Fig. 12. Pulmonary mean transit time

Pulmonary Mean Transit Time (Fig. 12)

Before nifedipine, the mean value of pulmonary mean transit time, expressed in cardiac cycles, was:

$$8.27 \pm 3.18 \text{ cardiac cycles.}$$

Five minutes after administration of nifedipine, pulmonary mean transit time was:

$$6.47 \pm 2.14 \text{ cardiac cycles.}$$

The difference was highly significant ($p < 0.001$).

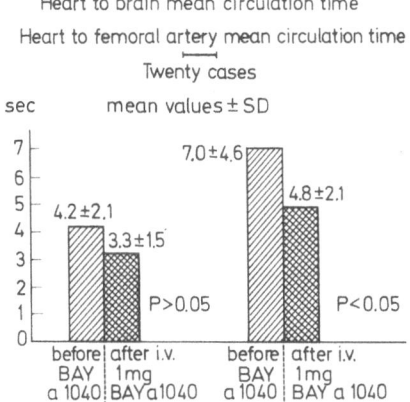

Fig. 13. Heart-to-brain and heart-to-femoral artery mean circulation times

Heart-to-Femoral Artery Mean Circulation Time (Fig. 13)

Before nifedipine, the heart-to-femoral artery mean circulation time (measured in seconds) was:

$$7.01 \pm 4.6 \text{ seconds.}$$

Five minutes after nifedipine it was:

$$4.84 \pm 2.17 \text{ seconds.}$$

The difference was significant ($p < 0.05$).

Heart-to-Brain Mean Circulation Time

Before nifedipine, the heart-to-brain mean circulation time (measured in seconds) was:

$$4.20 \pm 2.12 \text{ seconds.}$$

Five minutes after nifedipine, the heart-to-brain mean circulation time was:

$$3.39 \pm 1.5 \text{ seconds.}$$

The difference was not significant ($p > 0.05$).

Lack of significance of the change of mean heart-to-brain circulation time was probably due to the high heterogeneity of the sample in comparison to the number of cases observed.

This suggests that the action of the drug on the vascular bed of the brain differs from patient to patient, while in other vascular beds the drug action is more constant.

We also tried to perform a separate statistical analysis of the three groups of cases: i.e. cardiac patients with failure, cardiac patients without failure and noncardiac patients.

Because of the small number of patients studied in each group, we were not able to reach the level of significance.

However, our clinical observations suggest that changes of cardiac index and of systolic index are lesser in patients with cardiac failure; in fact, in three out of six patients with cardiac failure we could not observe any modification of these parameters after nifedipine.

In one of these patients, cardiac index increased dramatically after 5 days of therapy with intravenous strophantine.

This observation suggests that in patients with coronary disease and cardiac failure, it is advisable to use cardiocinetic therapy, together with coronary vasodilating drugs.

This research confirms that nifedipine undoubtly increases venous return and, if the cardiac pump is efficient, the drug also increases cardiac output and thereby contributes to increasing coronary blood flow. We know, however, that the primary direct action of nifedipine is the relaxation of smooth muscle, which is the predominant type of muscle on the coronary vascular bed.

In our patients, on acute i.v. injection of 1 mg of nifedipine, we never observed any significant change of blood pressure, either of systolic or of diastolic values.

The same applied to heart rate.

No patient showed any side-effects, except one alcoholic patient, who complained of flushing for a few minutes.

In contrast to clinical observations, we never observed headache in any patient who received the drug orally.

Abstract

The hemodynamic action of nifedipine (BAY a 1040) administered by intravenous injection was studied in twenty human subjects using radioactive tracer methods, including radiocardiography. The parameters studied included cardiac index, systolic index, pulmonary mean transit time, heart-to-brain and heart-to-femoral artery mean circulation times, heart rate and blood pressure. Intravenous injection of nifedipine caused a significant increase of cardiac index and systolic index, a significant decrease of pulmonary mean transit time and of heart-to-femoral artery mean circulation time.

Heart-to-brain mean circulation time, heart rate and blood pressure were not significantly modified (Table 3).

Table 3

Parameter	Before Nifedipine	After Nifedipine	Significance
Cardiac index	3.258 ± 1.49 lt.	3.917 ± 1.29 lt.	($p < 0.05$)
Systolic index	44.02 ± 17 cc	55.88 ± 18 lt.	($p < 0.05$)
Pulmonary mean transit time	8.27 ± 3.18 card. cycles	6.47 ± 2.14 card. cycles	($p < 0.001$)
Heart-to-brain mean circulation time	4.20 ± 2.12 seconds	3.39 ± 1.5 seconds	($p > 0.05$)
Heart-to-femoral artery mean circulation time	7.01 ± 4.6 seconds	4.84 ± 2.17 seconds	($p < 0.05$)
Heart rate	74 ± 16	77 ± 16	($p > 0.05$)

Acknowledgement. We are deeply indebted to Prof. G. VACCA, Director of the Clinical Biochemistry Department for computer processing of statistical data.

References

1. DONATO, L., GIUNTINI, C., LEWIS, M.L., DURAND, J., ROCHESTER, D.F., HARWEY, R.M., COURNAND, A.: Quantitative radiocardiography. I. Theoretical considerations. Circulation **26**, 174 (1962).
2. GIUNTINI, C., LEWIS, M.L., SALES LUIS, A., HARVEY, R.M.: A study of the pulmonary blood volume in man by quantitative radiocardiography. J. Clin. Invest. **42**, 1589 (1963).
3. GIUNTINI, C., OREN, V., LUBIN, E.: Simplified radiocardiography for obtained cardiac output and mean pulmonary transit time. Hour. Nucl. Biol. Med. **15**, 81 (1971).
4. HASHIMOTO, K., TAIRA, N., CHIBA, S., HASHIMOTO, K., JR., ENDOH, M., KOKUBUN, M., KOKUBUN, H., IIJIMA, T., KIMURA, T., KUBOTA, K., OGURO, K.: Cardiohemodynamic effects of BAY a 1040 in the Dog. Arzneim.-Forsch. **1**, 15 (1972).
5. HAYASE, S., HIRAKAWA, S., HOSOKOWA, S., MORI, N., ITO, H., KONDO, Y., HIEI, K., BANNO, S.: Basic and clinical studies on BAY a 1040 with special reference to its influence on the coronary systemic resistance and capacitance blood vessels. Jap. Circ. Jour. **35**, 903 (1971).
6. HAYASE, S., HIRAKAWA, S., HOSOKAWA, S., MORI, N., KANYAMA, S., IWASA, M.: Hemodynamic and therapeutic effect of BAY a 1040 on the patients with ischemic heart disease. Arzneim.-Forsch. **2**, 370 (1972).
7. LEWIS, M.L., GIUNTINI, C., DONATO, L., HARVEY, R.M., COURNAND, A.: Quantitative radiocardiography. III. Results and validation of theory and method. Circulation **26**, 189 (1962).
8. SCHNEIDER, K.W., JESSE, R.: Der Informationswert der Änderung der zentralen Hämodynamic nach Applikation eines O-Nitrophenyl-dihydropyridinderivates. Arzneim.-Forsch. **2**, 373 (1972).
9. VATER, W., KRONEBERG, G., HOFFMEISTER, F., KALLER, H., MENG, K., OBERDORF, A., PULS, W., SCHLOSSMANN, K., STOEPEL, K.: Zur Pharmakologie von 4-(2'-Nitrophenyl)-2,6-dimethyl-1,4-dihydropyridin-3,5-dicarbonsäuredimethylester (Nifedipine, BAY a 1040). Arzneim.-Forsch. **1**, 1 (1972).
10. WOCHNER, R.D., ADATEPE, M., VAN AMBURG, A., POTCHEN, E.J.: A new method for estimation of plasma volume with the use of the distribution space of indium-113 m-transferrin. J. Lab. & Clin. Med. **75**, 711 (1970).

Discussion Remarks

LOCHNER: Is there a slight stimulation of cardiac output or circulation because you measured a shortening of different circulation times?

ANGELINO: Yes. We have obtained an increase in cardiac output especially in those patients with cardiac disease but without cardiac failure. In patients with cardiac failure we have seen that the response to Adalat is not equal to that of patients with no cardiac failure. Patients with cardiac failure have a slight increase of cardiac output only. Therefore I believe that the association of strophanthin or digitalis to Adalat is very useful in patients with coronary disease and cardiac insufficiency.

Another finding was, that the increase in "heart-to-femoral artery time" and in "pulmonary mean transit time" was statistically significant. No significance was found in "heart-to-brain time".

The "transit pulmonary time" changes by adding digitalis to Adalat because it corresponds with cardiac failure. This time does not change with Adalat alone in patients with cardiac insufficiency.

Effect of Nifedipine (Adalat) on Myocardial Oxygen Extraction and Lactate Metabolism and ST-T Segment Changes in Patients with Coronary Insufficiency during Artificial Stimulation of the Heart

J. SCHAEFER, H.-J. SCHWARZKOPF, M. SCHOETTLER, and R. WILMS

Abteilung für Spezielle Kardiologie, Zentrum Konservative Medizin I
der Christian-Albrechts-Universität Kiel, Fed. Rep. Germany

In studying the effects of a drug on the coronary vascular system and on hemodynamics, experimental conditions should be as constant and reproducible as possible.—In our experience, the artificial stimulation of the heart with an electrode catheter provides stepwise increases in heart rate leading to reproducible changes in arterial and left ventricular pressure and stroke volume and keeping cardiac output relatively constant within a rate range of 80–140 beats/min. In addition, it is known that with increasing beating rate, myocardial oxygen and substrate demand rise in a linear fashion. This increased myocardial oxygen demand is normally met by an increase in coronary blood flow, while the resistance to coronary and myocardial blood flow drops.

Usually coronary-venous oxygen saturation, arterio-coronary venous oxygen difference, and lactate extraction remain constant. As long as the general and regional coronary vascular reserve is not fully used, this is also true for patients with a limitation of coronary reserve. If, however, myocardial oxygen and substrate demand increase with further increase in heart rate beyond this upper limit of functional coronary vascular capacity, oxygen and substrate extraction rise, and a decrease in lactate extraction or even lactate production occurs.

Within this pathophysiologic framework, it can be expected that 1. any drug that increases coronary or myocardial blood flow beyond the immediate myocardial demand may lead to an increase in coronary venous oxygen saturation and 2. any drug that influences myocardial general or regional oxygen demand may have an influence on lactate extraction beyond the limits of the respective coronary vascular reserve.

Materials and Methods

We studied 11 patients, aged 35–65 years, in whom a diagnosis of coronary insufficiency was assumed on clinical, anamnestic and electrocardiographic evidence. At the time of the study the patients were on no drug regimen.

In all patients a bipolar electrode catheter was inserted via an antecubital vein into the right atrium.

In addition, a bird's eye catheter was introduced into the coronary sinus under fluoroscopic control, taking care to pick up the efflux of the great vein. Serial determinations of arterial and coronary venous oxygen content and of lactate concentration were carried out at the spontaneous heart rate and during pacing-induced tachycardia before and up to 40 min after the sublingual administration of 20 mg nifedipine.

The ECG was monitored continuously on a 6 channel recorder (Hellige & Co., 78 Freiburg/Brsg., FRG.) during the test. The ST-T segments of leads, I, II, aVL, V4, V6 were measured during and up to ten beats after the cessation of stimulation.

Results and Discussion

A schematic presentation of the procedure of the investigation is shown in Fig. 1. The change in heart rate was about 50–60 beats/min, since the spontaneous heart rate was usually around 80/min. Successful stimulation was achieved by electrical square wave impulses of 2 msec duration. The blood samples, marked with stars, were drawn as double determinations 2 min after the respective change in rate, since it could be assumed that a new steady state had then occurred.

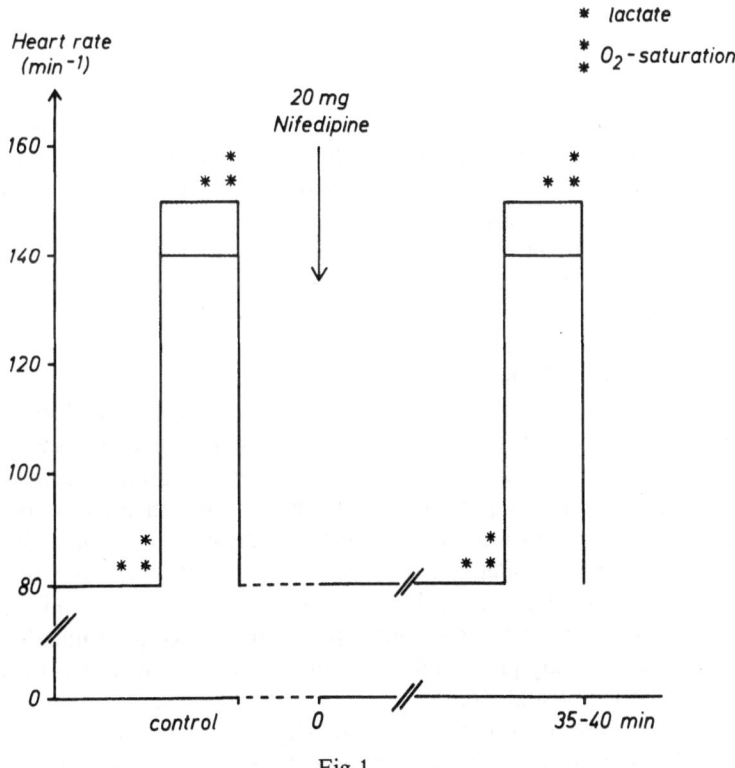

Fig. 1

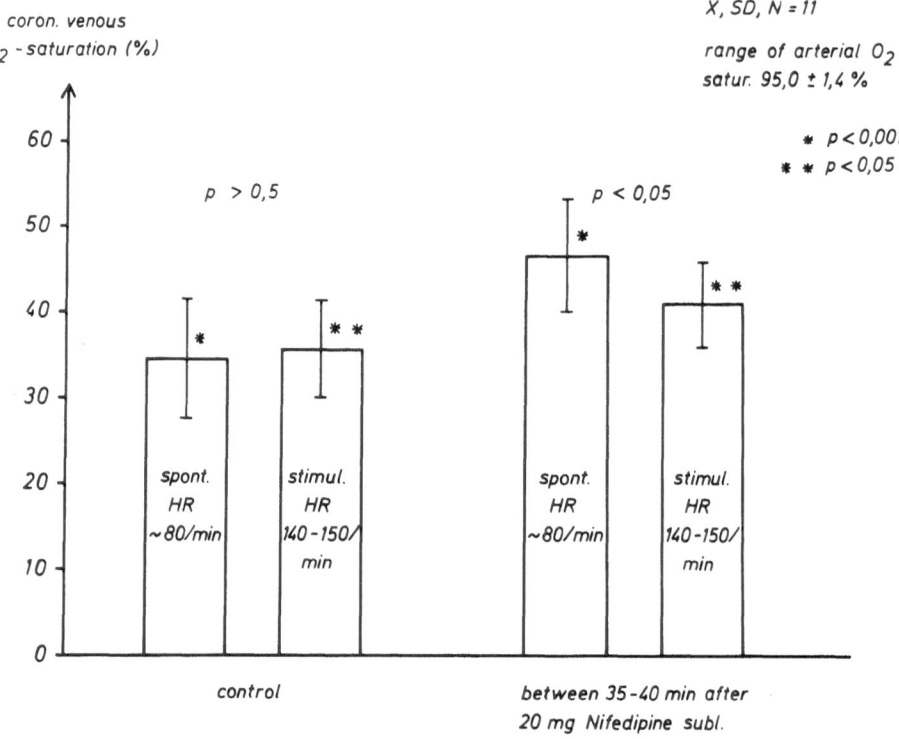

Fig. 2

In the group of patients studied, arterio-coronary venous oxygen saturation did not change significantly during pacing-induced tachycardia (PIT), as can be seen in the left part of Fig. 2. After the administration of nifedipine, however, there was a significant increase in coronary venous oxygen saturation at the spontaneous heart rate of 80/min. This increase is distinctly diminished during PIT, but the elevation of coronary venous oxygen saturation is still evident at a 0.05 confidence level compared to the values before nifedipine.

Coronary venous lactate concentration changed considerably during PIT as can be seen in Fig. 3. It increased from a mean value of 3.8 mg% at the spontaneous heart rate to 6.4 mg% during pacing. This is a meaningful increase, since the crossing of the shaded area indicates the occurrence of myocardial lactate production, because the range of arterial lactate concentration is surpassed.

After nifedipine (right part of Fig. 3), there is still an increase of coronary venous lactate concentration but it is much less distinct than before the administration of the drug. The difference is significant at the 0.05 confidence level.

Concurrent with the discussed changes in coronary venous and lactate concentration, the extent of ST-T segment depression declined after nifedipine during PIT (Fig. 4). Graphically presented is the sum of ST-T segment depression in mm in leads I, II, aVL, V 4, and V 6.

In addition: The occurrence and intensity of precordial anginal pain were diminished in 8 out of 11 patients, thus indicating an elevation of the pain thresh-

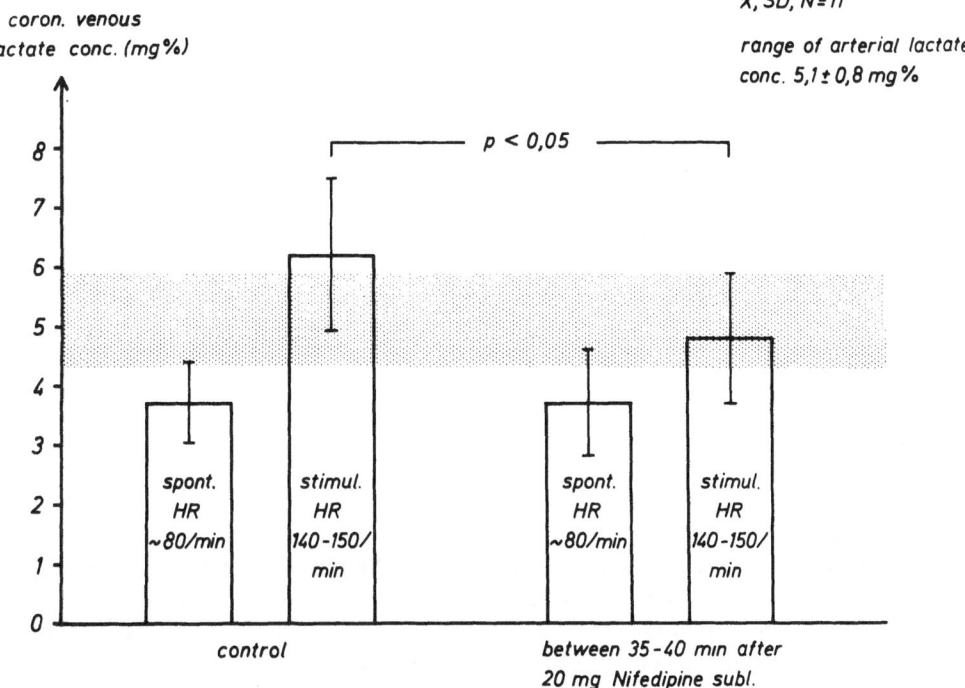

Fig. 3

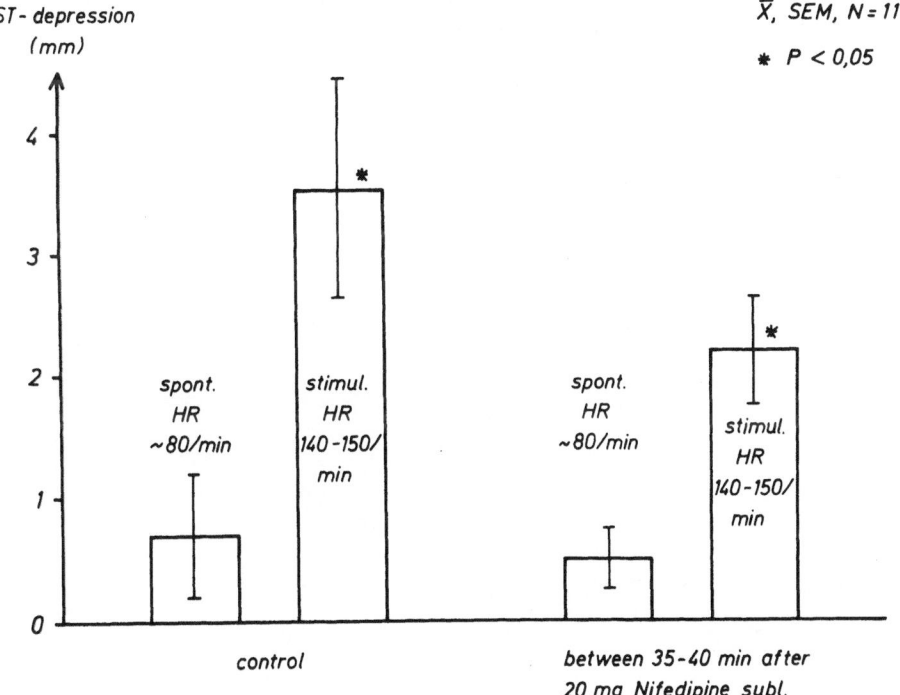

Fig. 4

old for PIT under nifedipine. In view of these and other published results that complement observations we have made in patients with bradycardic distur-bances of rhythm, we draw the following conclusions:

1. In patients with coronary insufficiency and thus a limitation of their coro-nary reserve, nifedipine may increase coronary venous oxygen content as an indication of increased coronary or myocardial blood flow.

2. The threshold for the occurrence of pain and lactate production during PIT is elevated by sublingually applied nifedipine.

The mechanism or mechanisms by which this is achieved remains unclear, but it appears as if nifedipine changes not only coronary blood flow but also myo-cardial blood flow distribution, thus improving the metabolic situation of the ischemic myocardium, without impeding too much, at least under *in situ* condi-tions, the contractile behavior of ventricular muscle.

Abstract

In 11 patients with coronary insufficiency the effect of 20 mg sublingually applied nifedipine on myocardial oxygen extraction, lactate metabolism and ST-T segment changes was studied before and during pacing-induced tachycardia (PIT). It could be shown, that under nifedipine the threshold for the occurrence of pain and lactate production is elevated during PIT and the extent of ST-T segment changes diminished. The increase in coronary venous oxygen saturation that was regularly observed during control heart rate was distinctly less during PIT, indicating a limitation of the coronary vascular reserve.

Hemodynamic Effect of Nifedipine (Adalat) in Patients Catheterized for Coronary Artery Disease

M. VAN DEN BRAND, W. J. REMME, G. T. MEESTER, I. TIGGELAAR-DE WIDT, R. DE RUITER, and P. G. HUGENHOLTZ

Faculteit der Geneeskunde, Erasmus Universiteit, Thoraxcentrum (Cardiologie), Rotterdam, Netherlands

Introduction

Previous investigations on the effect of Adalat on cardio-hemodynamics have shown the following results: There seems to be agreement on the fact that Adalat causes a definite fall in both systolic and diastolic systemic blood pressure. It also increases coronary blood flow, caused by a decrease in coronary resistance. Heart rate was shown to be higher or to remain stable in different studies, after the administration of the drug, as was the cardiac index. As far as contractility parameters are concerned, according to VATER et al. [2] there is primarily an inhibitory action on myocardial contractility. LICHTLEN [1] found an increase in peak dp/dt, together with an increase in heart rate and decrease in left ventricular end-diastolic pressure. It is not clear, whether these last effects are interrelated, i.e., is the higher peak dp/dt the result of a positive inotropic action of Adalat, independent of a concomitantly higher heart rate, or is it the result of the positive inotropic effect of the higher heart rate itself?

Also, we feel that contractility cannot be defined by the rate of rise of left ventricular pressure (LV peak dp/dt) alone, which is both preload- and afterload-dependent, but ought to be characterized by the measurement of Vmax.

Materials and Methods

To define in what way contractility and hemodynamic parameters are altered by Adalat at a fixed heart rate, we studied the effect of Adalat on 7 patients undergoing routine right- and left-heart catheterization for evaluation of coronary artery disease. The age of the subjects ranged from 38–56, all were male. The position of the catheters and the parameters measured are shown in Table 1.

A right atrial pacing electrode was introduced via an antecubital vein, and the atrium paced at a rate of 90 beats/min. A Swan-Ganz thermodilution catheter was positioned through the same vein with its injection site in the right atrium and the termistor in the pulmonary artery root. The catheter was used for cardiac output measurements by the thermodilution method.

Table 1. Positioning of catheters and measured parameters

Catheter	Position	Measured parameters
Bipolar stimulating	Right artrium	HR 90 beats/min.
Swan Ganz thermodilution	Pulmonary artery root	Cardiac index PA pressures
Tipmanoneter	Left ventricle	LV pressures peak dp/dt Vce Vmax TP
Gensini	Aorta	Ao pressures

Table 2. Catheterization data of 6 patients

	Three vessel coronary artery disease			Normal coronary arteries		
LVSP mmHg	120	140	135	125	164	142
LVEDP mmHg	13	10	11	9	14	4
Peak dp/dt mmHg/sec.	1540	2150	1870	1150	2015	1780
Vmax TP sec.$^{-1}$	54	51	55	37	43	59
APST + ± −	+	+	+	+	+	+
Ao S. P. mmHg	120	140	135	125	170	150
D. P. mmHg	70	90	80	85	120	90
PA S. P. mmHg	20	16	18	17	15	16
D. P. mmHg	10	8	7	10	7	8
Cardiac index l/min/m^2	2.3	2.9	4.3	4.0	3.3	2.9
Coronary obstructions %						
RCA	100	90	30	0	0	0
LAD	90	90	90	0	0	0
RCX	100	80	90	0	0	0

A tipmanometer catheter (Telco MMC, or Millar) was placed in the left ventricle via a brachial artery cutdown. It was used for measurements of left ventricular pressures, peak dp/dt, peak Vce and Vmax.

A Gensini catheter was introduced percutaneously in the aorta via a femoral artery according to the Seldinger technique for measurements of aortic pressures.

All parameters were measured before the sublingual administration of 20 mg of Adalat and at 10 min intervals for up to one hour after the drug was given. All calculations were performed on-line by a PDP-11 computer.

Before or after the Adalat study, an atrial pacing stress test was performed to see if inotropic intervention resulted in an increase of Vmax TP.

After the Adalat study left ventricular angiograms in the RAO position and coronary arteriograms in different projections were made. All coronary arteries were wide according to our experience. The catheterization data of 6 patients are shown in Table 2. The results from one patient with severe coronary artery disease were discarded because the experienced prolonged angina during catheterization which prompted us to give nitroglycerin after Adalat was administered.

The table shows that 3 patients had severe coronary artery disease with major obstructions in 2 or 3 coronary vessels, and 3 had normal coronary arteries.

There was a good reaction of the left ventricle during a pacing stress test. The other hemodynamic and contractility parameters were within normal limits, or showed borderline values in both groups.

Results

From our experiments we could not conclude any difference in the hemodynamic effects of Adalat in normal subjects and in patients with severe coronary artery disease. The results presented here were obtained by putting together all experimental subjects into a single group. The effect of the drug on the various parameters is shown in the following figures. The average value of the parameter per patient receiving the drug was calculated at various times after administration of the drug. The ratio of this value to the value of the parameter per patient in the control group was then calculated. The ratio was calculated in terms of per cent, hence at zero time the value of the ratio was 100% for all parameters.

From these, mean values and SEM were calculated. Comparisons between the different periods are evaluated using standard student t-test.

Left Ventricular Systolic Pressure

The effect on left ventricular systolic pressure is shown in Fig. 1. Twenty minutes after the administration of Adalat there was a moderate, but significant decrease in LVSP, which was still present after 60 min.

Aortic Systolic Pressure

The effect on aortic systolic pressure tended to be the same as on LVSP, with significant decreases in systolic aortic pressure of 10%, starting after 20 min (Fig. 2).

Aortic Diastolic Pressure

The aortic diastolic pressure also decreased about 10%. This was significant at 30–40 and 50 min (Fig. 3).

Left Ventricular End-Diastolic Pressure

The LVEDP tended to increase. Due to the great variations in individual patients, this increase was only significant at 30 min (Fig. 4).

Cardiac Index

As early as 10 min after the administration of Adalat there was an increase of about 15% in cardiac index, which was significant after 30 min. After one hour it was still significantly increased and even higher, about 25% (Fig. 5).

Peak dp/dt

The next two figures show the effect of Adalat on two contractility parameters. In Fig. 6, the effect on peak dp/dt in mm Hg/sec is shown. One has the impression that there is a slight rise in peak dp/dt value. It was not significant at any moment.

M. VAN DER BRAND et al.

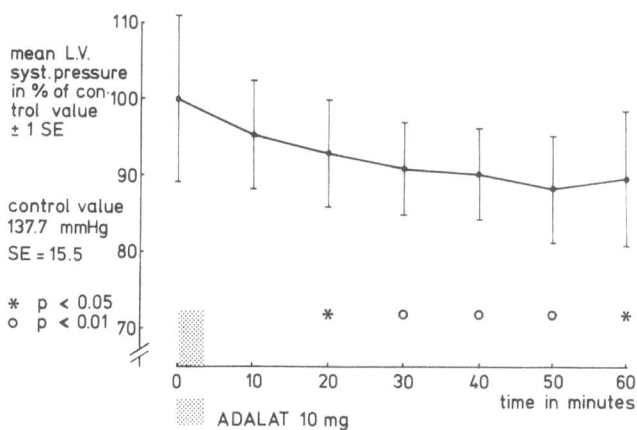

Fig. 1. Effect of Adalat, 20 mg s.l., on l.v. systolic pressure

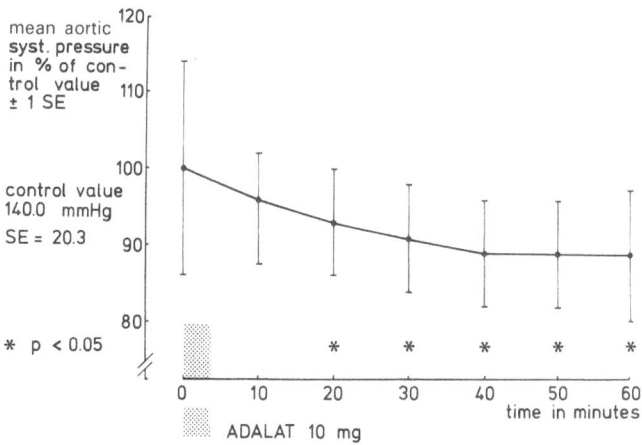

Fig. 2. Effect of Adalat, 20 mg s.l., on aortic systolic pressure

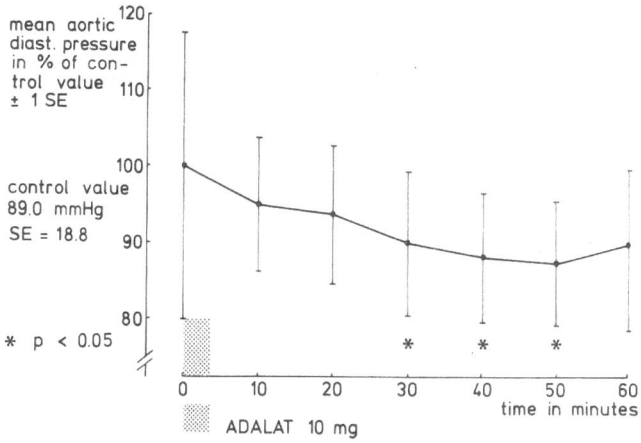

Fig. 3. Effect of Adalat, 20 mg s.l., on aortic diastolic pressure

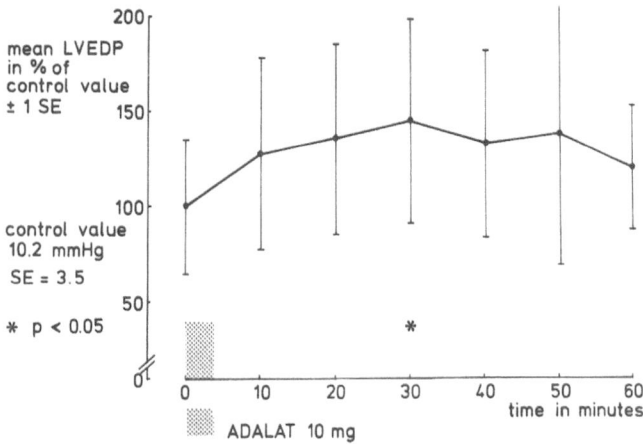

Fig. 4. Effect of Adalat, 20 mg s.l., on l.v. enddiastolic pressure

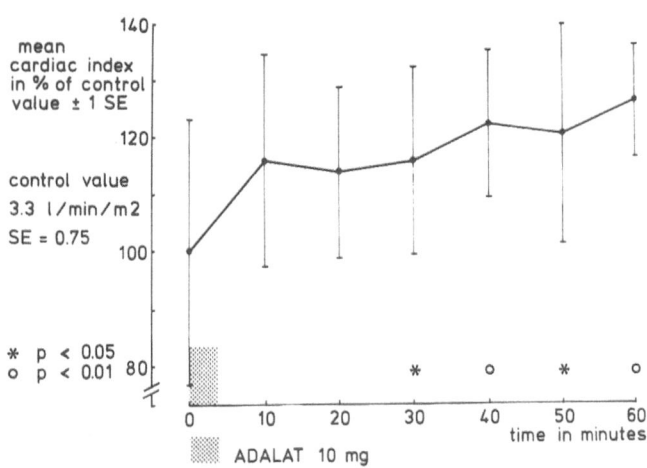

Fig. 5. Effect on Adalat, 20 mg s.l., on cardiac index

V max

The value of Vmax showed the same direction. It tended to go up, the rise being significant only after 60 min (Fig. 7).

In conclusion it can be said that Adalat has not produced any adverse reactions in our experimental setup.

The following effects were shown:

1. It dilates coronary arteries, at least that is the impression I got, looking at the coronary arteriograms.

2. There is a significant decrease in left ventricular systolic, aortic systolic and diastolic pressures, starting after 20 min and persisting throughout the study. These effects can be explained by the vasodilating effects of Adalat on the peripheral vascular beds.

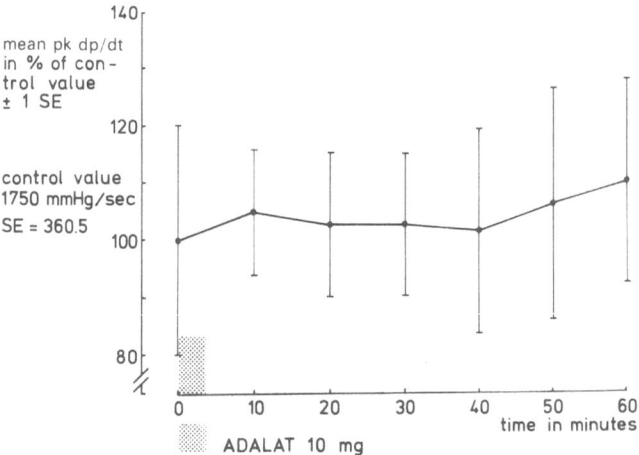

Fig. 6. Effect of Adalat, 20 mg s.l., on peak dp/dt

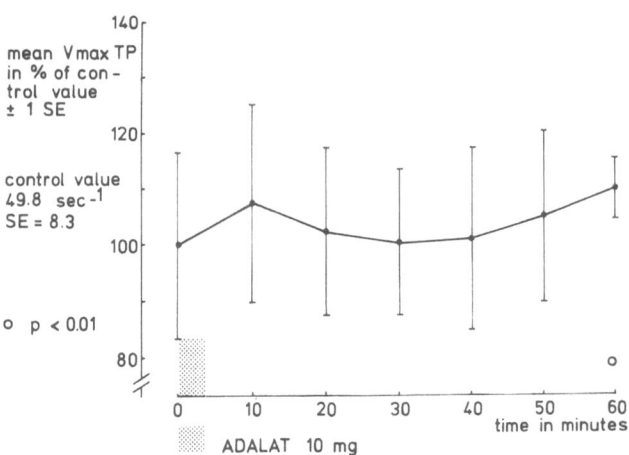

Fig. 7. Effect of Adalat, 20 mg s.l., on Vmax total pressure

3. There is a consistent rise in Vmax with significant changes after one hour, showing that Adalat has a positive inotropic effect on the heart.

4. Cardiac index is elevated from the beginning with significant increases after 30 min and lasting during the whole experiment.

5. Finally there is a slight elevation of LVEDP with a significant rise only after 30 min. This last effect could be explained by an increased venous return due to the higher cardiac output, combined with an unchanged compliance.

In Fig. 8, the overall effect on oxygen supply and consumption of the heart is shown. On the one hand, the higher contractility will increase oxygen consumption as does the rise in preload, while a decrease in afterload will definitely reduce oxygen consumption. On the other hand, the oxygen supply will be increased by the coronary dilatation and the higher cardiac output. A fall in perfusion pressure,

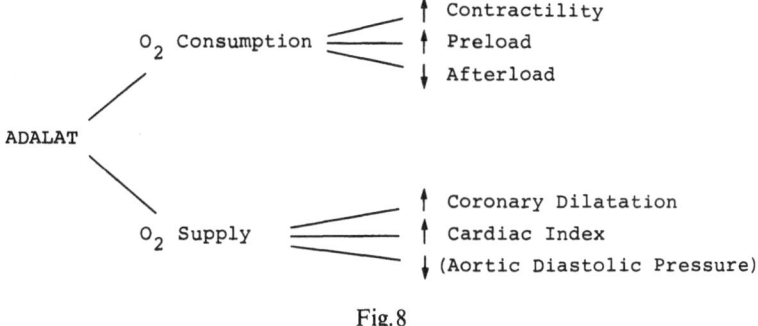

Fig. 8

however, might lead to a diminished oxygen supply to a region behind a critical coronary stenosis.

It would be tempting to philosophize about the overall results on net oxygen balance. This, however, has not been the aim of this study.

Abstract

In seven patients undergoing heart catheterization for coronary artery disease the hemodynamic effect of nifedipine, 20 mg sublingually given before any angiograms were made, was studied. The heart rate was kept constant at a rate of 90 beats per minute by means of a right atrial electrode catheter.

The following parameters were measured at 10 min intervals up to one hour after the administration of nifedipine: cardiac index (CI), pulmonary artery pressure (PA), left ventricular systolic pressure (LVSP), left ventricular end-diastolic pressure (LVEDP), contractility parameters derived from the isometric contraction (peak dp/dt, Vmax and Vce), and aortic pressure (AoP). All calculations were done by a PDP 11 computer.

Cardiac index was measured in duplo by means of a Swan-Ganz thermodilution catheter with the injection site in the right atrium and the thermistor in the pulmonary artery root. Pulmonary artery pressure was recorded by the same catheter.

Left ventricular systolic and end-diastolic pressures were recorded by a tip manometer catheter. Zero adjustment of the tip manometer pressures was effected either with their own fluid channel or through introducing the catheter percutaneously according to the Seldinger technique, via a femoral artery.

Mid-chest level in the supine position was taken as zero reference. Vce was calculated on line in a digital computer (PDP 11) from the pressure pulse (P) using the formula Vce $= dp/dt/KP$, where K is the stiffness factor of the series elastic element. In our laboratory K is set to 1, Vce is then expressed in sec^{-1}. By plotting the calculated Vce against its corresponding pressure, a pressure-load curve of the intact left ventricle can be obtained. Straight line extrapolation of the descending limb between peak Vce and p 80 mm Hg to zero pressure allows estimation of the hypothetical maximal intrinsic Vce or Vmax.

Aortic pressure was recorded through a percutaneously introduced Seldinger catheter.

At least one hour after administration of nifedipine an atrial pacing stress test was performed to measure the inotropic effect of pacing on the left ventricle.

Finally a left ventricular angiogram in the RAO position was made and coronary arteriograms were made in several projections.

The effect of nifedipine in patients with different stages of coronary heart disease is shown.

References

1. LICHTLEN, P.: 1st Internat. Nifedipine "Adalat" Symposium, p. 114. Tokyo: Tokyo Univers. Press 1975.
2. VATER, W., KRONEBERG, G., HOFFMEISTER, F., KALLER, H., MENG, K., OBERDORF, A., PULS, W., SCHLOSSMANN, K., STOEPEL, K.: Arzneim.-Forsch. (Drug Res.) **22**, 1 (1972).

Discussion Remarks

LYDTIN: Dr. V. D. BRAND, you showed the systolic pressure decreased over about 40–50 min. How long did you observe the pressure before the administration of the drug, and how long did you control your resting values? If you place a catheter in the left ventricle the sympathetic drive could increase slightly, which changes your resting values.

V. D. BRAND: The mean time between introducing the catheters and commencing the study was between 45 min to 1 hr. The left ventricular systolic pressure remained stable beforehand.

LICHTLEN: I think it is nice that somebody showed that the increase in dp/dt_{max}, which was seen by us and other people too, was obviously heart-rate dependent.

I have more difficulty in understanding that you found an increase in end-diastolic pressure because we all have seen a decrease in end-diastolic pressure. First, I wonder how this is possible in normal patients. I could agree that in coronary patients you might get an increase in end-diastolic pressure during pacing although you paced only up to 90 beats/min, provided the patients have big ventricules or akinetic areas. However, in normals, if you still agree that you also saw an increase in the inotropic state and not a decrease, then one would expect that you should get a decrease in end-diastolic pressure.

Second, there is a big difference between clinical and pharmacologic findings. The pharmacologists tell us that they see a decrease in the inotropic state, and we, by secondary beta-stimulation, see an increase. But I thought your data seemed to indicate a decrease in the inotropic state: V max either did not increase or only decreased 60 min later, and then only minimally, and all other contractility parameters decreased. Cardiac index increased secondarily as a result of the increase in venous return; thus I think your data could also be turned around.

V. D. BRAND: We either saw an LVdp elevation after Adalat or no change; it never went down. In all patients we did an atrial pacing stress test before the Adalat study and we saw in all that the left ventricular end-diastolic pressure went down when we paced up to 130, 140, and 150 beats/min. I cannot explain the fact that left ventricle end-diastolic pressure was the same or was higher after Adalat was given when we applied a pacing frequency of 90 beats/min. As far as contractility is concerned, of course we measure overall effects. This is a complex reaction of decrease in contractility and a corresponding elevation of contractility. So we measured these two processes at the same time with the net result being a slight elevation of both dp/dt and V max at a fixed heart rate of 90 beats/min. But I agree, it is minimal.

MCARTHUR: Mr. Chairman, Ladies and Gentlemen, there seems to be good evidence from the foregoing papers that exercise tolerance after administered nifedipine is increased. However, to be of use clinically it must be shown that the substance is active when administered chronically by the oral route. Beta-blockers have been shown to improve exercise tolerance when thus administered. Therefore, in a study in Glasgow we planned to compare the efficacy of nifedipine with that of propranolol.

It must be emphasized that this was a preliminary study. (We plan to go on to a double-blind study later.) We had five patients with stable angina, lasting more than one year, and angiographically proven coronary artery disease. Before treatment, we exercised them to onset of angina on a bicycle ergometer, then on escalating doses of nifedipine, and on escalating doses of propranolol.

The dosage regime for nifedipine was, for the first week, 10 mg t.i.d., up to 20 mg t.i.d. and 30 mg t.i.d. We stopped the drug once we had reached the 90 mg/day dose, if there were intolerable side effects, or if we were unable to demonstrate a significant increase in exercise tolerance.

With oral propranolol our dose schedule was 10 mg q.i.d. up to as much as 60 mg q.i.d. at weekly intervals. Our end point was the high dose, a heart rate of less than 60, the assumption being that they were then beta-blocked, the presence of intolerable side effects, or a significant decrease in exercise tolerance.

The results are as follows. The heart rate after nifedipine does not seem to change significantly. The maximum exercise tolerance measured as kpm did not change significantly with nifedipine. However, as expected, on propranolol the heart rate went down and maximum exercise tolerance increased. The average changes in the heart rate was +4% on nifedipine, −24% on propranolol. Exercise tolerance was on the average +12% on nifedipine, +48% on propranolol.

We also noted a high incidence of gastrointestinal side effects; four patients were so affected and this was dose-related, occurring at the 20-mg t.i.d. and 30-mg t.i.d. doses and sometimes being improved by reducing the dosage. Cardiovascular side effects were seen in three patients and did not appear to be dose-related, occurring in all patients at the 10-mg t.i.d. dosage. We also saw dizziness and pruritus.

Reluctantly we came to the conclusion that, in chronically administered oral nifedipine—and I must emphasize that there was no sublingual administration of nifedipine at any time—we were not able to demonstrate a significant change in exercise tolerance and we had a disturbingly high incidence of side effects.

Session IV

Clinical Pharmacology Efficacy

Chairmen: W. KAUFMANN (Köln), B. TABATZNIK (Baltimore)

Comparison of the Effects of Adalat with Other Substances on Myocardial Ischemia under Loading Conditions

H.-J. BECKER, M. KALTENBACH, and G. KOBER

Zentrum d. Inn. Medizin, Klinikum der Univ. Frankfurt, Fed. Rep. Germany

Critical evaluation of therapeutic results is complicated by a large number of factors, such as the subjective character of anginal pain and the variability in the natural course of the disease. Drugs with an analgetic or tranquillizing side effect may also relieve anginal pain without exerting any effect on the underlying coronary insufficiency. Therefore, we have for several years used for evaluation of antianginal drugs the influence of ST-depression under exercise as an objective parameter, providing strict criteria for interpretation. In our study, a particular step-test evaluation was used that has been shown to be of the same accuracy and reproducibility as the bicycle ergometer method [2].

Methods

Only patients with reproducible ST-segment depression due to coronary heart disease were included. All patients had a typical history of exertional retrosternal chest pain relieved by nitroglycerin. Most of the patients underwent selective coronary angiography, which invariably demonstrated severe obstructions of the coronary artery tree. Criteria used for a positive exercise test included: ST-depressions of at least 0.5 mm, either horizontal, descending or upwardly convex in shape. Ascending ST-depressions or isolated changes of T-waves were disregarded.

Not included were patients on digitalis, with electrolyte imbalance or with a WPW-syndrome, because of the possibility of a false positive reaction. Prior to exercise, an ECG was regularly taken in the upright position in order to exclude ST-depression induced merely by the autonomous nervous system and otherwise not necessarily distinguishable from a true ischemic reaction. The ECG was made before, during and after exercise (Fig. 1). Eighteen patients (17 male and one female) with history of angina pectoris and reproducible ST-segment depression under exercise were included in the group which received a single dose of nifedipine. The exercise tests were first performed without any drugs and were repeated 30 min after chewing 10 or 20 mg of nifedipine (Adalat).

Eleven male patients received long-term treatment over a period of six weeks. They were given 20 mg nifedipine 3 times per day. Before the drug treatment was

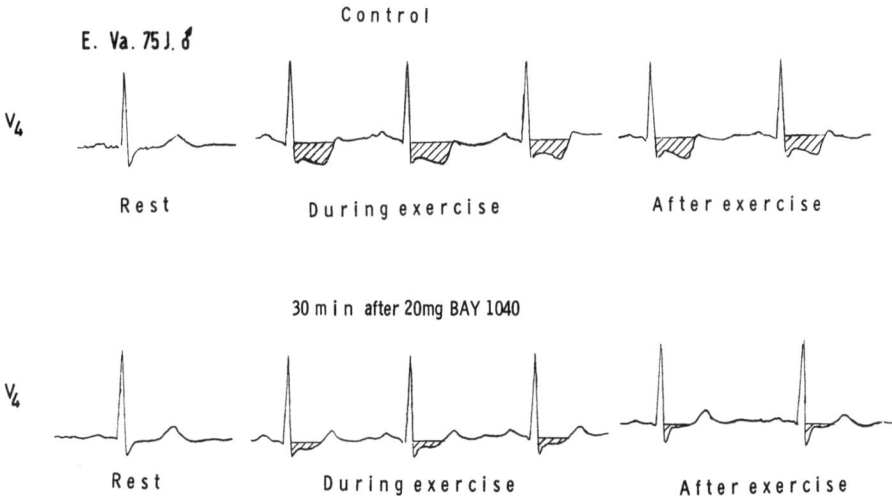

Fig. 1. Example for the improvement of ST-depression under exercise in a patient with proved coronary heart disease after administration of a single dose of 20 mg nifedipine

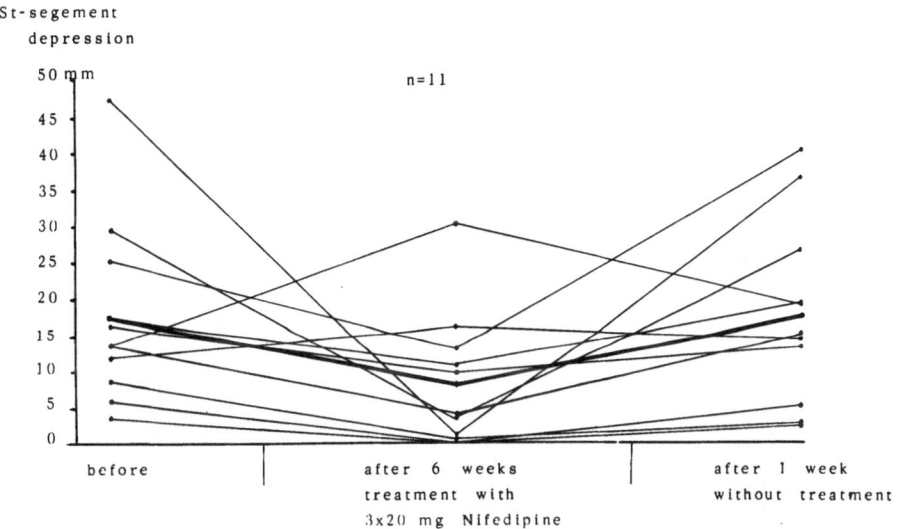

Fig. 2. ST-segment depression before, during and after long-term treatment with nifedipine. In the mean, the ST-depression improved during drug therapy (thick line)

startet, an exercise test was performed. After six weeks, the second exercise test was performed half an hour after administration of 20 mg nifedipine. After the sixth week, the treatment was interrupted, and a control test was performed one week later. The ST-segment depressions were measured every minute during exercise and over a five-minute period after exercise. From each minute the ST-depression of 4–5 beats was measured. Thereafter, the average ST-depression could be seen. The averages of each minute during exercise and those of a five-minute period after exercise were summed up. The sum was compared with the sum obtained under drug treatment and the mean value also.

Results

Forty-two exercise tests were performed before and after administration of a single dose of nifedipine (Table 1). The sum of the ST-depressions of all patients before treatment was 362.7 mm and after, 187.1 mm (mean value 17.2–8.9 mm). As a mean, the ST-segment depression after nifedipine was only 51.6% as compared with the control. Except one patient all showed an improvement of ischemic ST-depression under nifedipine. Therefore, only about half as much ST-depression was observed in the exercise ECG after nifedipine. Subjective statements on angina pectoris revealed in all 18 patients an improvement after the medication, i.e. less anginal pain during the second exercise test.

Table 1. Sum of ST-depressions before and after administration of a single dose of nifedipine in 42 exercise tests in 18 patients. 3 patients with 10 and 18 patients with 20 mg nifedipine. Pat. No. 11 showed a worse effect

No.	Name	Sex	Age	Dose (mg)	Control (mm)	Nifedipine (mm)
1	Do. R.	♂	57	20	7.5	4.8
2	Ch. O.	♂	59	20	15.3	9.2
3	En. G.	♂	58	20	17.5	12.8
4	Fi. D.	♂	63	20	64.2	34.1
5	Fi. A.	♂	46	20	28.6	20.3
6	Ge. F.	♂	64	20	3.7	0.9
7	Gü. J.	♂	50	20	7.5	5.0
8	He. I K.	♂	52	10	6.5	1.6
9	He. II K.	♂	52	20	13.3	5.4
10	Ho. I K.	♂	55	10	13.0	6.9
11	Ho. II K.	♂	55	20	11.3	19.8
12	Ke. K.	♂	47	20	19.6	0
13	Kep. W.	♂	62	20	26.8	13.5
14	Ma. I K.	♂	53	10	7.5	4.5
15	Ma. II K.	♂	53	20	5.5	1.4
16	Mi. E.	♀	64	20	3.2	1.0
17	Sa. W.	♂	47	20	7.6	1.8
18	Schö. J.	♂	63	20	9.9	6.5
19	Sei. S.	♂	59	20	36.8	11.1
20	Va. E.	♂	75	20	42.0	16.0
21	W. F.	♂	63	20	15.4	10.5
				Σ	362.7 = 100%	187.1 = 51.6%
				$\bar{x}$	17.2	8.9
				SEM	±3.3	±1.8

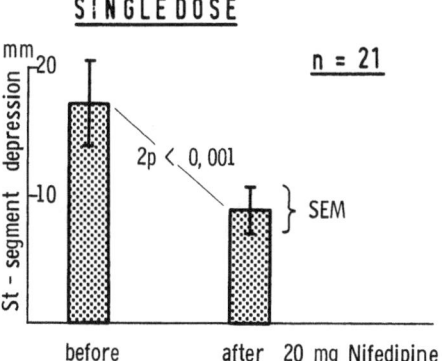

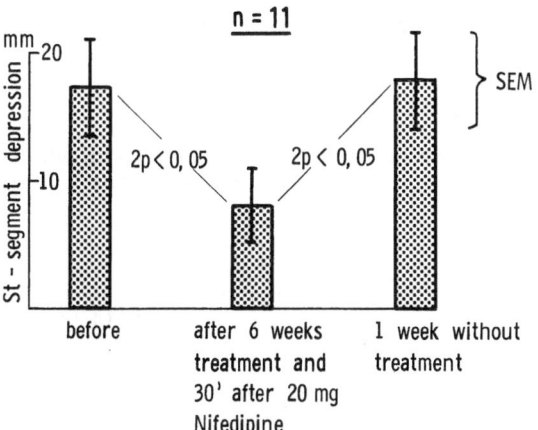

Fig. 3. Mean values of ST-depressions before and after a single dose of nifedipine, before, during and after long-term treatment with nifedipine

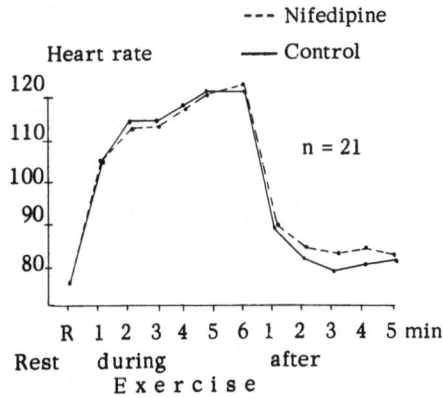

Fig. 4. Heart rate before and after a single dose of nifedipine. The heart rate was not influenced

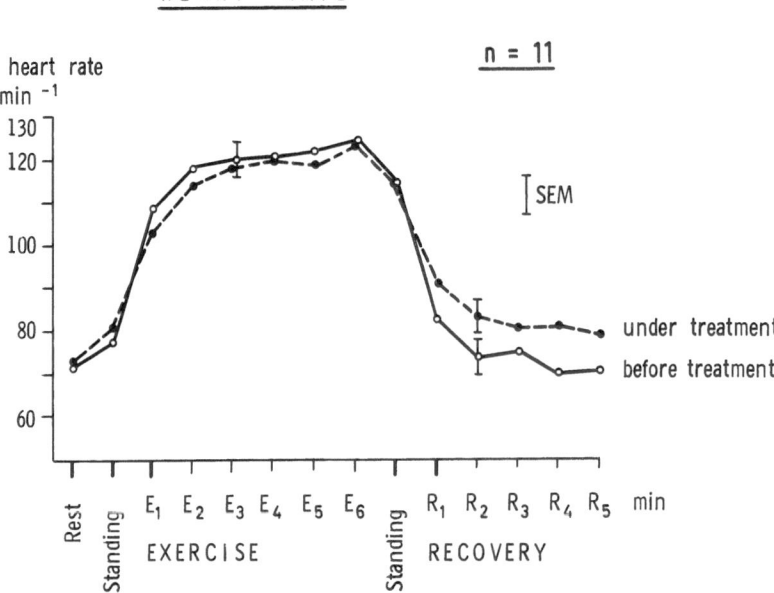

Fig. 5. Heart rate before and during long-term treatment with nifedipine. In the mean, the heart rate was not influenced

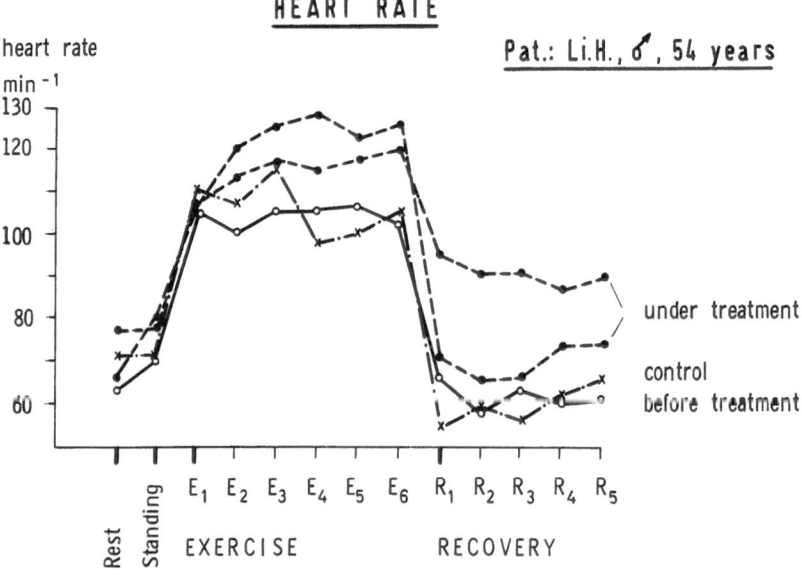

Fig. 6. Heart rate of one patient (No. 4) who showed no improvement of ST-depression under a chronic treatment. This figure shows that the patient had a higher heart rate under exercise after long-term treatment with nifedipine than during the control test. This phenomenon was reproducible and was the reason for the absence of improvement of ST-depression under the drug. Patient No. 6 showed the same effect

ST-SEGMENT DEPRESSION

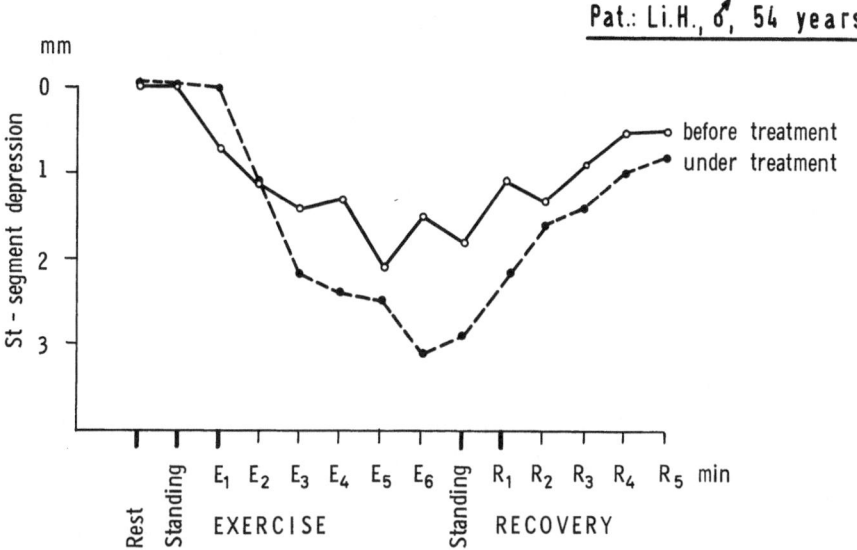

Pat.: Li.H., ♂, 54 years

before treatment
under treatment

Fig. 7. ST-depression before, during and after long-term treatment with nifedipine in a patient with a higher heart rate under drug therapy. The figure shows worse ST-depression under treatment than in the control tests. This was due to the higher heart rate. This phenomenon was an exception and not the rule

Table 2. Results before, during and after long-term treatment with nifedipine. One can see the improvement of ST-depression under the drug therapy except in two patients, who showed a worse effect (Nos. 4 and 6)

No.	Name	Sex	Age	ST-segment depression before treatment	After 6 weeks and 30′ after 20 mg nifedipine	Control— 1 week without treatment
1	St. W.	♂	44	13.1	3.8	15.3
2	Sch. W.	♂	40	25.2	13.7	40.9
3	Pe. H.	♀	59	16.1	9.8	13.3
4	Li. H.	♂	54	11.8	16.4	14.9
5	Kn. J.	♂	61	8.3	0.5	2.6
6	We. J.	♂	61	13.7	30.5	19.3
7	Z. R.	♂	55	29.5	3.3	26.7
8	Ja. W.	♂	52	5.6	0	2.5
9	Sp. D.	♂	59	47	1.0	36.5
10	Ol. W.	♂	50	3.2	0	5.3
11	Lu. A.	♂	63	17.3	11.1	19.5
			Σ	190.8	90.1	196.8
			$\bar{x}$	17.3	8.2	17.9
			SEM	±3.8	±2.9	±3.8

Long-Term Treatment

Thirty-three exercise tests were performed (Table 2). The beneficial effect of a single dose of 20 mg nifedipine remained even after treatment for a period of six weeks. The ST-segment depressions during the control tests before and after treatment were in the same range. The sum of the ST-segment depressions before treatment was 190.7 mm (100%); after six weeks of therapy and an additional dose of 20 mg nifedipine it was 90.1 mm (47.2%) and after one week without the drug, 196.8 mm. The corresponding mean values were 17.3 ± 3.8 SEM, 8.2 ± 2.9 SEM and 17.9 ± 3.8 SEM.

Discussion

The exercise tests reveal the remarkable antianginal effect of nifedipine, as is evident in the reduction of ST-segment depression from 100 to 51.6% after a single dose, and from 100 to 47.2% during chronic treatment over six weeks. The difference between the control test and the drug test after a single dose is highly significant ($2\,p < 0.001$).

The difference between the chronic test and the control test was significant too, but only at the 5% level, because two patients showed a paradox effect.

All patients noticed a release from or an improvement of anginal pain upon effort. In comparison to other antianginal drugs, the effect of nifedipine is similar to that of nitroglycerin, which produced the same improvement of ischemic ST-depression under exercise that we reported previously [1, 3, 4].

During chronic treatment with nifedipine, we have observed no severe side effects, even when the patients evidenced poor contraction of the ventricle (seen in the ventriculogram). The development of collaterals under chronic treatment could not be determined because it would have produced less ischemic ST-depression in the control test after the treatment. However, no tachyphylaxis was noted in the patients investigated.

Abstract

The effect of nifedipine on ischemic ST-segment depressions under exercise is reported in patients with proved coronary heart disease. Eighteen patients received a single dose and performed exercise tests before and after administration of the drug. Three of the patients repeated the tests after administration of a single dose of 10 or 20 mg nifedipine.

The ST-depression was less under nifedipine than in the control tests. The improvement was about 50% in comparison to the control tests. The improvement was similar to that seen after administration of nitroglycerin but less than that under beta-blockers. A beneficial effect of more than 50% could be demonstrated following chronic treatment with nifedipine. The development of collaterals within the six-week period was uncertain because the control tests after treatment showed the same ST-depression as before. Tachyphylaxis or severe side effects were not observed during the six-week period.

References

1. GRAEF, V., BECKER, H.-J., KOBER, G., KALTENBACH, M.: Evaluation of different anti-anginal drugs. In: KALTENBACH, M., LICHTLEN, P. (Eds.): Coronary Heart Disease. Stuttgart: Thieme 1971.
2. KALTENBACH, M.: Zur Beurteilung der Leistungsreserven von Herzkranken mit Hilfe von Arbeitsversuchen. Mannheim: Boehringer 1968.
3. KALTENBACH, M.: Assessment of antianginal substances by means of ST-depression in the exercise EKG. In: HASHIMOTO, K., KIMURA, E., KOBAYASHI, T. (Eds.): New Therapy of Ischemic Heart Disease, p. 126. Tokyo: Univ. Tokyo Press 1975.
4. KALTENBACH, M., BECKER, H.-J., VON KROCKOW, P., ZIMMERMANN, D.: Zur medikamentösen Behandlung der Angina pectoris. Verh. Dtsch. Ges. Inn. Med. München **73**, 591 (1967).

Discussion Remarks

TABATZNIK: Dr. BECKER, could you clarify one point? Did you exercise your patients to maximum capacity or was it the same work load under different conditions?

BECKER: We tested the work load where the ischemia occurred and then we always used the same work load in the following tests. Before entering the study the patients performed two or three exercise tests to determine the work load limits up to an ST-depression.

LYDTIN: Dr. BECKER, did you measure blood pressures during exercise tests and were they different under nifedipine?

BECKER: We did not measure blood pressures because our special exercise test makes it impossible to do so.

SCHÄCKE: Dr. BECKER, I have a question. If I understand your explanation correctly, you add the ST-depression from several ECG leads, and do not consider those with ascending ST-elongation. Can you comment on the order of magnitude of variations in individual values within the comparison groups?

BECKER: The measured values are fully comparable because the patients were stressed equally before and during medication, so that no variation in measured values was found in individual groups—always the same.

Left Ventricular Hemodynamics in Patients at Rest before and after Nifedipine (Adalat)

G. KOBER, H.-J. BECKER, and M. KALTENBACH

Zentrum der Inneren Medizin, Klinikum der Universität, Frankfurt, Fed. Rep. Germany

Angina pectoris is caused by a regional disproportion between blood supply and demand, which is removed by antianginal agents.

Theoretically, a favorable effect can be expected from the improvement of blood flow to the ischemic region and, on the other hand, from a reduction of heart work.

Thus, one can distinguish the different coronary therapeutics with regard to their site of action and the alterations caused in the cardiovascular system. From nitroglycerin, very complex modifications of circulatory parameters are known, which are important for the antianginal action [2]. The aim of this study was to contribute to the clarification of the mechanism of action of nifedipine, a recently developed antianginal drug.

The action of nifedipine on left ventricular hemodynamics at rest was compared with that of nitroglycerin in 16 patients in supine position during diagnostic left heart catheterization. Some of the patients investigated were suffering from valve diseases, the others from coronary heart disease. None of them had signs of congestive heart failure or ischemic chest pain at the beginning or during the drug

Table 1. Average values from pressure curves after 0.8 mg nitroglycerin and 10 mg nifedipine. $N = 16$

	LV enddiast.	LV syst.	Ao syst.	Ao diast.	Ao $\bar{p}$	dp/dt max	dp/dt max[a] p	Heart rate[a] min
Control	13	127	124	76	99	1578	87	79
2 min after nitroglycerin	12	119	117	77	97	1565	107	73
5 min after nitroglycerin	9	114	113	76	92	1567	103	81
10 min after nitroglycerin	9	116	116	78	93	1669	108	78
Control	16	129	131	81	99	1679	90	80
2 min after nifedipine	17	126	126	80	99	1449	77	77
5 min after nifedipine	16	125	124	81	100	1572	88	77
10 min after nifedipine	15	121	120	77	97	1648	99	80
15 min after nifedipine	13	121	118	75	95	1632	101	80

[a] $n = 10$.

examination. Both medications were given sublingually: nitroglycerin, 0.8 mg and nifedipine, 10 mg.

Left ventricular and aortic pressure and left ventricular maximal dp/dt were measured over a period of 10 min after the administration of nitroglycerin and one hour later for 15 min after nifedipine. Heart rate was obtained from the ECG. In addition, a quotient was obtained from dp/dt max and the simultaneously developed left ventricular pressure to minimize the effect of the variant initial values. For technical reasons, it was not possible to measure $dp/dt:P$ with the help of an electronic device.

In each patient, nitroglycerin was given first and nifedipine, second. The diagnostic left heart catheterization was performed in the time between administration of the two substances. This examination caused the different control values that were observed before the administration of nitroglycerin and nifedipine. Randomization was not possible because of the relatively long-lasting effect of nifedipine.

Results

Table 1 shows the mean values of the measured data 2, 5, 10 min and, in the case of nifedipine also 15 min, after the application of the drug. A statistically significant alteration of heart rate did not occur. Both drugs caused a decrease of systolic and diastolic left ventricular pressure and of systolic and mean aortic pressure. Max dp/dt increased slightly after nitroglycerin and remained unchanged or decreased slightly after nifedipine. The quotient dp/dt max:P increased with both agents.

Figure 1 is a diagram of the behavior of the measured parameters. It is evident that the effect of nifedipine begins later and continues longer than that of nitroglycerin. Considering the higher enddiastolic left ventricular pressure before the administration of nifedipine in relation to the initial value before nitroglycerin, the effect of nifedipine on lowering these values is less obvious. The enddiastolic pressure, possibly elevated as a result of the angiographic procedures, was reduced due to nifedipine only to the initial values measured at the beginning of the catheterization, before the administration of any of the drugs.

Discussion

As with nitroglycerin, the effectiveness of nifedipine in angina pectoris could be demonstrated by means of exercise tests [5]. While the beneficial effect on ST-segment depression during exertion is one of the most reliable criteria for the antianginal activity of a drug, the ECG did not allow any conclusions with regard to the mode of action. The changes of left ventricular hemodynamics showed that the action of nifedipine on circulation can to some extent be compared with that of nitroglycerin. The antianginal action of nifedipine must be at least partially based on a reduction of heart work caused by a decrease of peripheral resistance, lowering of blood pressure and of left ventricular enddiastolic pressure and a

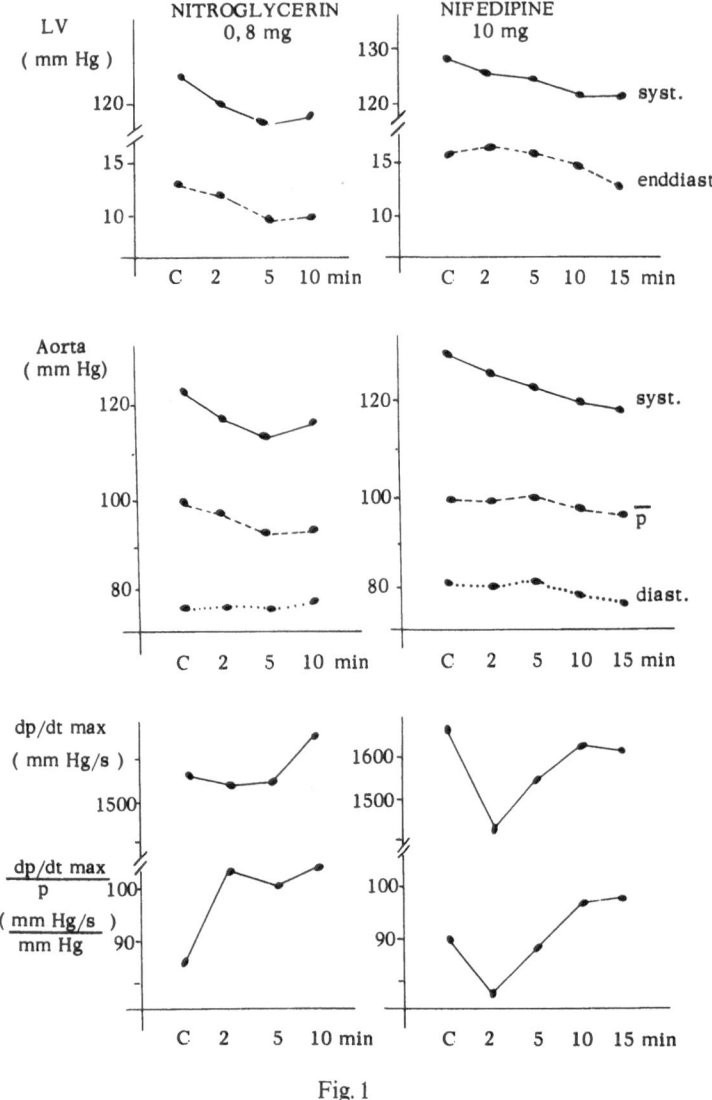

Fig. 1

reduction of left ventricular wall tension. The decrease of left ventricular filling pressure may be of importance for the perfusion of the inner layers of the left ventricular wall due to an increase of transmural coronary vascular pressure [7].

The measurements of left ventricular contractility showed no clear signs of a negative inotropic effect of nifedipine in patients without signs of left ventricular failure and with normal left ventricular contractility at rest. The different findings in other investigations and in experiments on isolated papillary muscles [1] can possibly be explained by the different doses administered. The increase of total coronary blood flow in animals and patients observed by some investigators [3, 8] is probably of no importance for the therapeutic mechanism because of the metabolically maximum dilatation of the vessels in the ischemic region [6] and the failing antianginal effect of pure coronary dilating drugs [6]. The ischemic region would not benefit from this increase in total coronary blood flow, which would only lead to an increase of blood flow to non-ischemic areas and thus to a superfluous additional perfusion of these regions.

Abstract

Exercise tests in patients with coronary heart disease showed a favorable effect of nifedipine on the exercise tolerance, exertional angina pectoris and the ST-segment depression in the ECG. It was the aim of the following examinations to define the action of nifedipine on the hemodynamics in humans in relation to nitroglycerin, which is, to date, the most common drug in the therapy of acute anginal attack. Nitroglycerin 0.8 mg and nifedipine 10 mg were given sublingually in 16 patients during diagnostic left heart catheterizations. Left ventricular and aortic pressures and left ventricular contractility were measured continuously for 10 min after nitroglycerin and 15 min after the administration of nifedipine. After both medications a similar decrease of systolic and diastolic pressures in the aorta and the left ventricle was observed. Simultaneously an increase of left ventricular contractility occurred. It is concluded, that the hemodynamic action of nifedipine is like that of nitroglycerin and that the antianginal activity is based on this "nitroglycerin-like" mechanism. The increase of myocardial blood flow after the administration of nifedipine, observed by some investigators, is probably a therapeutic mechanism of less importance because of the failing anti-anginal effect of pure coronary dilating drugs. It is not clear how much of the increase of left ventricular contractility is caused by reflex and other mechanisms, but as in nitroglycerin this effect should be of no therapeutic importance.

References

1. FLECKENSTEIN, A., TRITTHART, H., DÖRING, H. J., BYON, K. J.: Arzneim.-Forsch. (Drug Res.) **22**, 22 (1972).
2. KALTENBACH, M., LICHTLEN, P., FRIESINGER, G. C.: Coronary Heart Disease, 2nd International Symposium at Frankfurt 1972. Stuttgart: Thieme 1973.
3. KOCHSIEK, K., NEUBAUR, J.: Arzneim.-Forsch. (Drug Res.) **22**, 353 (1972).
4. LEE, R. J., BAKY, S. H.: J. Pharmacol. Exp. Ther. **184**, 205 (1973).
5. LOOS, A., KALTENBACH, M.: Arzneim.-Forsch. (Drug Res.) **22**, 358 (1972).
6. PITT, B., CRAVEN, P.: Cardiovasc. Res. **4**, 176 (1970).
7. SALISBURY, P. F., CROSS, C. E., RIEBEN, P. A.: Amer. Heart J. **66**, 650 (1963).
8. VATER, W., KRONEBERG, G., HOFFMEISTER, F., KALLER, H., MENG, K., PULS, W., OBERDORF, A., SCHLOSSMANN, K., STOEPEL, K.: Arzneim.-Forsch. (Drug Res.) **22**, 1 (1972).

Discussion Remarks

v. D. BRAND: I would like to ask Dr. KOBER why he states that the effect of Adalat and nitroglycerin are similar because the only thing I can see is that the heart rate goes up, and, in his experiment, the left ventricular end-diastolic pressure goes down. The effect of nitroglycerin at least is due to a reduction in left ventricle end-diastolic pressure and end-diastolic volumes with a lower wall stress and a lower oxygen consumption.

KOBER: We did not measure end-diastolic volume of the left ventricle in patients under Adalat. But we were able to show that in both drugs there is a parallel decrease in peripheral resistance and a fall in arterial and in left ventricular end-diastolic pressure. We have not compared other parameters and deduce an effect of Adalat similar to nitroglycerin with respect to hemodynamic data only.

FLECKENSTEIN: With regard to several clinical papers one remark seems to be necessary: The beneficial influences of Adalat in patients with coronary disease may be different in patients with or without digitalis and the influence of Adalat on the hemodynamic parameters may also change due to such differences in the pretreatment of the patients. In other words, digitalized and nondigitalized patients should not be placed in the same test group.

BECKER: No patients on digitalis are included in this study.

LOCHNER: Dr. KOBER, the decrease of left ventricular end-diastolic pressure is an important point. Did you see this when the heart rate stayed more or less constant or did you see this only when the heart rate was increased at the same time?

KOBER: In our experiments the heart rate remained on the same level and the end-diastolic pressure went down slightly.

Adalat and Beta Blockers; the Mechanism Studied with Two Series of Work Tests in Two Groups of Patients with Angina Pectoris

L.-G. EKELUND and J.-H. ATTERHÖG

Department of Clinical Physiology, Karolinska Sjukhuset, Stockholm, Sweden

Two groups consisting respectively of ten male patients, mean age 57 years (Table 1), and 13 patients (10 men and 3 women), mean age 56 years (Table 2), with a stable angina pectoris performed standardized exercise tests after double-blind randomized administration of 10 mg Adalat and 50 mg metoprolol, respectively. Metoprolol is a selective β_1-blocking drug without intrinsic effect.

The two groups were similar, but the ten patients in the group receiving Adalat had higher exercise tolerance. There was no difference in respect to earlier infarctions, treatment with digitalis, heart volume and so on.

We shall now describe the reactions of the two groups following the exercise tests in terms of some of the variables looked at in this study. First, we shall consider two major determinants of left ventricular oxygen consumption (Table 3), heart rate and blood pressure. In subjects at rest, Adalat caused a 13% increase in heart rate and a slight, 10% decrease in systolic blood pressure (Fig. 1). The increase in heart rate is definitely secondary to the decrease in blood pressure. Metoprolol caused a similar decrease in systolic blood pressure of 12%, but the heart rate decreased 23%, as could be expected.

In standing subjects, Adalat caused an increase in heart rate of 10% and a decrease of 13% in systolic blood pressure that did not differ from the orthostatic

Table 1. Some clinical data for the Adalat group

Patient	Age years	Duration of ang. pect. years	Previous myocardial infarction	Blood press. syst/diast mm Hg	Digitalis
1	60	5	+	100/60	+
2	60	3	+	150/90	−
3	64	3	+	150/60	−
4	56	2	+	140/70	+
5	65	7	−	150/90	−
6	69	4	+	150/90	−
7	44	1	−	150/100	−
8	51	4	+	125/90	−
9	59	2	−	170/100	−
10	45	2	+	145/90	−

Table 2. Some clinical data for the Metoprolol group

Patient	Age years	Duration of ang. pect. years	Previous myocardial infarction	Blood press. syst/diast mm Hg	Digitalis	Heart volume ml/m²
1	54	1	+	120/65	+	580
2	60	3	+	150/80	−	330
3	66	11	+	125/80	+	450
4	61	11	+	130/75	−	400
5	64	7	+	130/75	−	420
6	59	4	+	120/85	−	440
7	60	8	+	90/65	+	440
8	56	12	−	125/80	−	480
9	63	14	+	135/80	−	460
10	56	0.5	−	100/55	−	460
11	59	10	+	110/65	−	380
12	63	10	−	140/80	−	460
13	51	2	−	110/70	−	missing

Table 3. The main determinants of myocardial oxygen consumption

Major
Factors affecting systolic wall stress
    Systolic intraventricular pressure
    Ventricular size, configuration, and thickness
Factors determining fraction of time systolic wall stress is exerted
    Heart rate
    Ejection time
Inotropic state of myocardium, influence of catecholamines
Minor
    External contractile element work and extent of fiber shortening, stroke volume
    Activation energy for depolarization and electromechanical coupling.

reaction after placebo. The corresponding changes after metoprolol were −26% for heart rate and −6% for systolic blood pressure (Fig. 1).

During exercise at comparable loads for each individual, Adalat—as at rest—increased heart rate by 8% and decreased systolic blood pressure by 7% (Fig. 2). The rate-pressure product was thus unchanged. Metoprolol, on the other hand, decreased heart rate by 22% and systolic blood pressure by 14%, causing a decrease in the rate-pressure product of 31% (Fig. 2).

Both drugs increased exercise tolerance significantly, Adalat by 51% expressed as total work and by 25% expressed as the highest work load sustained for 6 min (W_b). The corresponding increases for metoprolol were 25% and 9% (Fig. 3).

At the end of exercise, heart rate was 13% higher after Adalat with an unchanged systolic blood pressure, so that the rate-pressure product was increased by 11%. Metoprolol caused a decrease in final heart rate of 24% and a decrease in blood pressure of 13%. The rate-pressure product accordingly was decreased by 33% (Fig. 4).

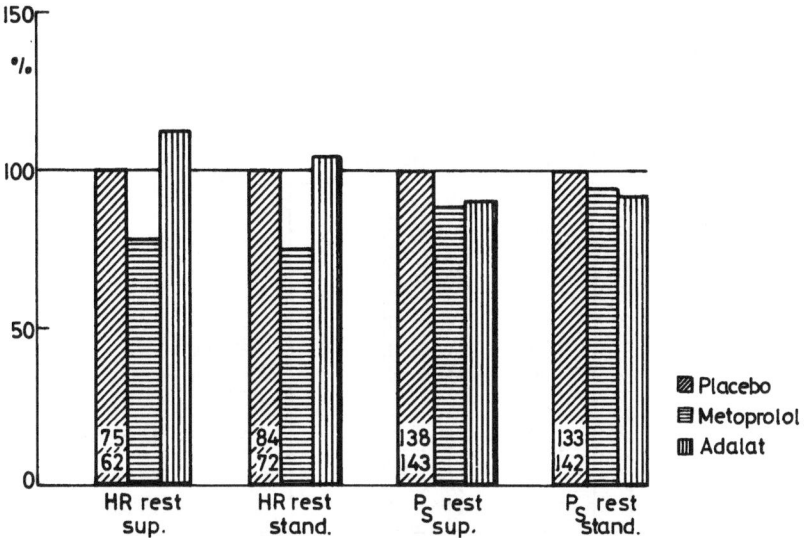

Fig. 1. Heart rate (HR) at rest, supine and standing, brachial artery pressure *(P_S)* at rest, supine and standing. Values expressed as % of placebo-values (absolute values inside the bars)

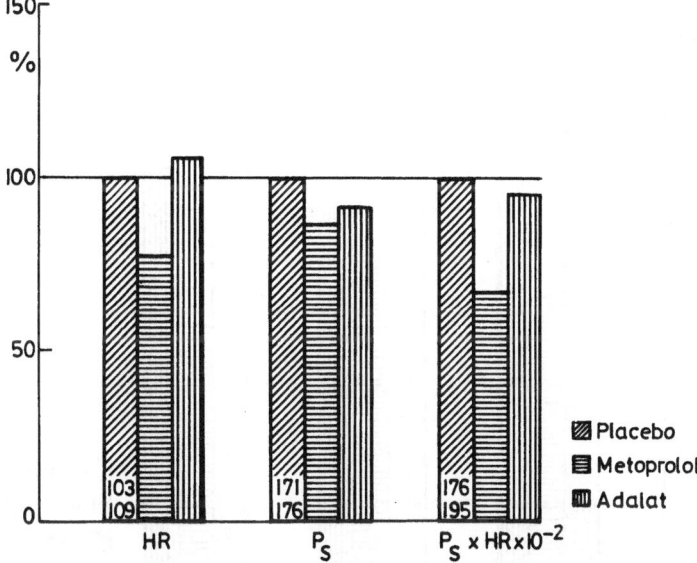

Fig. 2. Heart rate (HR), brachial artery pressure *(P_S)* and rate-pressure product $(P_S \times HR \times 10^{-2})$ at comparable individual loads (absolute values inside the bars)

The decrease in rate-pressure product at the end of exercise after metoprolol administration is in line with the values of 20–30% reported in studies with other beta blockers. The decrease is clearly explained by the slight increase in heart volume and by an increase in filling pressures observed after administration of beta blockers.

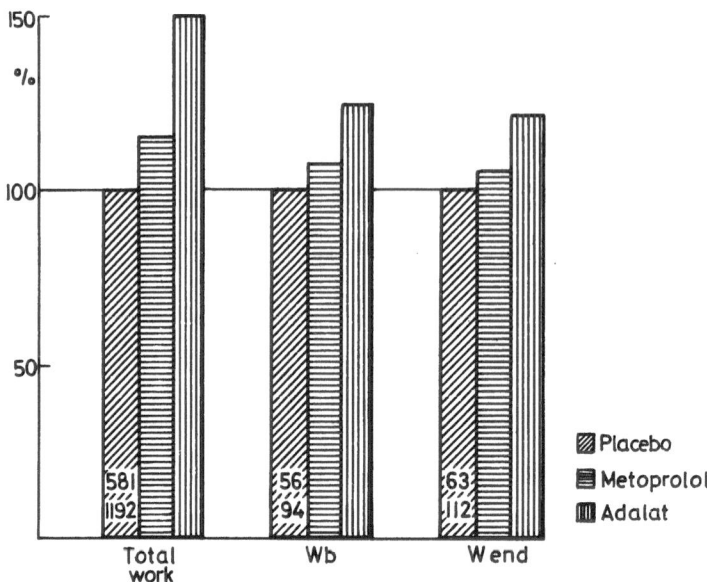

Fig. 3. Total work at end, watt min, W_b (watt) and work load at end of exercise (absolute values inside the bars)

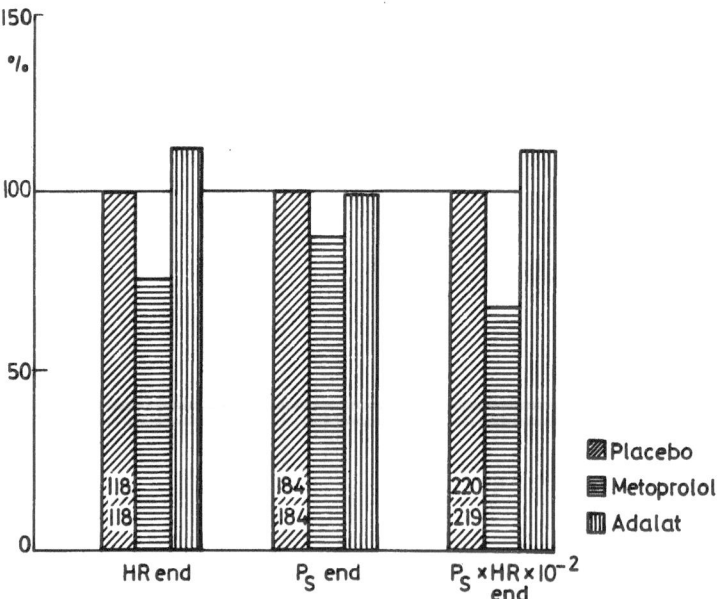

Fig. 4. Heart rate, brachial artery pressure and rate-pressure product at end of exercise

The changes in the variables after Adalat are of much the same type as those reported after nitroglycerin, but the doses used here do not seem to have any significant effect on the capacity vessels. The marked increase in exercise tolerance, despite only a slight increase in rate-pressure product at the end of exercise, may indicate a better regional utilization of the available coronary flow and perhaps a decrease in heart volume.

In neither the Adalat nor the metoprolol patients were there any changes in atrio-ventricular conduction time measured at rest.

A very interesting observation is that in four of the Adalat patients [1, 3, 5, 8], a beta blocker, alprenolol, had been tested repeatedly with a standardized exercise test without any positive effect. After Adalat, three of them [1, 3, 5] increased their exercise tolerance by an average of 95% expressed as total work and by 45% expressed as W_b.

A combination of a beta blocker and Adalat could be of value, because a synergistic action has been reported for both beta blockers and nitroglycerin. A beta blocker could counteract the increase in heart rate observed after administration of Adalat. In that case, however, one would have to consider the negative inotropic effects of both drugs.

Abstract

Two groups of patients with typical angina pectoris have been studied with stepwise increasing exercise tests in a standardized manner. One group of ten patients was studied after double-blind administration of placebo and Adalat (10 mg). The other group of thirteen patients was studied after double-blind administration of metoprolol (50 mg), a new selective beta-blocker, without any intrinsic effect. Both drugs gave a significant increase in the exercise tolerance. The two drugs gave, however, different reactions in heart rate and systolic blood pressure both at rest and during exercise and the two drugs will be compared with respect to the different actions on the measured variables. Three patients who did not respond to a beta-blocker, but did respond to Adalat, will be discussed separately.

Adalat (Nifedipine) under Loading Conditions

G. MCILWRAITH

King's College Hospital, London, Great Britain

Introduction

Exercise tests are frequently used in order to assess antianginal drugs. The basic assumption is, that as angina is precipitated by exertion, any medication which significantly increases exercise tolerance should be of value in the treatment and prevention of angina. The method used has been to exercise a patient under constant conditions from rest until angina is induced. The work loads and the time to induce angina when on placebo are compared with those when on the drug under test.

At King's College Hospital in London we decided to carry out an acute study exercising a small number of patients with angina. Our intention was to establish that nifedipine was more effective than placebo in increasing exercise tolerance before proceeding to a chronic double-blind trial on a larger number of patients. More than that, we wished to be able to quantify any difference in effect between drug and placebo. A survey of the literature on exercise testing and, in particular, of the cardiovascular response to loading strongly suggested that this second aim could only be achieved by single-stage tests in which the work load from rest to the onset of angina is unaltered and the same for both drug and placebo. It had been our previous experience, however, that when single-stage tests were used, untrained patients showed considerable fluctuations in time to angina. Yet with repeated exercising of the same patients, highly reproducible results could be obtained. We therefore devised and carried out our study in the following way.

Method

The exercise apparatus used was a motor-driven treadmill. It was adjustable for speed and slope and controlled by a console. It had an emergency stop button for the patient and a safety harness.

Each patient was seen for five consecutive mornings or afternoons. On each day they were exercised to the onset of angina. This was carried out four to seven times each day with rest periods of not less than 20 min in between. Their electrocardiographs were carefully monitored throughout by radiotelemetry. The first three days were spent in training and finding the most suitable speed and slope which, from rest, would repeatedly induce angina after 60–100 sec. On day 4 each patient was given a placebo capsule after the first exercise but he was told that it could be either nifedipine or placebo and that the selection was double-blind. He was asked to break the capsule with the teeth and keep the fluid contents in the mouth as long as possible so as to aid buccal absorption. Exercising was then repeated as on previous days up to another six times at the same speed and at the same slope. The times to the onset of angina were recorded. Day 5 was the same as day 4 except that half the patients had placebo capsules and the other half had nifedipine. This selection was genuinely double-blind.

Patients

Eighteen patients were tested of whom 14 were male. The age range was from 43 to 71 years. The duration of anginal symptoms was from 5 months to 8 years and all had ischemic ECG's at rest or on exercise. No traces showed left bundle branch block or left ventricular hypertrophy including those of two patients who were hypertensive. No patient had aortic valve disease and none had ever been in failure. During the test week the only cardiac treatment was trinitrin and they were not allowed to smoke.

Results

Four patients did not complete the study. One of them went into ventricular fibrillation during his third exercise on the first day and was immediately cardioverted. Three others improved so much with training that angina could not regularly be induced even with maximal exercising. The 14 who completed the study are divided equally into two groups depending on whether their second capsule was placebo or nifedipine.

After the first exercise, group A patients received placebo capsules on day 4 and nifedipine on day 5, whereas the group B patients received placebo both days. The results of a typical group A patient on placebo show that the times to the onset of angina all fall within narrow limits and the longest time after the capsule is only eight seconds longer than the base time (Table 1). On the fifth day the base time falls within the previous day's range, but all subsequent times are far longer

Table 1. Group A patient		
	Day 4	Day 5
1	105 seconds Capsule	112 seconds Capsule
2	110	185
3	113	190
4	111	190
5	100	170
6		165
7		175

Table 2. Group B patient		
	Day 4	Day 5
1	80 seconds Capsule	88 seconds Capsule
2	80	88
3	84	70
4	72	95

Table 3. Mean values of log (maximum time ÷ base time)

	A			B		
	Day 4	Day 5		Day 4	Day 5	
Mean	0.094 (1.24)	0.214 (1.64)	Difference 0.120	0.059 (1.15)	0.075 (1.19)	Difference 0.016

Bracketed values are antilogarithms of mean.
Difference of differences = 0.104.
Standard error is ± 0.039, t-value 2.68, 12° freedom, 5% value of t is 2.18.

and some are almost doubled. In contrast, the group B patient shows little fluctuation on either day although times on day 5 are slightly more than on day 4 (Table 2). The results were calculated as follows: For each patient, for both day 4 and day 5, we calculated the percentage improvement of the best time after the capsule over the precapsule times. We then compared the percentage improvements of day 4 and 5 and compared the means of both groups. Table 3 shows the mean percentage improvement after capsule in group A patients to be 24% on day 4 (placebo) and 64% on day 5 (nifedipine). In group B patients, the percentage improvements were 15% and 19% on days 4 and 5 respectively with the patients having placebo both days. The differences between these groups were statistically significant. The 5% value of t was 2.18.

Abstract

Fourteen patients completed a double-blind exercise study in which nifedipine was found to cause a significantly greater improvement on exercise tolerance than placebo.

Discussion Remarks

TABATZNIK: Dr. MCILWRAITH, how long is the action of nifedipine in your studies?

MCILWRAITH: We wanted to see the length of action of nifedipine when taken orally and chewed, in other words, whether there was some buccal absorption as well as gastrointestinal absorption. In practice, however, we gave this up because we found that after patients had been doing repeated exercises for—in some cases—as long as 3–4 hrs, they had had enough, and did not want to go on. There is also the point, of course, that perhaps we entered into different physiologic periods. We started them at 9 a.m. and by noon or 2 p.m. other factors might influence exercise tolerance.

TABATZNIK: So you really have no direct answer to that at present. Could you give me some idea of the average slope of the treadmill and the speed of the treadmill inasmuch as you got your patients up to angina within 1–2 min. I imagine they were working hard at that point.

McIlwraith: The first three days were used as practice days. I would select, depending on age, sex, height, and personal evaluation, a slope of between 8 and 12 degrees. Most older females would take 8 degrees; a relatively healthy young man would take 12 degrees. I would start off at 2 km/hour with a stepwise test to find the speed that would induce angina. Thereafter I would test the patient at that speed right from the beginning. Patients would start off at 2 km/hour and if angina had not been induced by 3 min, we would go to 4, and, if necessary, 6 km/hour. If they got angina at 6 km/hour after 3 min or thereabouts, the next test would be at 6 km/hour from the start.

Results of a Comparative Study with Adalat: Phonomechano-Cardiograms in Normal Persons and Patients with Coronary Heart Disease

R. J. ESPER, R. A. MACHADO, R. A. NORDABY, and H. J. BIDOGGIA

Service of Cardiology, Military Central Hospital, Buenos Aires, Argentina

The duration of the phases of the left ventricular systole depends intrinsically on the condition of the myocardium and its contractile synergy as varied by means of the preload, afterload and heart rate (HR) (Fig. 1) [5, 7–9, 11, 15, 18, 21, 23, 26–29, 32, 43, 53, 55, 61, 66, 72, 73, 75–80, 82, 83, 85, 86].

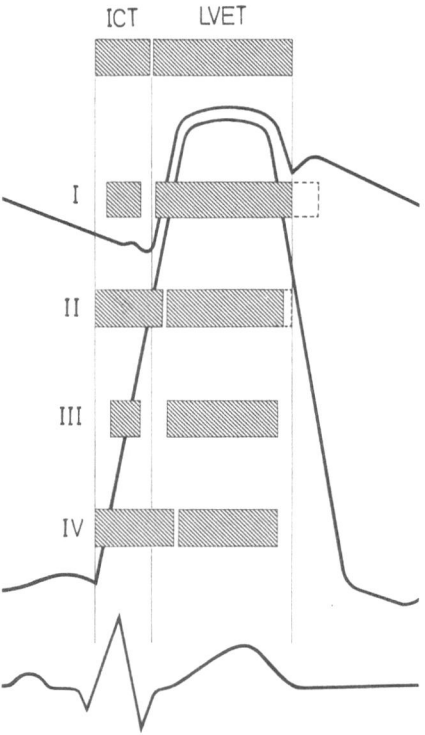

Fig. 1. Modifications in the duration of the isovolumic contraction time (ICT) and left ventricular ejection time (LVET) with the independent increments of preload (I), afterload (II), heart rate under the action of inotropic drugs (III) and heart rate with a diminished contractility of the left ventricle (IV)

Coronary artery disease decreases the efficiency of the heart as a muscle and/or as a "pump". Sometimes, however, in the early stages of the disease, these alterations are not sufficiently evident to be detected in basal conditions [1, 13, 14, 25, 31, 37, 42, 54, 58–60, 71, 74].

Isometric exercise provides an effective and sustained increment of the afterload which, by creating a state of stress in the heart, may demonstrate in many cases these deficiencies [2, 24, 30, 41, 45, 47, 49, 50–52, 56].

A drug that is considered to be a vasodilator of the coronary arteries, which simultaneously improves oxygen uptake by the tissues, is thought to normalize a pathological response, even in basal conditions or during overload [34–36, 44, 46, 63].

These facts induced us to study the duration of the phases of the left ventricular systole at rest and during the performance of an isometric exercise (handgrip test), in a group of coronary patients, before medication and after administration of nifedipine (BAY a 1040, Adalat), by evaluating its supposed beneficial action in the coronary circulation.

As a control, a similar study was performed in normal subjects, with the purpose of setting aside erroneous interpretations made from secondary effects.

Materials and Methods

The normal group was composed of 10 males, aged from 20–30 years, without demonstrable pathology, as determined clinically, radiologically and electrocardiographically. The group with coronary artery disease consisted of 20 patients, 18 male and 2 female, ranging in age from 41 to 58. They were not overweight and diabetes was excluded in every case. Except for one case with hypertension and rest values of 190/110, the others were within normal values and suffered no other illness that could have any cardiovascular involvement. No one presented left bundle branch block. The coronary disease was diagnosed clinically, radiologically, electrocardiographically and hemodynamically. In all cases, coronariography and ventriculography were performed.

They did not receive any type of drug therapy, including digitalis [33, 63, 64, 81]. Sedatives were suspended 48 h before the study, and smoking, coffee or tea were suspended 12 h prior to the test.

Each patient performed isometric exercises twice: after administration of a placebo and after administration of 20 mg of nifedipine. Four groups were established:

N.—Normal patients after the administration of placebo
Nn.—Normal patients after the administration of nifedipine
C.—Coronary patients after the administration of placebo
Cn.—Coronary patients after the administration of nifedipine
The same methodology was used in all cases.

For the isometric exercise, the conventional dynamometers offered no comfort and the rubber balloons opposed uneven resistance, depending upon which segment was grasped [76]. For that reason, an original dynamometer was used,

designed by one of the authors (H.B.), adapting a comfortable handle to a spring
scale with lineal response (Fig. 2).

We based our calculations on figures that represent 50% of the total effort,
because smaller loads (25%) did not evoke changes in the heart rate (HR) and
arterial pressure (AP) large enough to be considered statistically. On the other
hand, greater loads produced exhaustion. The test lasted 3 min, because the
changes of HR and AP evoked during this period were statistically significant,
even between the 2nd and 3rd minutes. It was not prolonged because most of the
patients could not tolerate longer times.

The tests were performed after 10 h of fasting and always between 8:00 and
8:30 a.m. [81] in a half darkened environment and after a restperiod of at least
30 min. The patients were instructed several days before, in order to become
familiarized with the method.

Lying in a supine position, having previously been connected to a polygraph,
the subject took 2 capsules containing the placebo, which he broke with his teeth
and absorbed sublingually. Twenty minutes later, with normal breathing, a basal
register was obtained. Then the maximum strength the patient could develop with
one hand was measured in three consecutive tries, choosing the one that did not
correspond with the electrocardiographic lead used. After a 5-minute restperiod,
he was told to maintain for 3 min an effort equal to 50% of the average of the

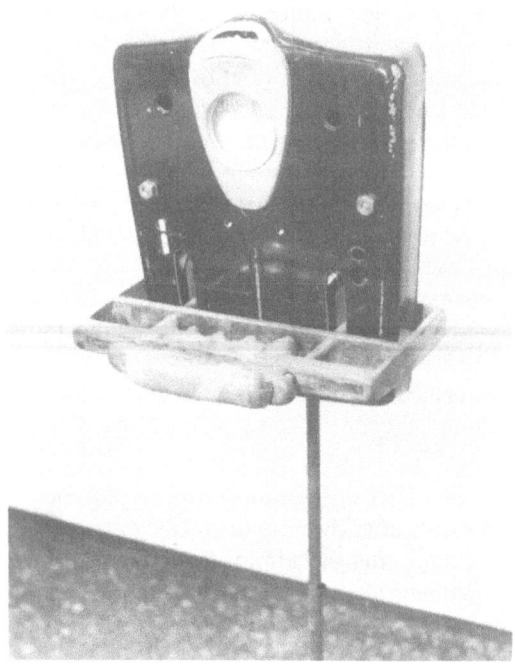

Fig. 2. Original dynamometer designed for the performance of the isometric exercise (handgrip test)

three previous loads. The patient controlled his own effort by looking directly at the scale.

The data were recorded at the first, second and third minutes from the beginning of the test. Caution was taken to maintain normal breathing during the recording in order to avoid the test of Valsalva. The systolic and diastolic arterial pressures were taken simultaneously with a mercury manometer by the usual technique, during the restperiod and while the reactions were being recorded. The HR was obtained from electrocardiographic records.

At the end of the experiment, and after a restperiod of 5–10 min, 20 mg of nifedipine in 2 capsules were administered in the same way as the placebo. Twenty minutes later, the experiment was repeated in the same form.

The data were obtained with an Electronics for Medicine DR 8 machine, with 8 channels, at a speed of 100 mm/s.

The earliest electrocardiographic lead which would allow easier detection of the beginning of the QRS was taken (real beginning of the QRS) [12].

There were 2 beams recorder of phonocardiograms with cut frequencies between 120 and 500 Hz., situated in the apex and mesocardio areas. The carotidogram was always taken on the right carotid, with the head slightly extended. A funnel, 2.3 cm in diameter and 0.5 cm deep, was firmly inserted; it was connected by a 10 cm long rigid (polyethylene) pipe, with an internal diameter of 0.3 cm, to a transducer of variable inductance, model Statham P.M.5. A 3-way switch was interposed in the pipe [19, 38, 39].

The carotidogram was considered to be satisfactory when it fulfilled the following requirements [15, 18]:

a) An upstroke and carotid notch easily recognizable and sufficiently clear for a correct measuring;

b) Diastolic fall sustained and constant, not allowing more than one slight presystolic rebound, caused by the proximity of an energetic venous pulse;

c) Carotid notch always situated at a higher level than that of 50% of the greatest height of the pulse wave.

This type of wave always proved to be the one with less differentiation and to be the most suitable, when compared to intravascular tracings [3, 4, 6, 15, 18, 20, 76].

In each determination a minimum of 10 beats were recorded, so that the measurements were always made from more than 5 beats, at least.

The parameters were evaluated according to the following considerations [5, 15, 18, 74, 76, 85].

Electromechanical Systole (ES)

The ES extends from the actual beginning of the QRS until the first important oscillation of the aortic component of the second sound (A 2) [44]. It includes the electropressure delay (from the arrival of the electrical stimulus until the elevation of the intraventricular pressure), the isovolumic contraction time and the left ventricular ejection time. Included also is the beginning of the ventricular diastole

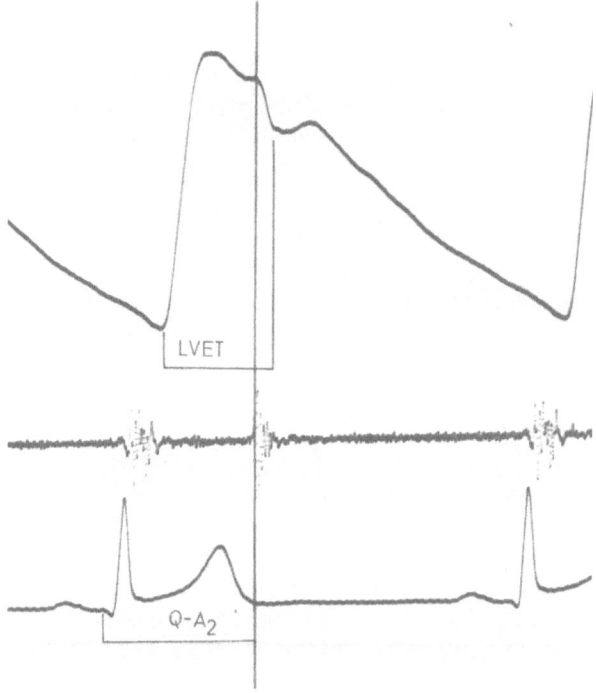

Fig. 3. Methodology for the measurement of the systolic time intervals of the left ventricle.
Electromechanical systole (Q-A$_2$); ejection time (LVET)

until the closure of the aortic valves; this latter interval is impossible to measure
at the present time (Fig. 3) [10, 48, 59, 62, 85].

Left Ventricular Ejection Time (LVET)

It extends from the upstroke until the notching of the carotidogram. It reflects
the real ejection period of the left ventricle [16, 32, 53, 57, 59, 61, 65, 68, 82, 83, 85].
The pre-ejection period was determined from the difference of the following:
Pre-Ejection Period (PEP)
PEP = ES-LVET.
It represents the time of the electropressure delay plus the isovolumic contrac-
tion time [17, 40, 57, 65, 68, 69, 84].

PEP/LVET Ratio

Because it is not influenced by the HR, this index, according to WEISSLER [85]
reflects with more accuracy small, isolated deviations of each one of the components.
One of the authors obtained and measured the records, another the arterial
pressure and a third, the statistic calculations. The fourth analyzed and evaluated
the results and elaborated the conclusions.

Statistical Methodology

Determination of the statistical significance of the different values found in the present study was done by means of student "t" test.

To determine intergroup differences between normal subjects and coronary patients, this test was applied to the difference of the average. Intragroup changes were evaluated by applying the student "t" test to the difference obtained from each pair of individual values. The differences were considered significative whenever $p < 0.05$.

Snedecor was mainly followed for comparing the different functions of regression between themselves [67, 70].

A Hewlett-Packard computer, model 9810-A, with statistical block, was used.

Results

As stated in Materials and Methods, the results obtained were grouped as follows:

N.—Normal subjects after the administration of placebo
Nn.—Normal subjects after the administration of nifedipine
C.—Coronary patients after the administration of placebo
Cn.—Coronary patients after the administration of nifedipine
The following parameters were considered and compared as follows:

1. Heart rate (HR)
2. Systolic arterial pressure (sAP)
3. Diastolic arterial pressure (dAP)
4. Left ventricular ejection time (LVET)
5. Pre-ejection period (PEP)
6. Electromechanic systole (ES)
7. PEP/LVET ratio.

1. Heart Rate (HR)

The mean values and deviations for the HR in the four groups are given in Table 1.

In all groups a significative increment of HR was found between rest and the 3rd minute of exercise (Table 1).

During rest, the HR was higher with nifedipine, as much so in normal subjects ($p < 0.005$) as in coronaries ($p < 0.001$). Nevertheless the increment of the HR between rest and the 3rd minute of exercise was similar before and after administration of nifedipine, to the same degree in normal subjects ($p > 0.40$) as in the coronaries ($p > 0.60$).

If we compare groups N and C in another way, we see that the respective values of the HR are alike, during rest and in each minute of exercise (Table 2). The same is true for the Nn and Cn groups.

Table 1. Heart in beats/min

Group N	Rest	1 min	2 min	3 min
Mean	80.8	93.5	96.6	98.7
s.d.[a]	11.3	15.4	17.9	14.0
s.e.[b]	3.6	4.9	5.7	4.4
		80.8→98.7	$(p<0.001)$	
Group Nn				
Mean	97.0	106.3	112.3	119.2
s.d.	14.1	11.5	11.7	11.8
s.e.	4.5	3.6	3.7	3.7
		97.0→119.2	$(p<0.0005)$	
Group C				
Mean	79.2	91.6	96.8	100.4
s.d.	14.0	18.1	18.6	21.1
s.e.	3.1	4.1	4.2	4.7
		79.2→100.4	$(p<0.001)$	
Group Cn				
Mean	95.4	106.9	112.5	115.3
s.d.	22.0	26.0	27.4	26.2
s.e.	4.9	5.8	6.1	5.9
		95.4→115.3	$(p<0.001)$	

[a] s.d. Standard deviation.
[b] s.e. Standard error of the mean.

Table 2. Comparison of the HR in the N and C groups and in the Nn and Cn groups

HR	Rest	1 min	2 min	3 min
Group N	80.8	93.5	96.6	98.7
Group C	79.2	91.6	96.8	100.4
p	$p>0.70$	$p>0.70$	$p>0.975$	$p>0.80$
Group Nn	97.0	106.3	112.3	119.2
Group Cn	95.4	106.9	112.5	115.3
p	$p>0.80$	$p>0.90$	$p>0.98$	$p>0.60$

From the foregoing, we concluded that at least two independent factors exist, which are able to produce tachycardia. On the one hand, the handgrip test causes a significant increment of HR, independently of the administration of nifedipine. On the other hand, the drug, which increases the HR during the rest period in both normal subjects and in coronary patients, does not affect the increment of the HR during exercise.

2. Systolic Arterial Pressure (sAP)

The data obtained are presented in Table 3.

Table 3. sAP in mm Hg

Group N	Rest	1 min.	2 min	3 min
Mean	121.0	128.5	132.0	133.5
s.d.	11.0	12.9	11.6	12.7
s.e.	3.5	4.1	3.7	4.0
	121.0→133.5	$(p<0.001)$		
Group Nn				
Mean	115.0	122.5	127.0	132.5
s.d.	14.3	13.8	16.4	19.8
s.e.	4.5	4.4	5.2	6.3
	115.0→132.5	$(p<0.01)$		
Group C				
Mean	133.7	148.7	154.2	161.1
s.d.	17.9	23.1	24.8	22.5
s.e.	4.1	5.3	5.7	5.2
	133.7→161.1	$(p<0.001)$		
Group Cn				
Mean	120.5	131.6	138.2	141.8
s.d.	19.8	29.8	30.8	32.2
s.e.	4.5	6.8	7.1	7.4
	120.5→141.8	$(p<0.001)$		

In the four groups, a significant increment ($p<0.001$, groups N, C and Cn; $p<0.01$, groups Nn) of sAP was found between rest and the 3rd minute of exercise.

Between groups N and Nn, during rest, the sAP was lower after nifedipine was administered, but no statistically significant levels were reached ($0.05<p<0.10$). In these groups, the middle increment of sAP between rest and the 3rd minute of exercise was 12.5 mm Hg before receiving nifedipine, and 17.5 mm Hg after receiving the drug. There were no statistically significant differences ($p>0.30$) between the two values.

Comparing C and Cn during rest, it could be seen that, as in normal subjects, the sAP was lower after administration of nifedipine (120.5 mm Hg) than before (133.7 mm Hg): these values were statistically significant ($p<0.001$). The middle increment of sAP between rest and the 3rd minute of exercise was 27.4 mm Hg before administration of nifedipine, and 21.3 mm Hg after ($p<0.05$).

Tension-Time Index (T.T.I.)

T.T.I. = HR × sAP

In order to establish the utility of the 3rd minute of isometric exercise as a test of the overloading, the variations of the T.T.I. between the 2nd and 3rd minutes of handgrip were compared in both the normal and coronary groups, prior to the administration of the drug; the increment of the index was very significant ($p < 0.001$). For that reason, we prolonged the test through the 3rd minute; however the exhaustion experienced by the majority of individuals during and at the end of the 3rd minute made it impossible for us to prolong the exercise any further.

3. Diastolic Arterial Pressure (dAP)

The results obtained are presented in Table 4.

In the four groups a significant increment ($p < 0.001$) of the dAP between rest and the 3rd minute of exercise was verified.

In normal subjects at rest, the dAP was lower after administration of nifedipine (70.0 mm Hg) than before (77.5 mm Hg) ($p < 0.05$). The middle increment of

Table 4. dAP in mm Hg

Group N	Rest	1 min	2 min	3 min
Mean	77.5	84.0	87.5	89.5
s.d.	9.5	8.1	8.6	8.0
s.e.	3.0	2.6	2.7	2.5
		77.5→89.5	($p < 0.001$)	
Group Nn				
Mean	70.0	76.5	85.5	84.5
s.d.	11.8	13.1	13.0	13.2
s.e.	3.7	4.2	4.1	4.2
		70.0→84.5	($p < 0.001$)	
Group C				
Mean	89.2	97.1	103.2	106.3
s.d.	11.8	13.5	12.7	14.6
s.e.	2.7	3.1	2.9	3.4
		89.2→106.3	($p < 0.001$)	
Group Cn				
Mean	80.5	87.1	90.0	91.8
s.d.	12.9	12.8	12.5	11.5
s.e.	3.0	3.0	2.9	2.6
		80.5→91.8	($p < 0.001$)	

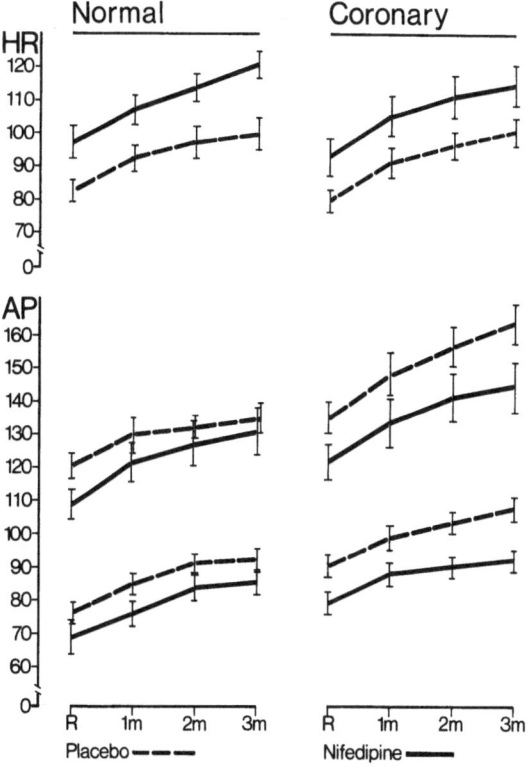

Fig.4. Variations of heart rate (HR), systolic and diastolic arterial pressure (AP), in normal subjects and in coronary artery disease patients, before and after nifedipine

the dAP between rest and the 3rd minute of exercise was 12 mm Hg prior to administration of nifedipine and 14.5 mm Hg after; these values were not statistically significant ($p < 0.30$).

In the coronaries during rest, as in the normal subjects, the dAP was lower after administration of nifedipine (80.5 mm Hg) than before (89.2 mm Hg); both sets of values were equally statistically significant ($p < 0.001$). The middle increment of dAP between rest and the 3rd minute of exercise was 17.1 mm Hg prior to administration of nifedipine and 11.3 mm Hg with the drug ($p < 0.02$) (Fig.4).

4. Left Ventricular Ejection Time (LVET)

Table 5 contains the mean values and their deviations in the different groups.

In all groups, a progressive shortening of the LVET between rest and the 3rd minute of isometric exercise was observed. This shortening was statistically significant in the four groups (Table 5).

Group N

A high degree of correlation was found between the duration of the LVET and the HR, both during rest and during the 3rd minute of exercise. The correspond-

Table 5. LVET (in msec)

Group N	Rest	1 min	2 min	3 min
Mean	245.0	240.0	237.5	237.0
s.d.	13.1	15.8	16.9	17.2
s.e.	4.2	5.0	5.3	5.4
		245.0→237.0	($p<0.05$)	
Group Nn				
Mean	240.0	234.5	230.0	226.0
s.d.	16.2	16.4	14.1	14.9
s.e.	5.1	5.2	4.5	4.7
		240.0→226.0	($p<0.001$)	
Group C				
Mean	240.0	231.8	230.5	229.3
s.d.	21.1	22.6	21.5	19.9
s.e.	4.7	5.0	4.8	4.5
		240.0→229.3	($p<0.001$)	
Group Cn				
Mean	237.3	230.5	225.5	221.5
s.d.	22.0	23.8	22.8	25.2
s.e.	4.9	5.3	5.1	5.6
		237.3→221.5	($p<0.001$)	

ing functions of linial regression of this period in the HR were obtained. During rest:

LVET = 321.7–0.95 HR $r = -0.82$
                              $p < 0.005$

During the 3rd minute of exercise:

LVET = 339.8–1.04 HR $r = -0.85$
                              $p < 0.005$

Group Nn

A high degree of correlation was found between the duration of the LVET and the HR during rest, calculating the function of regression:

LVET = 333.0–0.96 HR $r = -0.83$
                              $p < 0.005$

During the 3rd minute of exercise, the degree of correlation found was not statistically acceptable ($r = -0.62, 0.05 < p < 0.10$), not calculating the function of regression.

Group C

A correlation exists between the duration of the LVET and the HR. The function of regression at rest was:

LVET = 321.2–1.03 HR $r = -0.68$
                                        $p < 0.001$

In the 3rd minute of exercise, the line of regression is given by:

LVET = 283.4–0.54 HR $r = -0.57$
                                        $p < 0.01$

Group Cn

A correlation was noted between the duration of LVET and HR: the function of regression at rest was:

LVET = 302.0–0.68 HR $r = -0.68$
                                        $p < 0.001$

In the 3rd minute of isometric exercise, the regression was:

LVET = 307.9–0.75 HR $r = -0.78$
                                        $p < 0.001$

N and C

Given the very slight differences observed in each experiment between the HR reached by each group (Table 2), we decided to compare directly the magnitude of the LVET in both groups (similarly, we compared the resting systolic intervals in these two groups). The LVET was always lower between the coronaries than between the normal subjects, but the difference was not statistically significant.

No significant difference in the grades of the respective regression lines was found, either at rest or during the 3rd minute of exercise (Fig. 5).

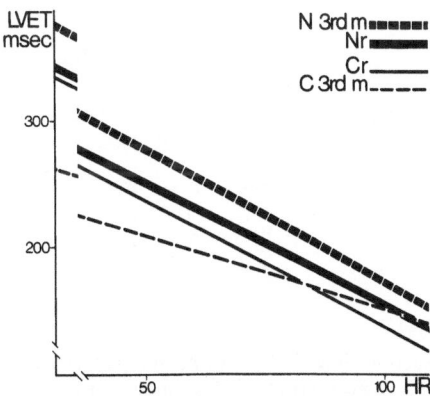

Fig. 5. Left ventricular ejection time (LVET) in normal subjects (N) and in coronary artery disease patients (C), at rest (r) and during the 3rd minute of handgrip test

Nn and Cn

Considering the close adjustment existing at each stage between the HR reached by each group under the action of nifedipine (Table 2), we made a direct comparison of the values obtained for the LVET in each of these groups. The same procedure was followed for the other systolic time intervals measure. In this case, the LVET was, at each step, lower in the coronaries than in the normal subjects; here also, no significant differences were found.

N and Nn

The respective values of LVET were lower during the action of nifedipine, with significant differences only in the 3rd minute of exercise (Table 6). For better interpretation of these results, the evident tachycardiac action of nifedipine should be borne in mind, since the LVET necessarily has a tendency to become shorter under the action of the drug. To "separate" this tachycardiac effect on the LVET induced by nifedipine, we analyzed the functions of regression.

Table 6. Comparison of the LVET in groups N and Nn

LVET	Rest	1 min	2 min	3 min
Group N	245.0	240.0	237.5	237.0
Group Nn	240.0	234.5	230.0	226.0
p	$p>0.10$	$p>0.10$	$p>0.05$	$p>0.025$

The lines of regression for rest may be considered statistically as parallels. Resulting significant ($p<0.05$) their difference in highness, being above the line corresponding to the same subjects after having received nifedipine (Fig. 6).

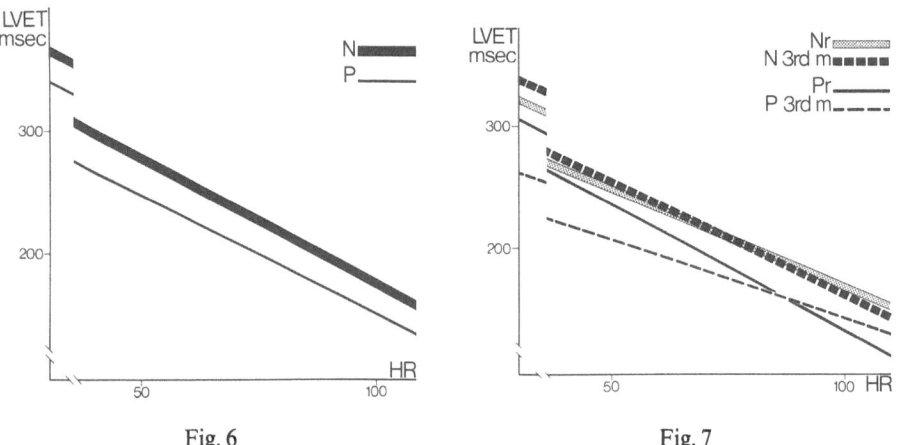

Fig. 6   Fig. 7

Fig. 6. Left ventricular ejection time (LVET) in normal subjects at rest, after administrating placebo (P) and after nifedipine (N)

Fig. 7. Left ventricular ejection time (LVET) in coronary artery disease patients at rest (r) and during the 3rd minute of hadgrip test, after administrating placebo (P) and after nifedipine (N)

During the first minute of exercise, the situation of the lines was alike, although the significance of the difference in height disappears. In the last minute of exercise, as was pointed out, there was no good correlation between LVET and HR in the Nn group, because comparisons in that stage of the test were not performed.

C and Cn

Similarly in the normal control group, LVET was lower during the action of nifedipine, but in no stage of the test were the differences significant (Table 7). The tachycardiac action of nifedipine must also be considered when interpreting the results in coronary patients.

Table 7. Comparison of the LVET in groups C and Cn

LVET	Rest	1 min	2 min	3 min
Group C	240.0	231.8	230.5	229.3
Group Cn	237.3	230.5	225.5	221.5
p	$p>0.10$	$p>0.60$	$p>0.10$	$p>0.05$

The lines of regression during rest may be considered statistically als parallels, the line corresponding to nifedipine being above the line representing the situation before administration of the drug.

Although the difference in height is not statistically significant, it probably is indicative of a tendency that must be considered in every case in future studies (Fig. 7).

5. Pre-Ejection Period (PEP)

The results are shown in Table 8.

Group N

The PEP underwent an irregular shortening ($p>0.10$) between rest and the 3rd minute of exercise. Otherwise, no acceptable statistical correlation was obtained between this period and HR, either at rest ($r= -0.35$, $p>0.30$) or during the 3rd minute of exercise ($r= -0.23$, $p>0.50$). For this reason we did not consider the respective functions of regression within and between the four groups.

Group Nn

In this group the PEP was shortened significantly between rest and the 3rd minute of exercise ($p<0.05$).

Group C

Similarly to group N, there was an irregular shortening ($p>0.05$) between rest and the 3rd minute of exercise. The degree of correlation found between PEP and HR at rest was $r= -0.37$, $p>0.10$. Here again there was no acceptable correlation, as was the case in the group of normal subjects in the 3rd minute only, we had $r=0.45$, $p<0.05$).

R. J. Esper *et al.*

Table 8. PEP (in msec)

Group N	Rest	1 min	2 min	3 min
Mean	83.5	78.5	79.5	79.5
s.d.	11.3	14.7	15.4	15.5
s.e.	3.6	4.7	4.9	4.9
	83.5→79.5	$(p>0.10)$		
Group Nn				
Mean	78.0	75.0	69.5	67.5
s.d.	13.0	12.5	10.1	12.5
s.e.	4.1	3.9	3.2	4.0
	78.0→67.5	$(p<0.05)$		
Group C				
Mean	95.0	95.5	91.5	89.5
s.d.	13.5	18.3	16.9	16.9
s.e.	3.0	4.1	3.8	3.8
	95.0→89.5	$(0.05<p<0.10)$		
Group Cn				
Mean	77.3	76.8	74.3	73.8
s.d.	15.5	18.6	18.4	15.3
s.e.	3.5	4.2	4.1	3.4
	77.3→73.8	$(p>0.20)$		

Group Cn

Again the shortening observed between rest and the 3rd minute was not significant $(p<0.20)$.

N and C, Nn and Cn

Before administration of nifedipine the PEP was always smaller in the normal group than in the coronaries, reaching statistical significance during rest and in the first minute of exercise (Table 9). After administration of the drug, no difference could be demonstrated between the two groups (Table 9).

N, Nn and C, Cn

In all cases the PEP was lower after the administration of nifedipine (Table 10). As was mentioned previously for the LVET, the tachycardia induced by nifedipine must be considered when interpreting the results.

Table 9. Comparison of the PEP in groups N, C and Nn, Cn

PEP	Rest	1 min	2 min	3 min
Group N	83.5	78.5	79.5	79.5
Group C	95.0	95.5	91.5	89.5
p	$p < 0.05$	$p < 0.02$	$0.05 < p < 0.10$	$0.10 < p < 0.20$

PEP				
Group Nn	78.0	75.0	69.5	67.5
Group Cn	77.3	76.8	74.3	73.8
p	$p > 0.80$	$p > 0.70$	$p > 0.40$	$p > 0.20$

Table 10. Comparison of the PEP in groups N, Nn and C, Cn

PEP	Rest	1 min	2 min	3 min
Group N	83.5	78.5	79.5	79.5
Group Nn	78.0	75.0	69.5	67.5
p	$p < 0.02$	$0.20 < p < 0.30$	$p < 0.02$	$p < 0.025$

PEP				
Group C	95.0	95.5	91.5	89.5
Group Cn	77.3	76.8	74.3	73.8
p	$p < 0.001$	$p < 0.001$	$p < 0.001$	$p < 0.001$

6. Electromechanical Systole (ES)

The corresponding results are in Table 11.

In the four groups, a significant shortening of ES was observed between rest and the 3rd minute of exercise (Table 11).

Group N

A statistical correlation was found between ES and HR at rest:

ES = 433.3–1.3 HR $r = 0.77$
                                     $p < 0.01$

During the 3rd minute:

ES = 444.1–1.29 HR $r = -0.69$
                                     $p < 0.05$

Group Nn

Similarly to the N group, there was a correlation between ES and HR at rest:

ES = 417.5–1.03 HR $r = -0.68$
                                     $p < 0.05$

During the 3rd minute:

ES = 441.5–1.24 HR $r = -0.82$
                                     $p < 0.005$

Table 11. ES (in msec)

Group N	Rest	1 min	2 min	3 min
Mean	328.5	318.5	317.0	316.5
s.d.	19.0	24.7	26.3	26.1
s.e.	6.0	7.8	8.3	8.3
	328.5→316.5	$(p<0.01)$		
Group Nn				
Mean	318.0	309.5	299.5	293.5
s.d.	21.4	16.9	17.4	18.0
s.e.	6.8	5.4	5.5	5.7
	318.0→293.5	$(p<0.005)$		
Group C				
Mean	335.0	327.3	322.0	318.8
s.d.	24.6	26.4	24.9	25.1
s.e.	5.5	5.9	5.6	5.6
	335.0→318.8	$(p<0.001)$		
Group Cn				
Mean	314.5	307.3	299.8	295.3
s.d.	25.9	32.2	33.2	35.8
s.e.	5.8	7.2	7.4	8.0
	314.5→295.3	$(p<0.001)$		

Group C

Again we obtained statistical correlation between ES and HR in subjects at rest:

ES = 443.4–1.37 HR $r = -0.78$
                                    $p<0.001$

For the 3rd minute of exercise:

ES = 410.1–0.91 HR $r = -0.76$
                                    $p<0.001$

Group Cn

Correlation was also obtained between ES and HR at rest:

ES = 398.4–0.88 HR $r = -0.75$
                                    $p<0.001$

For the 3rd minute we found:

ES = 424.3–1.12 HR $r = -0.82$
                                    $p<0.001$

N, C and Nn, Cn

In neither situation (before and after administration of nifedipine) were significant differences found between the groups of normal and coronary subjects.

N and Nn

In each stage of the test, the ES was lower after the administration of nifedipine, without being statistically significant in the 1st minute of isometric exercise (Table 12).

Table 12. Comparison of ES between N and Nn

ES	Rest	1 min	2 min	3 min
Group N	328.5	318.5	317.0	316.5
Group Nn	318.0	309.5	299.5	293.5
p	$p<0.025$	$p>0.10$	$p<0.05$	$p<0.02$

C and Cn

After the administration of nifedipine, the ES was always less under the action of the drug in the coronary group as well as in the normal group, reaching statistical significance in all stages (Table 13).

As was mentioned for the other intervals, the tachycardiac action of nifedipine must be considered when interpreting the results obtained for N and Nn and C and Cn.

Table 13. Comparison of ES between C and Cn

ES	Rest	1 min	2 min	3 min
Group C	335.0	327.3	322.0	318.8
Group Cn	314.5	307.3	299.8	295.3
p	$p<0.001$	$p<0.001$	$p<0.001$	$p<0.001$

7. Pre-Ejection Period/Left Ventricular Ejection Time Ratio (PEP/LVET)

The results obtained are given in Table 14.

Group N

The PEP/LVET ratio fell in the first minute of exercise, then rose again in the second and third minutes. None of these fluctuations were statistically significant.

Group Nn

A progressive fall was observed as the experiment proceeded; it was not statistically significant.

Table 14. PEP/LVET ratio

Group N	Rest	1 min	2 min	3 min
Mean	0.341	0.327	0.335	0.336
s.d.	0.047	0.059	0.062	0.064
s.e.	0.015	0.019	0.019	0.020
Group Nn				
Mean	0.326	0.322	0.303	0.300
s.d.	0.057	0.064	0.048	0.061
s.e.	0.018	0.020	0.015	0.019
Group C				
Mean	0.399	0.417	0.402	0.394
s.d.	0.068	0.096	0.092	0.086
s.e.	0.015	0.021	0.021	0.019
Group Cn				
Mean	0.329	0.336	0.330	0.333
s.d.	0.075	0.085	0.079	0.059
s.e.	0.017	0.019	0.018	0.013

Group C

The PEP/LVET ratio rose during the first minute of exercise, then fell. These fluctuations, too, were not statistically significant.

Group Cn

No significant variations of the ratio were observed as the test proceeded.

N and C

The values of the ratio were always lower in normal subjects than in coronary patients, reaching statistical significance at rest, and in the 1st and 2nd minutes of exercise (Table 15).

Table 15. Comparison of the PEP/LVET in Groups N and C

LVET/PEP	Rest	1 min	2 min	3 min
Group N	0.341	0.327	0.335	0.336
Group C	0.399	0.417	0.402	0.394
p	$p<0.025$	$p<0.02$	$p<0.05$	$0.05<p<0.10$

Nn and Cn

After the administration of nifedipine, the ratio continued to be lower in normal subjects throughout the entire experiment; at no point were the differences significant (Table 16).

Table 16. Comparison of the PEP/LVET in Groups Nn and Cn

LVET/PEP	Rest	1 min	2 min	3 min
Group N	0.326	0.322	0.303	0.300
Group Cn	0.329	0.330	0.330	0.333
p	$p > 0.90$	$p > 0.30$	$p > 0.30$	$p > 0.10$

N and Nn

During the whole experiment, the respective values of the ratio were lower after administration of nifedipine, reaching significant levels only in the 2nd minute of the test (Table 17).

Table 17. Comparison of the PEP/LVET in groups N and Nn

LVET/PEP	Rest	1 min	2 min	3 min
Group N	0.341	0.327	0.335	0.336
Group Nn	0.326	0.322	0.303	0.300
p	$0.05 < p < 0.10$	$p < 0.60$	$p < 0.02$	$0.05 < p < 0.10$

C and Cn

After the administration of nifedipine, the ratio throughout the test was, as in the normal subjects, always lower; this time, however, the differences were highly significant (Table 18).

Table 18. Comparison of the PEP/LVET in groups C and Cn

LVET/PEP	Rest	1 min	2 min	3 min
Group C	0.399	0.417	0.402	0.394
Group Cn	0.329	0.336	0.330	0.333
p	$p < 0.001$	$p < 0.001$	$p < 0.001$	$p < 0.001$

In contrast to the situation in systolic intervals, which are affected by the HR, it has been demonstrated that HR does not affect the PEP/LVET ratio [16, 52, 73, 84]; this fact is of fundamental importance in interpreting the results obtained for groups N and Nn and for groups C and Cn.

Secondary Effects

Nifedipine produced headache in 3 of 10 normal subjects (30%) and in 4 of the 20 coronaries (20%).

In the coronary group, the trouble was transitory and cleared up spontaneously within a short period of time (20–30 min); in the normal group, however, it persisted with a tolerable intensity throughout the day.

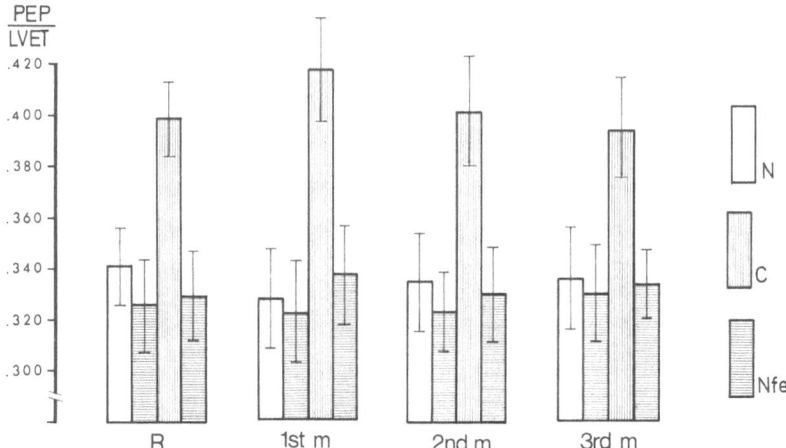

Fig. 8. PEP/LVET ratio in normal subjects (N) and in coronary artery disease patients (C), before and after administrating nifedipine (Nfe), at rest and during each minute of handgrip test

Two of the three normal subjects took 500 mg of acetylsalicylic acid in the afternoon. In two, the headache disappeared; and in the third, it invariably lasted until bedtime.

Discussion

Our first task was to analyse the efficiency of the isometric exercise in producing an overload of the left ventricle. The increases in the HR, sAP and dAP (Tables 1, 3, 4) were statistically significant, not only when the rest values were compared with those from the final minute of effort, but also when those from the 2nd and 3rd minutes of the test (T.T.I.) were compared. Otherwise the increments of each parameter were similar in the four groups, i.e. independent of the action of nifedipine, so that the isometric exercise can be considered to have a comparative value as an overload producer.

Nifedipine produced a tachycardiac effect as well as systolic and diastolic hypotension in normal subjects and in coronary patients; the changes were significant (Tables 1, 3, 4). The increments in the patients, response to the isometric exercise after administration of the drug were similar to those observed in the group receiving placebos, permitting us to evaluate the action of the isometric exercise before and after nifedipine. The increases of HR, sAP, and dAP were statistically comparable and independent of the action of the drug, though the absolute values at rest or during the exercises were influenced by nifedipine, in normals as well as in coronaries.

As expected logically, the tachycardia shortened the LVET in all groups. Therefore, for a correct interpretation, we will refer to the LVET "corrected" for HR.

In the coronary group, LVET was always lower than in the normal group. However, the difference increased during the isometric exercise because, while in the normals the LVET becomes longer during the isometric effort, in the coronaries it becomes shorter (Fig. 5). Although these results were not statistically significant, a strong tendency was observed, which probably would be increased with the addition of future cases.

After nifedipine, the LVET was prolonged in the N and in the C groups, both at rest and during the exercise. In the normal group at rest, a prolonged LVET was significantly greater after nifedipine; in the coronaries, it exhibited a similar tendency.

The PEP was always lower in the normal group than in the coronary group. In both cases it was shortened after nifedipine (Nn and Cn), though to a greater degree in coronaries (Cn) than in normals (Nn).

Because ES includes the PEP and the LVET, its variations are not specific. Thus differences between N and C, and between Nn and Cn were not found. Even when, after nifedipine, the ES was always shortened in relation to the placebo groups, in normals and in coronaries, it was necessary to note the limits of the increase of HR for its correct evaluation.

The PEP/LVET ratio is the most sensitive method for detecting small deficiencies in the contractile capacity of left ventricle. The ratio was always lower in the normals than in coronaries before and after the administration of nifedipine, but the differences were not significant. Of considerable interest, however, is its decrease in the Cn group as compared to the C group; the reduction at rest was highly significant, and at each minute of the isometric exercise, the data suggest an increment in the contractility of the left ventricle in the coronaries under the action of nifedipine (see Fig. 8).

Conclusions

The isometric exercise produced an increment of HR, sAP and dAP in all groups, thus proving to be an effective method of overloading the left ventricle.

Nifedipine produced in all cases tachycardia and systolic and diastolic hypotension.

The LVET "corrected" for the HR was always lower in the coronary patients than in the normal group and was prolonged in every case after nifedipine.

The PEP, always higher in coronaries than in normals, was shortened after nifedipine, though to more significant degree in the C group than in the N group.

The ES, even though shortened after the drug, has no specificity for its correct evaluation.

The PEP/LVET ratio proved to be the more reliable index. In the N group it was lower than in the C group. After nifedipine, it was lower in both groups, Nn and Cn, but in this case, the values were highly significant.

Abstract

Ten normal men and twenty with coronary artery disease, as demonstrated clinically, radiologically, electrocardiographically, hemodynamically and cineangiographically, performed a 50% total capacity isometric handgrip test for a period of three minutes.

The following systolic time intervals were measured to evaluate the left ventricular function: Left ventricular ejection time, pre-ejection period, total electromechanical systole and PEP/LVET ratio.

Simultaneous readings of heart rate and blood pressure were taken to prove the usefulness of isometric contraction in producing a cardiac load.

The test was repeated after administering 20 mg of nifedipine (BAY a 1040, Adalat) sublingually, a drug considered to be a coronary and systemic vasodilator, with a beneficial effect on myocardial cellular metabolism.

The effect of the drug on the different systolic time intervals was processed statistically. The most significant variation obtained was a shortening of the PEP/LVET ratio under the effects of nifedipine, more accentuated in patients with coronary artery disease than in normal subjects.

References

1. AGRESS, C. M., *et al.*: Comparison of the ejection time-heart rate relationships in normal and ischemic subjects. Jap. Heart J. **6**, 497 (1965).
2. AMENDE, I., KRAYENBUEHL, H. P., RUTISHAUSER, W., WIRZ, P.: Left ventricular dynamics during handgrip. Brit. Heart J. **34**, 688 (1972).
3. ARANOW, W. S.: Isovolumic contraction and left ventricular ejection time. Amer. J. Cardiol. **26**, 238 (1970).
4. ARANOW, W. S., BOWYER, A. F., KAPLAN, M. A.: External isovolumic contraction time and left ventricular ejection time/external isovolumic contraction time ratios at rest and after exercise in coronary artery disease. Circulation **43**, 59 (1971).
5. BASSINGTHWAIGHTE, J. B., BURCHEL, H. B.: Duration cardiac systole in children with femoral arteriovenous fistulas. Amer. Heart J. **83**, 732 (1972).
6. BENCHIMOL, A.: A study of the period of isovolumic relaxation in normal subjects and in patients with heart disease. Amer. J. Cardiol. **19**, 196 (1967).
7. BRAUNWALD, E. (Ed.): On the difference between the heart's output and its contactile state. Circulation **43**, 171 (1971).
8. BRAUNWALD, E., ROSS, J., JR., SONNENBLICK, E. H.: Mechanisms of contraction of the normal and failing heart. Boston: Little, Brown and Co. 1968.
9. BRAUNWALD, E., SARNOFF, S. J., STAINSBY, W. N.: Determinants of duration and mean rate of ventricular ejection. Circulation Res. **6**, 319 (1958).
10. BUSH, C. A., LEWIS, R. P., LEIGHTON, R. F., FONTANA, M. E., WEISSLER, A. M.: Verification of systolic time intervals and the apexcardiogram by micromanometer catheterization of the left ventricle and aorta. (Abstr.) Circulation **42**, III-121 (1970).
11. CINGOLANI, H. E., MATTIAZZI, A. R., MOREYRA, A. E., LARDANI, H.: Evaluación de la función miocárdica. Medicina **33**, 423 (1973).
12. CUESTA SILVA, M. A., RICCI, G. J., PEROSIO, A. M. A.: Factores de error en fonomecanocardiografia. I: Derivados de la falta de análisis del electrocardiograma. Rev. Argent. Cardiol. **38**, 241 (1970).
13. DIAMOND, G., FORRESTER, J.: Effect of coronary artery disease an acute myocardial infarction on left ventricular compliance in man. Circulation **45**, 11 (1972).
14. DIAMONT, B., KILLIP, T.: Indirect assessment of left ventricular performance in acute myocardial infarction. Circulation **42**, 579 (1970).
15. ESPER, R. J.: Tiempos sistólicos del ventriculo izquierdo. Rev. Argent. Cardiol. **41**, 451 (1973).
16. ESPER, R. J., *et al.*: Variaciones del carotidograma en la estenosis aórtica. Comunicado en el VIII Congreso Argentino de Cardiologia, Córdoba (1969).
17. ESPER, R. J., BIDOGGIA, H., MACHADO, R. A., NORDABY, R. A.: Tiempos sistólicos del V.I. en normales y coronarios durante el ejercicio isometrico. En Prensa.

18. ESPER, R. J., MADOERY, R. J.: Progresos en Auscultación y Fonomecanocardiografia. Buenos Aires: Lopez libreros enditores, S.R.L. 1974.

19. FABIAN, J., EPSTEIN, E. J., CULSHED, N.: Duration of phases of left ventricular systole using indirect methods. I. Normal subjects. Brit. Heart J. **34**, 874 (1972).

20. FABIAN, J., EPSTEIN, E. J., CULSHED, N., MCKENDRICK, C. S.: Duration of phases of left ventricular systole using indirect methods. II. Acute myocardial infarction. Brit. Heart J. **34**, 882 (1972).

21. FEIL, H. S., KATZ, L. N.: Clinical observation on the dynamics of ventricular systole. II. Hypertension. Arch. Intern. Med. **33**, 321 (1924).

22. FISHER, M. L., NUTTER, D. O., JACOBS, W., SCHLANT, R. C.: Hemodynamic responses to isometric exercise (handgrip) in patients with heart disease. Brit. Heart. J. **35**, 422 (1973).

23. FRANK, O. (translated by CHAPMAN, C. B., WASSERMAN, E.): On the dynamics of cardiac muscle. Amer. Heart J. **58**, 282, 467 (1959).

24. GAASH, W. H., QUINONES, M. A., WAISSER, E., THIEL, H. G., ALEXANDER, J. K.: Alterations in left ventricular contractile state during isometric exercise in patients with coronary artery disease. Amer. J. Cardiol. **29** (Abstr.): 264 (1972).

25. GARRARD, C. L., JR., WEISSLER, A. M., DODGE, H. T.: The relationship of alterations in systolic time intervals to ejection fraction in patients with cardiac disease. Circulation **42**, 455 (1970).

26. GARROD, A. H.: On some points connected with the circulation of the blood, arrived at from a study of the sphygmograph-trace. Proc. Roy. Soc. **23**, 140, 1874-S.

27. GLEASON, W. L., BRAUNWALD, E.: Studies on the first derivative of the ventricular pressure pulse in man. J. Clin. Invest. **41**, 80 (1962).

28. GLEASON, W. L., BRAUNWALD, E.: Studies of the first derivative of the ventricular pulse pressure on left ventricular dp/dt. Amer. J. Physiol. **216**, 185 (1969).

29. GREENFIELD, J. C., JR., HARLEY, A., THOMPSON, H. K., et al.: Pressure-flow studies in man during atrial fibrillation. J. Clin. Invest. **47**, 2411 (1968).

30. GROSSMAN, W., MACLAURIN, S. B., SALTZ, J. A., PARASKOS, J. A., DALEN, J. E., DEXTER, L.: Changes in the inotropic state of the left ventricle during isometric exercise. Brit. Heart. J. **35**, 697 (1973).

31. HALPERN, B. L., HODGES, M., DAGENAIS, G. R., FRIESINGER, G. C.: Left ventricular pre-ejection period and ejection time in patients with acute myocardial infarction. (Abstr.) Circulation **40**, 100 (1969).

32. HARLEY, A., STARMER, C. F., GREENFIELD, J. C., JR.: Pressure-flow studies in man: Evaluation of the duration of the phases of systole. J. Clin. Invest. **48**, 895 (1969).

33. HARRIS, W. S., SCJOENFELD, C. D., BROOKES, R. H., WEISSLER, A. M.: Effects of beta adrenergic blockade on the hemodynamic responses to epinephrine in man. Amer. J. Cardiol. **17**, 484 (1966).

34. HASHIMOTO, K., TAIRA, N., CHIBA, S., HASHIMOTO, K., JR., ENDOH, M., KOKUBUN, M., KOKUBUN, H., IIJIMA, T., KIMURA, T., KUBOTA, K., OGURO, K.: Cardiohemodynamic effects of BAY a 1040 in the dog. Arzneim. Forsch. (Drug Res.) **22**, 15 (1972).

35. HAYASE, S., HIRAKAWA, S., MORI, N., KANYAMA, S., IWASA, M.: Hemodynamic and therapeutic effect of BAY a 1040 on the patients with ischemic heart disease. Arzneim.-Forsch. (Drug Res.) **22**, 370 (1972).

36. HIRAKAWA, S., ITO, H., KONDO, Y., WATANABE, I., HIEI, K., BANNO, S., HAYASE, S.: Coronary circulation, systemic resistance and capacitance blood vessels of dogs as affected by BAY a 1040. Arzneim.-Forsch. (Drug Res.) **22**, 345 (1972).

37. HODGES, M., HALPERN, B., FRIESINGER, G. C., GAGENAIS, C. R.: Left ventricular pre-ejection time period and ejection time in patients with acute myocardial infarction. Circulation **45**, 933 (1972).

38. HOOD, E. P., JR., RACKLEY, C. E., ROLETT, E. L.: Wall stress in the normal and hypertrophied human left ventricle. Amer. J. Cardiol. **22**, 550 (1968).

39. HOUSTON, J. D., ATKINS, J. M., BLOMQVIST, C. G.: Cardiovascular responses to isometric forearm contraction (Abstr.) Clin. Res. **18**, 70 (1970).

40. INOUE, K., YOUNG, G. M., GRIERSON, A. L., SMULYAN, H., EICH, K. H.: Isometric contraction period of the left ventricle in acute myocardial infarction. Circulation **42**, 79 (1970).

41. Jacobs,W.P., Nutter,D.O., Siegel,W., Schlant,R.C., Hurst,J.W.: Hemodynamic responses to isometric handgrip in patients with heart disease. Circulation **42** (suppl. III-169) (1970).

42. Johnson,A.D., O'Rourke,R.A., Karkiner,J.S., Burian,C.: Effect of myocardial revascularization on systolic time intervals in patients with left ventricular dysfunction. Circulation **45** (suppl. I-91) (1972).

43. Katz,L.N., Feil,H.S.: Clinical observations on the dynamics of ventricular systole. I. Auricular fibrillation. Arch. Intern. Med. **32**, 672 (1923).

44. Kimura,E., Mabuchi,G., Kikuchi,H.: The clinical effect of 4-(2'-nitrophenyl)-2,6-dimethyl-3,5-dicarbomethoxy-1,4-dihydropyridine (BAY a 1040) on angina pectoris evaluated by sequential analysis. Arzneim.-Forsch. (Drug Res.) **22**, 365 (1972).

45. Kivowitz,C., Marcus,H., Donoso,R., Ganz,W., Swan,H.J., Parmley,W.M.: Evaluation of cardiac performance with a handgrip dynamometer in patients with heart disease. The grip test. Circulation **42**, (suppl. III-122) (1970).

46. Kobayashi,T., Ito,Y., Tawara,I.: Clinical experience with a new coronary-active substance (BAY a 1040). Arzneim.-Forsch. (Drug Res.) **22**, 380 (1972).

47. Krayenbuehl,H.P., Rutishauser,W., Schoenbeck,M., Amede,I.: Evaluation of left ventricular function from isovolumic pressure measurements during exercise. Amer. J. Cardiol. **29**, 323 (1972).

48. Kumar,S., Spodick,D.H.: Study of the mechanical events of the left ventricle by atraumatic techniques: Comparison of methods of measurement and their significance. Amer. Heart J. **80**, 401 (1970).

49. Lind,A.R.: Cardiovascular responses to static exercise (Isometric, anyone?). Circulation **41**, 173 (1970).

50. Lind,A.R., McNichol,G.: Circulatory responses to substained handgrip contractions performed during other exercise, both rhythmic and static. J. Physiol. (London) **192**, 595 (1967).

51. Lind,A.R., Taylor,S.H., Humphreys,P.W., Kennelly,B.M., Donald,K.W.: The circulatory effects of sustained voluntary muscle contraction. Clin. Sci. **27**, 229 (1964).

52. Lindqvist,V.A., Spangler,R.D., Blount,G.S., Jr.: A comparison between the effects of dynamic and isometric exercise as evaluated by the systolic time intervals in normal man. Amer. Heart J. **85**, 227 (1973).

53. Lombard,W.P., Cope,O.M.: The duration of the systole of the left ventricle of man. Amer. J. Physiol. **77**, 263 (1926).

54. Margolis,C.: Significance of ejection period/tension period as a factor in the assessment of cardiac function and as a possible diagnostic tool for the uncovering of silent coronary heart disease: Study of 111 cases. Dis. Chest. **46**, 706 (1964).

55. Mason,D.T.: Usefulness and limitations of the rate of rise of intraventricular pressure (dp/dt) in the evaluation of myocardial contractility in man. Amer. J. Cardiol. **23**, 516 (1969).

56. Mullins,C.B., Leshin,S.J., Mierzwiak,D.S., Mattheus,O.A., Blomqvist,G.: Isometric exercise (handgrip) as a stress test for evaluation of left ventricular function. Circulation **42** (suppl. III-122) (1970).

57. Oreshkow,V.: Indirect measurement of isovolumetric contraction time on the basis of polygraphic tracing (apexcardiogram, carotid tracing and phonocardiogram). Cardiologia **47**, 315 (1965).

58. Perloff,J.K., Reichek,N.: Value and limitation of systolic time intervals (pre-ejection period and ejection time) in patients with acute myocardial infarction. Circulation **45**, 929 (1972).

59. Perloff,J.K., Talano,J.V., Ronan,J.A.: Técnicas incruentas en el infarto agudo de miocardio. Progresos en las enfermedades cardiovasculares **11**, 468 (1971).

60. Perry,J.M., Jr., Garrard,C.L.: Systolic time intervals: Relation to severity of coronary artery disease and left ventricular dysfunction. Circulation **42** (suppl III-121) (1970).

61. Peserico,E.: The influence of mechanical factors of the circulation upon the heart volume. J. Physiol. **65**, 146 (1928).

62. Robinson,B.: The carotid pulse. II. Relations of external recording to carotid, aortic and branchial pulses. Brit. Heart J. **25**, 61 (1963).

63. SAWAYAMA,T., OCHIAI,M., MARUMOTO,S., MATSUURA,T., NIKI,J.: Influence of amyl nitrite inhalation on the systolic time intervals in normal subjects and in patients with ischemic heart disease. Circulation **40**, 327 (1969).

64. SCHLANT,R.C.: Normal physiology of the cardiovascular system. In: HURST,J.W., LOGUE,R.B. (Eds.): The heart, 2nd ed., New York: MacGraw-Hill Book Co. 1970.

65. SHAH,P.M., SLODKI,S.J.: The Q-II interval. A study of the second heart sound in normal adults and in systemic hypertension. Circulation **29**, 551 (1964).

66. SHAVER,J.A., KROETZ,F.W., LEONARD,J.J., et al.: The effect of steady-state increases in systemic arterial pressure on the duration of left ventricular ejection time. J. Clin. Invest. **47**, 217 (1968).

67. SNEDECOR,G.W.: Métodos estadisticos. Compañia Editorial Continental S.A., Méjico, 1970 (5a Edición).

68. STAFFORD,R.W., HARRIS,W.S., WEISSLER,A.M.: Left ventricular systolic time intervals as indices of postural circulatory stress in man. Circulation **41**, 485 (1970).

69. TAFUR,E., COHEN,L.S., LEVINE,H.R.: The normal apexcardiogram. Its temporal relationship to electrical, acoustic and mechanical cardiac events. Circulation **30**, 381 (1964).

70. TORANZOS,F.I.: Estadistica. Editorial Kapelusz, Buenos Aires, Argentina, 1968 (3a Edición).

71. TOUTOUZAS,P., GUPTA,D., SAMSON,R., et al.: Q-second sound interval in acute myocardial infarction. Brit. Med. J. **31**, 462 (1969).

72. WALLACE,A.G., MITCHELL,J.H., SKINNER,N.S., SARNOFF,S.J.: Duration of the phases of left ventricular systole. Circ. Res. **12**, 611 (1963).

73. WALLACE,A.G., SKINNER,N.S., JR., MITCHELL,J.H.: Hemodynamic determinants of the maximal rate of rise of left ventricular pressure. Amer. J. Physiol. **205**, 30 (1963).

74. WEISSLER,A.M., HARRIS,W.S., SCHOENFELD,C.D.: Systolic time intervals in heart failure in man. Circulation **37**, 149 (1968).

75. WEISSLER,A.M., HARRIS,W.S., SCHOENFELD,C.D.: Bedside technics for the evaluation of ventricular function in man. Amer. J. Cardiol. **23**, 577 (1969).

76. WEISSLER,A.M., HARRIS,L.C., WHITE,G.D.: Left ventricular ejection time index in man. J. Appl. Physiol. **18**, 919 (1963).

77. WEISSLER,A.M., GAMEL,W.G., GRODE,H.E., COHEN,S., SCHOENFELD,C.D.: Effect of digitalis on ventricular ejection in normal human subjects. Circulation **29**, 721 (1964).

78. WEISSLER,A.M., KAMEN,A.R., BORNSTEIN,R.S., SCHOENFELD,C.D., COHEN,S.: Effect of deslanoside on the duration of the phases of ventricular systole in man. Amer. J. Cardiol. **15**, 153 (1965).

79. WEISSLER,A.M., LEWIS,R.P., LEIGHTON,R.F.: The systolic time intervals as a measure of left ventricular performance in man. In: YU,P.N., GOODWIN,J.F. (Eds.): Progress in Cardiology. Philadelphia: Lea & Febiger 1972.

80. WEISSLER,A.M., PEELER,R.G., ROEHLL,W.H., JR.: Relationships between left ventricular ejection time, stroke volume and heart rate in normal individuals and patients with cardiovascular disease. Amer. Heart J. **62**, 367 (1961).

81. WEISSLER,A.M., SHYDER,J.R., SCHOENFELD,C.D., COHEN,S.: Assay to digitalis glycosides in man. Amer. J. Cardiol. **17**, 768 (1966).

82. WIGGERS,C.J.: Studies on the consecutive phases of the cardiac cycle. I. The duration of the consecutive phases of the cardiac cycle and the criteria for their precise determination. Amer. J. Physiol. **56**, 415 (1921).

83. WIGGERS,C.J.: Studies on the consecutive phases of the cardiac cycle. II. The laws governing the relative durations of ventricular systole and diastole. Amer. J. Physiol. **56**, 439 (1921).

84. WILLEMS,J., DE GEEST,H., KESTELOOT,H.: On the value of apexcardiography for timing intracardiac events. Amer. J. Cardiol. **28**, 59 (1971).

85. WILLEMS,J., KESTELOOT,H.: The left ventricular ejection time. Its relation to heart rate, mechanical systole and some anthropometric data. Acta Cardiol. a22, 401 (1967).

86. WILLEMS,J., ROELANDT,J., DE GEEST,H., KESTELOOT,H., JOOSSENS,J.V.: Left ventricular ejection time in elderly subjects. Circulation **42**, 37 (1970).

Myocardial Circulation under Adalat in Different Phases of Coronary Diseases

H. Heeger, P. Kahn, and E. Aldor

Hanusch Hospital, Vienna, Austria

To test the effect of Adalat on myocardial blood perfusion, we treated 24 patients with coronary heart disease of different degree prior to coronarography according to Judkins with 20 mg Adalat sublingually.

Coronary blood flow was always determined before coronarography. Blood supply to the myocardium was assessed by the method developed by Ross et al. [4]. As indicator we used ^{133}xenon, which was selectively injected into the left coronary artery.

In contrast to other data in the literature [1, 5, 6], for blood-flow values in the left coronary artery at rest, we found in coronary patients at rest different blood-flow rates, depending on the extent of existing postnecrotic fibrosis [2]. The latter was determined by myocardial scintigraphy.

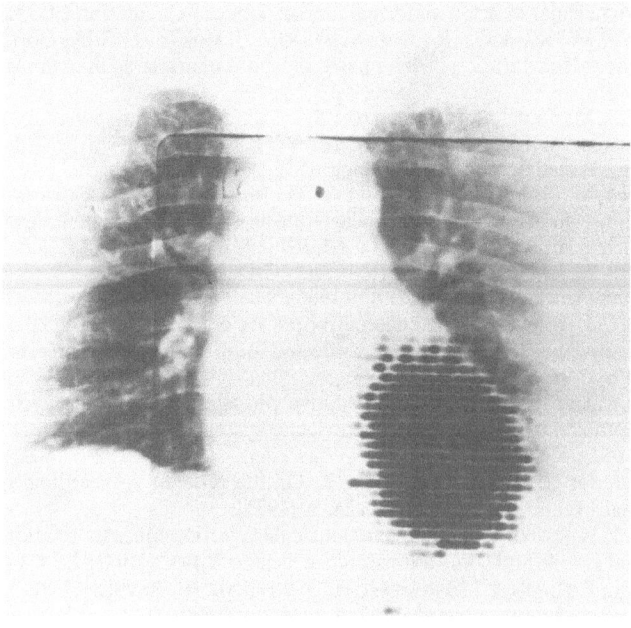

Fig. 1. Normal scintigram of the left coronary artery

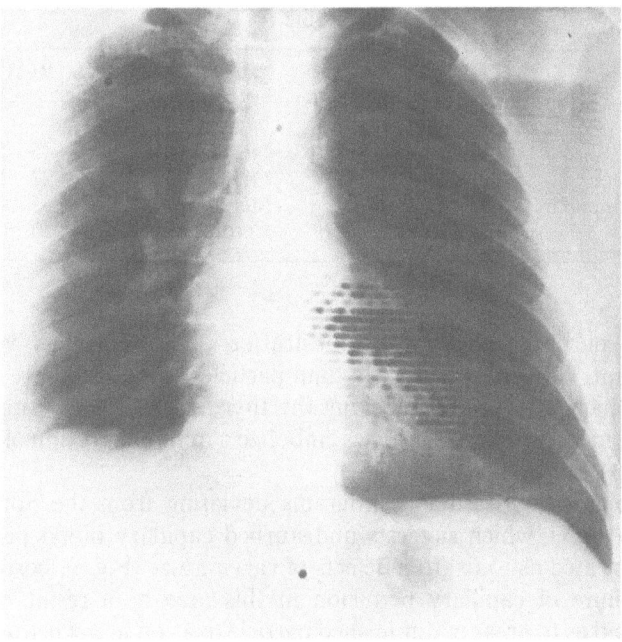

Fig. 2. Fixation defect in the left coronary scintigram; transmural anterior wall infarction

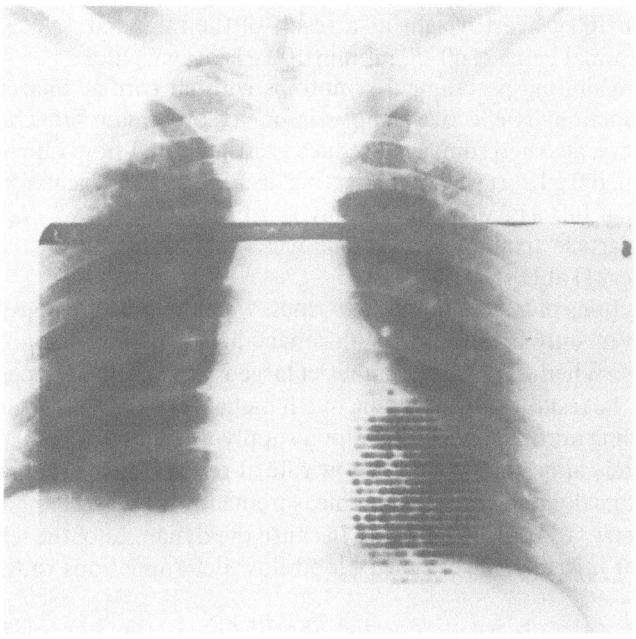

Fig. 3. Diminished particle fixation in the left coronary scintigram

Table 1

	LCA		RCA
Normal CBF	60—70 ml/min/100 g	Normal CBF	45—50 ml/min/100 g
Ant. wall infarct	30—45	Occlusion	22—34
Stenosis without infarct	50—60	Stenosis	35—45
Cardiomegaly	60—90	Cardiomegaly	50—65

For this purpose, following demonstration of the coronary vessels with a contrast agent, 200–300 µCi of [131]iodine particles (Hoechst) were injected into the left coronary artery, after blocking the thyroid gland with Lugol's solution. The injected macro-albumin particles embolize a minimal portion of the coronary capillaries [3].

Alterations in myocardial scintigrams deviating from the normal uniform blackening (Fig. 1), which suggests undisturbed capillary blood perfusion, have been differentiated as to fixation defects of varying size (Fig. 2), corresponding to complete failure of capillary perfusion in this area as a result of transmural infarction, and as to areas of diminished particle fixation in the perfusion area of a stenotic coronary branch (Fig. 3), indicating fibrosis localized mainly in the subendocardial myocardial layers in chronic angina pectoris.

A comparison of the results of coronary flow measurement, coronarography and myocardial scintigraphy shows in the area of the left coronary artery after transmural infarction a reduction of blood flow at rest (Table 1) to values between 30–45 ml/min/100 g heart weight as a result of the infarcted myocardial defect, against the normal value of 60–70 ml/min/100 g heart weight.

Patients exhibiting pectanginal symptoms without cardiac infarction, i.e. patients with functionally effective stenosis in one or both main branches of the left coronary artery, also had somewhat reduced resting blood-flow values of between 50–60 ml/min/100 g heart weight, indicating decrease of the vascular lumen due to subendocardial fibrosis, which in the myocardial scintigram was apparent as a diminished particle fixation. Conditions were similar in the area of the right coronary artery (Table 1).

The reductions of resting blood-flow rates, which in part are considerable, are found, however, only as long as the coronary heart disease has not yet led to cardiomegaly. When the heart becomes enlarged as a result of hypertrophy and dilatation of the residual myocardium, much higher flow rates are again recorded, often pretending normal myocardial blood supply.

Immediately after measuring the flow rate at rest, we gave each patient 20 mg Adalat sublingually and repeated the measurements, without changing the measuring geometry, at 5, 15, and 30 min. Because the dynamics of the left ventricula were of major interest, we restricted blood-flow determinations to the left coronary artery.

Throughout the observation period, the ECG was simultaneously obtained, and central aortic pressure and pressure in the left coronary artery were determined.

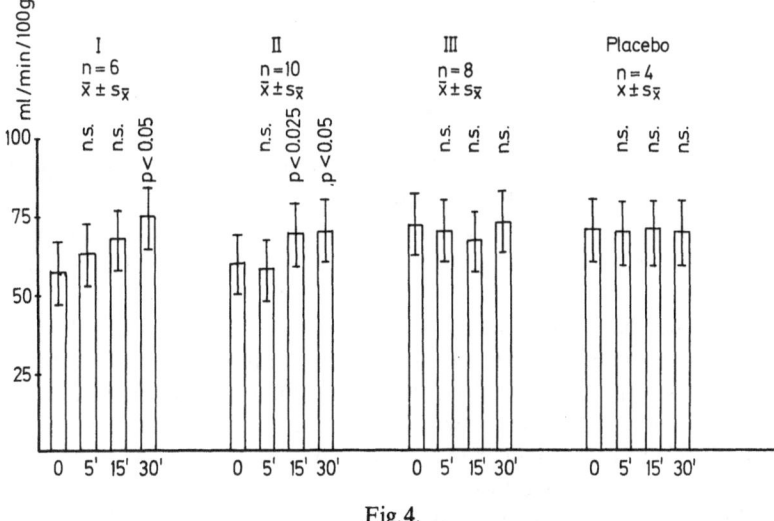

Fig. 4.

According to the increase in blood flow achieved, we divided our patients into three groups (Fig. 4).

The first group included patients in whom the flow rate increased by 30–40% or more, which we consider to be a normal response to the administered dose.

Patients in the second group showed an increase in coronary blood flow of between 15 and 30%.

In the third group, we included all patients in whom no or only a slight increase of up to 10% occurred.

Further differentiation of the patients within each group was based on the course of the blood-flow increase during the 30-minute observation period.

Normally, blood flow increased progressively, the highest flow rate being recorded at the end of the 30-minute observation period.

Within their group, patients with more severe myocardial damage achieved the maximum increase earlier, after 15 sometimes even after 5 min. They maintained this flow rate until the end of the 30-minute period, but in patients with damage of the highest category, the value fell back to base line earlier. Regularly connected with this phenomenon was a decrease of the mean central aortic pressure by 15–25 mm Hg; in dilated hearts showing little flow increase the decrease was as much as 40 mm Hg.

A pressure decrease does not seem to be a conditio sine qua non for the effect of Adalat. In one case we found an increase in blood supply, although the blood pressure did not fall. Such a rise may, however, be smaller without the extracardial effect of the substance.

To verify our test results, we conducted similar studies on 4 other patients with stenosing coronary sclerosis after administration of 2 placebos. Neither changes of the central aortic pressure nor of the measured blood-flow rates were found.

According to the results of this experimental series, the action of Adalat appears to be less dependent on the extent of coronary stenoses than on the functional condition of the myocardium. There exists, for example, no essential difference between the extent and localization of coronary lesions in group 2 and group 3 patients. Differences prevail, however, in the myocardial scintigrams. The patient not responding or only slightly responding to Adalat (group 3) show in general extensive defects of blood supply. One has to bear in mind that myocardial scintigraphy reveals only irreversible lesions of the myocardium, which often are the cause of cardial dilatation and therefore increased oxygen consumption, but which certainly cannot be modified by Adalat.

On the other hand, an infarction scar shown in the myocardial scintigram, unless its extent exceeds a critical limit, need not in any way cause a disturbance of the heart's contractility. As long as the residual myocardium is adequately supplied with blood, the blood-flow values at rest being reduced in relation to the myocardial defect, scarred hearts can be expected to respond with a normal increase in myocardial blood flow.

In addition, especially in the case of extensive myocardial fibrosis, we must assume the existence of *ischemic although still viable muscle areas* that on their part influence contractility but are not visible in the myocardial scintigram. These still reversible myocardial lesions are, in our opinion, significant for the effect of Adalat. If, besides infarct scars or fibroses of the heart muscle, such regional ischemias are present, the coronaries have already undergone compensatory metabolic dilatation. In such cases, only a slight possibility for medical enhancement of blood flow remains and eventually it will cease altogether.

In those cases in which, in the wake of coronary heart disease, cardiac dilatation occurred with increase in enddiastolic left-ventricular pressure, the heart's increased need for oxygen, which can be readily proved by Laplace's law, leads to increased blood flow at rest and thereby to maximum metabolic dilatation of the coronaries, so that only a limited flow increase is still possible.

Thus it can be said that when the effect of Adalat on myocardial blood flow is slight, it is suggestive of the existence of ischemic damage of the heart that may be the greater, the less response there is to a coronary dilator. Consequently, it can be expected that clinical application of Adalat will be especially effective in the pre-infarction stage, in which myocardial function is still well maintained, and that it will influence ischemic damage to the heart muscle to the extent that, it is reversible. The increased action observed with Adalat also suggests such temporary control of myocardial ischemia. Thus, a good correlation also exists for physical tolerance as measured by ergometric work; it grew in relation to the increase of myocardial blood flow effected by Adalat. On the other hand, in advanced scarring and chronic ischemia of the heart muscle, a therapeutic benefit can basely be expected any longer.

To conclude: Nifedipine is a coronary-active substance that, in coronary heart disease, permits the achievement of a substantial enhancement of myocardial blood supply as long as myocardial function is still largely preserved, probably by influencing myocardial ischemia. In advanced myocardial fibrosis and scarring, however, no essential increase of blood flow or improvement of ventricular function can be expected.

Abstract

In order to investigate the effect of Adalat on the myocardial blood flow we sublingually administered 20 mg Adalat each to 24 patients with coronary heart disease. The myocardial blood flow was measured by ^{133}xenon before and 5, 15, and 30 min after Adalat administration. Thereafter, the extent of the coronary disease was determined by coronary angiography, laevocardiography and perfusion scintigraphy. According to the extent of the achieved increase of the coronary blood flow we saw three different groups of patients:

1. a group of patients with an increase of 30–40% which can be considered as a normal reaction
2. a group of patients with an increase of 15–30% and
3. a group of patients with no or only a slight increase of 10% maximum.

A further classification of the patients could be made according to the increase of the coronary blood flow during the investigational period of 30 min after the administration of Adalat. This increase lasted the shorter the more the myocardium was damaged.

The effect of increasing the coronary blood flow depends on the functional state of the myocardium. Under Adalat, there might possibly be a temporary removal of the chronic myocardical ischemia. Therefore, Adalat is a coronary active substance, from which a considerable increase of the myocardical blood flow can be expected, especially in the pre-infarct state and under a still relatively good function of the myocardium.

References

1. CONTI,C.R., PITT,B., GUNDEL,W.D., FRIESINGER,G.C., ROSS,R.S.: Circulation **42**, 815 (1970).
2. HEEGER,H., ALDOR,E., KAHN,P.: Med. Klinik. **69**, 787 (1974).
3. HEEGER,H., KAHN,P., ALDOR,E., TURNHEIM,E.: Wien. Z. inn. Med. **84**, 13 (1973).
4. ROSS,R.S., UEDA,K., LICHTLEN,P.R., REES,J.R.: Circulation. Res. **15**, 28 (1964).
5. ROWE,G.G., THOMSON,J.H., STEMLING,R.: Circulation **39**, 139 (1969).
6. SULLIVAN,J.M., GORLIN,R.: Circ. Res. **21**, 919 (1967).

Discussion Remarks

LOCHNER: You said that the duration of the rise in coronary blood flow under Adalat depended on the severity of myocardial changes or damage. Have you expatiated upon this or furnished an explanation?

HEEGER: There is a misunderstanding here. We found that the rise in coronary blood flow under Adalat was *smaller* the more the heart muscle was damaged.

LOCHNER: My question was: Can you explain this?

HEEGER: We believe that when there are no longer dilatable vessels, then no further rise in blood flow is possible. In these cases also, in a long-term study, we saw no effect, whereas in patients who already had a resting blood flow increase, the described action of Adalat could be found. On the other hand, in these damaged hearts we could not establish clinically an increase in output.

Lichtlen: As I see it, group 3 in your last slide—those without an increase in coronary blood flow—had the highest resting flow. Why? If they were patients with isolated occlusions, e.g., an isolated occlusion of the ramus descendens and a normal circumflex, then one could imagine it. But in the case of patients with diffuse coronary sclerosis, then one would think that in spite of the flow there would not be much increase. Put another way, if there were isolated occlusions— which I partly assume on the basis of scintigraphy—there is no reason for an abnormal increase of flow.

Heeger: In group 3 there were only two or three vascular disorders and almost all had cardiac lesions. In addition, these patients all had enlarged hearts and signs of cardiac dilatation. For this reason I believe these cases had increased myocardial blood flow.

Session V

Clinical Aspects: Hemodynamics, Onset and Duration

Chairmen: H.Lydtin (München), P.F. Angelino (Cuneo)

Coronary and Left Ventricular Dynamics under Nifedipine in Comparison to Nitrates, Beta-Blocking Agents and Dipyridamole

P. LICHTLEN

Department of Internal Medicine, Division of Cardiology,
Medical University Hannover, Fed. Rep. Germany

Relief from angina pectoris, i.e. improvement of myocardial ischemia by means of medication, can be achieved in at least two ways:

1. by reducing the oxygen demand of the myocardium in general, thereby lessening the need for an increase in flow in the poststenotic, potentially ischemic areas of the myocardium, and

2. by increasing flow, mainly collateral flow to the ischemic area.

It is therefore necessary to understand the alterations of coronary dynamics leading to angina and thereby the mode of action of the antianginal drugs on the coronary system.

Angina develops whenever regional coronary flow drops below a critical level and anaerobic metabolism prevails (Fig. 1). Due to the low tissue oxygen pressure, the coronary arteriolar bed is maximally dilated in the underperfused area; poststenotic flow is maintained mainly through collaterals, blood being diverted from normal areas with a higher resistance toward the ischemic, low-resistance zone. Under conditions of increased oxygen demand, for instance during exercise, blood flow toward the normal areas becomes maximal due to a marked decrease of arteriolar resistance. This might reduce or even reverse collateral flow, thus rendering the poststenotic area truly ischemic.

This presentation is based on this pathophysiologic concept of angina and therefore concentrates mainly on the coronary effect of some antianginal drugs.

Methods

Using the xenon-residue-detection technique [7, 9], resting myocardial blood flow was recorded in 107 coronary patients undergoing coronary and left ventricular angiography before and after administration of nitroglycerin (0.4 mg, sublingually) and isosorbidedinitrate (5 mg, sublingually) as well as various beta-blocking agents (propranolol 0.07 mg/kg i.v., prindolol 0.01 mg/kg i.v., practolol 0.5 mg/kg i.v.), dipyridamole (0.5 mg/kg i.v.) and nifedipine (20 mg sublingually). All studies were performed not earlier than 30 min after angiography; they were combined with the recordings of right and left ventricular hemodynamics. For the

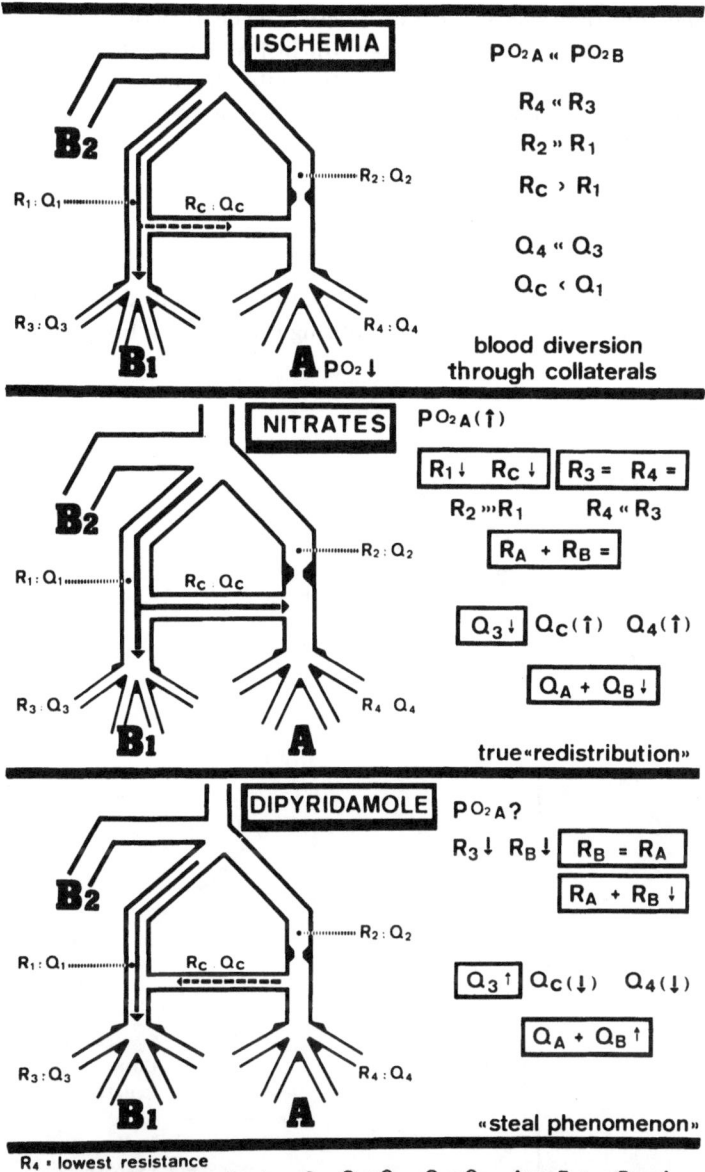

Fig. 1. Behavior of local coronary flow (Q) and resistance (R) in the normal (B_1, B_2) and the poststenotic areas (A). The situation is demonstrated for ischemia, medication with nitrates and dipyridamole. R_c collateral resistance, Q_c collateral flow, Q_3 and R_3 arteriolar flow and resistance in the normal area, Q_4 and R_4 in the poststenotic, potentially ischemic area. (From LICHTLEN [6])

nitrates, dypridamole and nifedipine, coronary dynamics were registered not only at rest, but also during exercise, comparing two exercise periods of equal work load, one representing the control period; all recordings began after the fifth minute of exercise, when a steady state had been reached. Furthermore, the effect of isosorbidedinitrate was studied at different levels of work load, the patients being subjected to three exercise periods, the last with a significantly higher load. For beta-blocking agents, flow studies were limited to rest; during exercise, only left ventricular hemodynamics were recorded. Methodological details have been described elsewhere [2, 6].

Results

1. Nitrates

Nitrates, when administered sublingually, were found to decrease global myocardial blood flow at rest [2] as well as during exercise [6]. Figure 2 contains the

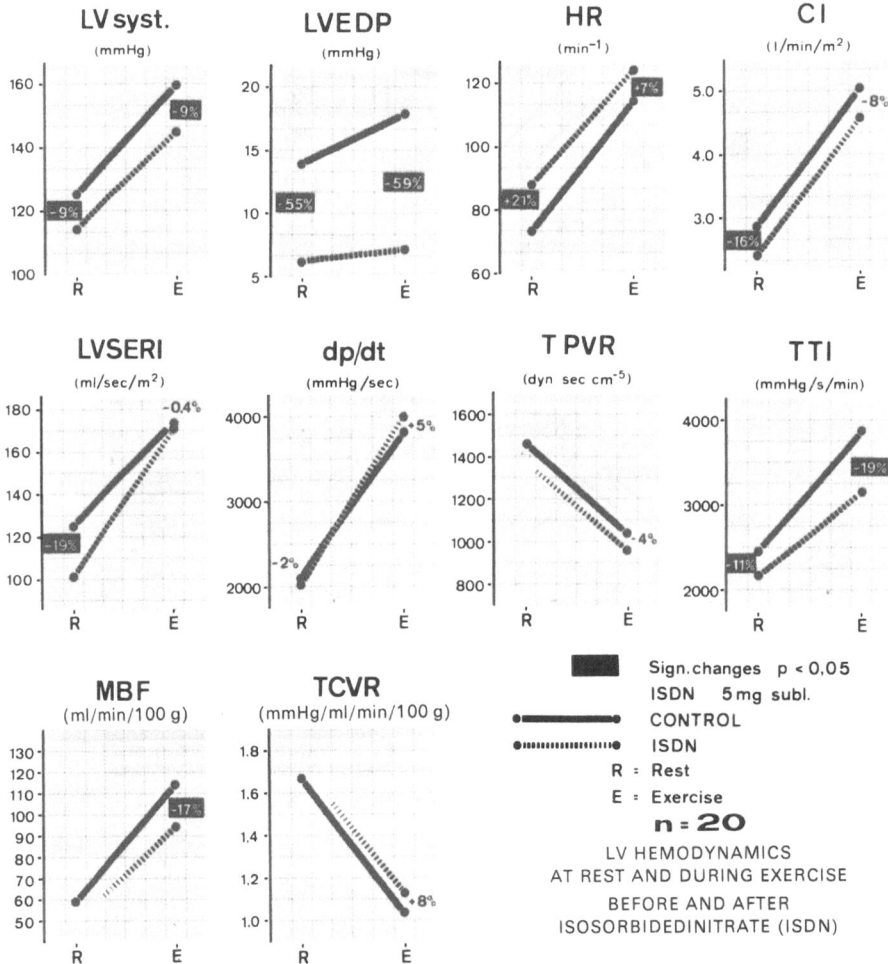

Fig. 2. Left ventricular and coronary dynamics at rest and during exercise before and after administration of isosorbidedinitrate. *LVsyst* left ventricular systolic pressure, *LVEDP* left ventricular enddiastolic pressure, *HR* heart rate, *CI* cardiac index, *LVSERI* left ventricular systolic ejection rate index, *TPVR* total peripheral vascular resistance, *TTI* tension-time-index, *MBF* myocardial blood flow, *TCVR* total coronary vascular resistance

findings from 20 patients undergoing two periods of exercise (bicycle ergometry) with identical work loads at an interval of approx. 10 min. The average work load amounted to approx. 65 watt, corresponding to a body oxygen consumption of approx. 940 ml/min. The nitrate led to a significant decrease in left ventricular systolic and enddiastolic pressure, cardiac index, stroke volume and stroke work index. Heart rate and dp/dt max showed a mild increase; peripheral resistance remained unchanged. The tension-time-index decreased significantly whereas the rate-pressure-product revealed only an insignificant reduction of -4%. This would suggest that myocardial oxygen consumption (MVO_2) did not change or decreased mildly, an excellent correlation being found between the rate-pressure-product, coronary flow and MVO_2 during exercise [5]. Myocardial blood flow was significantly lower during equal exercise (-17%), however—most importantly—coronary resistance remained unchanged after nitrates when work load, i.e. oxygen demand, was kept constant.

In order to further analyze the behavior of coronary resistance under nitrates, a number of patients were submitted to two exercise periods of different work

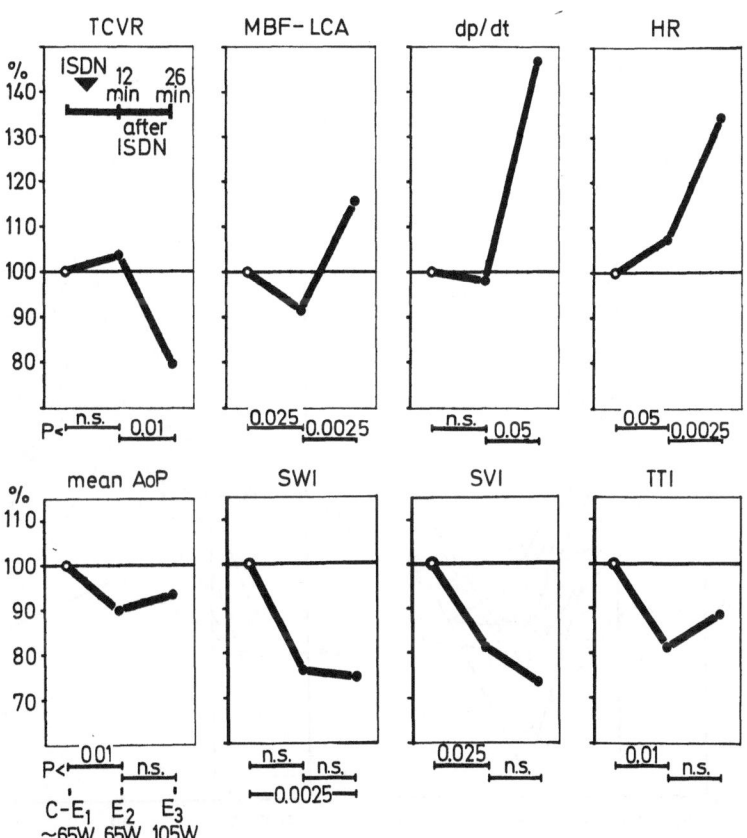

Fig. 3. Effect of isosorbidedinitrate (ISDN) during exercise. C-E_1 control exercise, E_2 exercise of equal load after ISDN, E_3 exercise of higher work load. The value of the control exercise represents 100%. Abbreviations as in Fig. 2, (see text). (From LICHTLEN [6])

loads (Fig. 3). First, a control exercise test was performed, then 5 mg isosorbidedinitrate were administered sublingually followed by an exercise period of equal
work—usually 65 watt—after which a third exercise period with a significantly
higher work load was carried out. Under equal work load (65 watt), there was
again a mild, yet significant decrease of myocardial blood flow; the higher load of
105 watt, however, resulted in a marked increase of myocardial blood flow. Under
equal work load, resistance remained unchanged; the increase of work and oxygen demand was, however, accompanied by a significant decrease (-23%) of
coronary resistance.

These changes of myocardial blood flow and resistance with higher work load
again followed closely the further rise of the rate-pressure-product, tension-time-
index and dp/dt max, i.e. the increase of MVO_2.

From these data, one has to conclude that nitrates, when administered sublingually, do not lead to substantial coronary arteriolar dilatation; in contrast, the
arteriolar bed is still capable of dilating further following the increased oxygen
demand, i.e. of reacting fully to beta-stimulation.

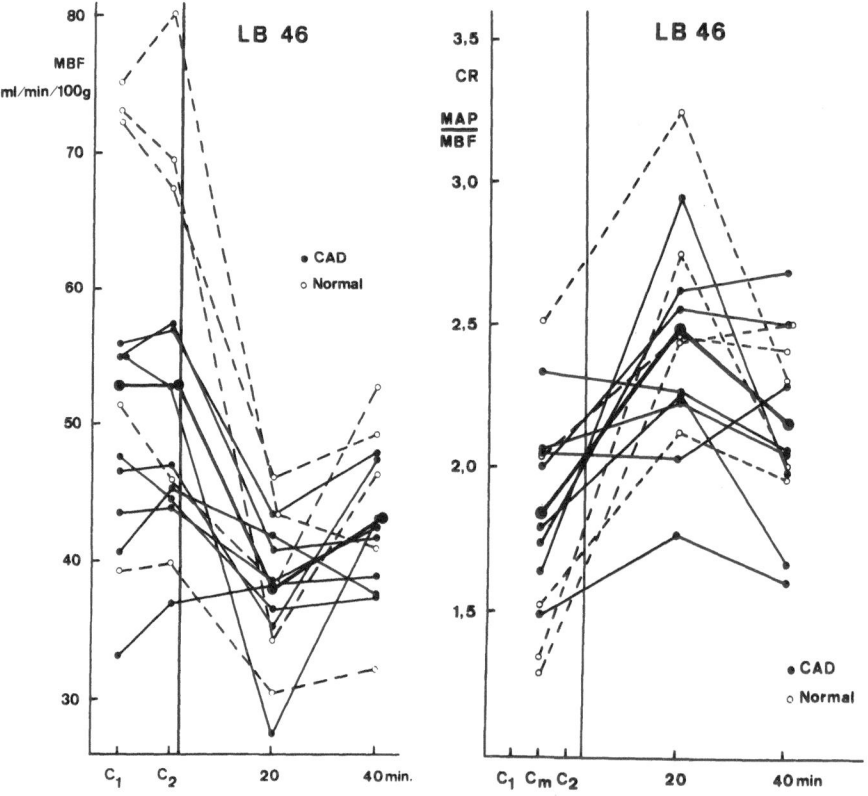

Fig. 4. The effect of prindolol (LB 46), 1 mg i.v., on myocardial blood flow (MBF) and total
coronary resistance (CR) at rest. C_1 and C_2 represent two control measurements at an interval
of 10 min

2. Beta-Blocking Agents

Beta-blocking agents also lead to a decrease of myocardial blood flow [8]. This is shown in Fig.4, demonstrating—as a typical example—the behavior of resting myocardial blood flow and resistance after intravenous administration of 1 mg prindolol. Two control recordings were followed by measurements 20 and 40 min after prindolol. There was a significant drop of myocardial blood flow in normal subjects as well as in patients with severe coronary artery disease, averaging 21%. However, in contrast to nitrates, this decrease of flow was accompanied by a significant increase of coronary resistance, amounting to 25%. Furthermore, MVO_2 was found to decrease by approx. 30% as did the rate-pressure-product and the tension-time-index [8] (Fig. 5). Thus, beta-blocking agents clearly reduce oxygen demand in the normal myocardium and probably also in the poststenotic potentially ischemic area. In addition, the increase of coronary resistance, probably due to the overwhelming action of the coronary alpha-receptors, might help shift blood from the normal toward the ischemic areas, where coronary arteriolar dilatation obviously still prevails due to the strong dilatory effect of hypoxia.

3. Dipyridamole

In contrast to nitrates and beta-blocking agents, the administration of dipyridamole results in a marked increase of resting coronary flow, accompanied by a

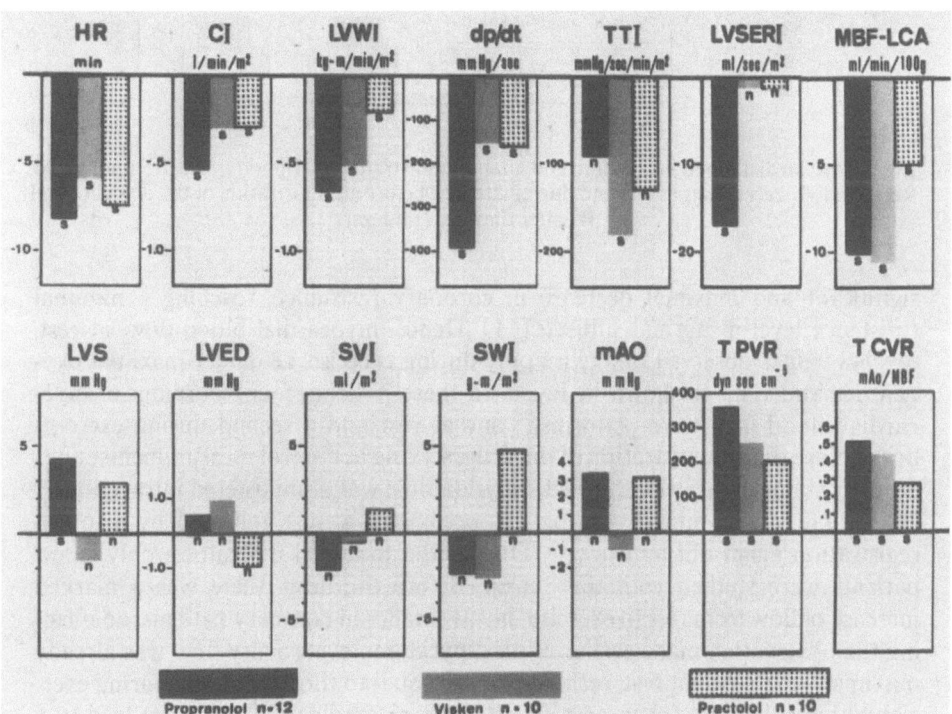

Fig. 5. Left ventricular and coronary dynamics after propranolol (0.07 mg/kg i.v.), prindolol (Visken) (0.01 mg/kg i.v.) and practolol (0.5 mg/kg i.v.). The columns represent the differences in comparison to the control values. Abbreviations as in Figs. 2 and 3. (From MOCCETTI [8])

MYOCARDIAL BLOOD FLOW ¹³³Xenon

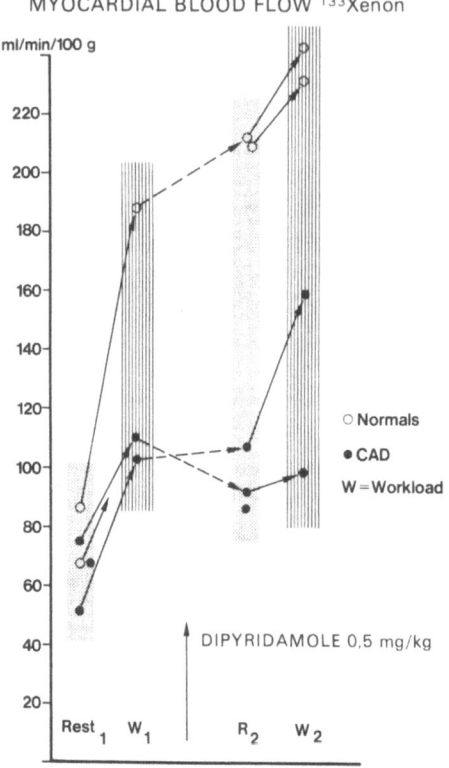

Fig. 6. Myocardial blood flow before and after administration of dipyridamole (0.5 mg/kg i.v.). Rest₁ and W_1 recordings at rest and during exercise before administration of the drug, R_2 and W_2 after the drug (see text)

significant and maximal decrease in coronary resistance, reaching a minimal resistance level in normal subjects [11]. Hence, myocardial blood flow, at rest, reaches values observed otherwise only during exercise, i.e. under maximal oxygen demand. This is shown in Fig. 6. In these patients, four recordings of myocardial blood flow were performed: one at rest and a second during exercise, both before the administration of the drug, serving as control measurements; after a steady state had been established, dipyridamole was administered intravenously (0.5 mg/kg), and a third recording was performed at rest, followed by a fourth registration again during exercise. Due to the technical difficulties, only a few patients were studied with this set-up. Before the drug, there was a marked increase of flow from rest to exercise; it was smaller in coronary patients, confirming the observation made earlier. With dipyridamole, coronary flow was already maximally increased at rest, reaching values equal to those observed during exercise without the drug. Thus, exercise after dipyridamole usually did not lead to a further or marked increase of flow. Based on these results, one has to conclude that the administration of dipyridamole, in contrast to nitrates or beta-blocking agents, is followed by maximal coronary arteriolar dilatation. Thus, any increase of myocardial oxygen demand, for instance during exercise, does not lead to a further decrease in coronary resistance. Obviously, this drug produces a kind of "luxury perfusion", mainly in normal areas of the myocardium; on the other hand, this maximal dilatation might lead to a diversion of blood from the post-stenotic areas to the normal zones of lower resistance, thus reversing collateral flow and producing a "steal phenomenon" similar to the mechanism of angina during exercise discussed at the beginning of this paper. Indeed, several laboratories have reported the occurrence of angina during exercise after administration of dipyridamole. It should be added that in a group of 10 patients studied at rest, no changes of the rate-pressure-product and tension-time-index were found; thus, an increase of myocardial oxygen consumption with this drug, as reported by another group using the argon-method to record myocardial blood flow, seems rather unlikely [11].

4. Nifedipine

Based on our study, nifedipine was found to have an action differing from that of beta-blocking agents, nitrates and dipyridamole. Figure 7 illustrates changes of resting myocardial blood flow and resistance in 8 patients. Fifteen min after sublingual administration of 20 mg nifedipine, a mild, yet significant increase of +18% in resting myocardial blood flow from an average of 45 to 56 ml/min/100 g was observed, accompanied by a significant 24% decrease of coronary resistance from 2.26 to 1.67 units. This effect was most pronounced in patients with mild coronary disease and normal resting flow values; it was minimal in patients with severe, triple vessel disease and extremely high resting resistance values.

These changes were accompanied by a mild, yet significant decrease of left ventricular systolic and enddiastolic pressure as well as of stroke volume and stroke work index. Heart rate, tension-time-index, rate-pressure-product and dp/dt max, however, revealed a significant 10–20% increase. From these data, one would conclude that overall myocardial oxygen consumption did not change much or increased only slightly [4].

In order to further analyze the behavior of the arteriolar bed, myocardial blood flow was studied during exercise, i.e. bicycle ergometry (Fig. 8). Prior to the administration of nifedipine, a significant 11% increase of myocardial blood flow from rest (50 ml/min/100 g) to exercise (105 ml/min/100 g) was observed, following closely the increase in rate-pressure-product; however, when exercise was repeated with an equal work load, nifedipine did not lead to a further change of flow. At the same time, from rest to exercise, coronary resistance decreased from 1.92 to 1.25 units, that is −41%, yet again, no change was seen after nifedipine, i.e. from the first control- to the second exercise period.

Exercise was followed by a slight reduction of left ventricular systolic and enddiastolic pressure whereas heart rate and dp/dt max again showed a significant, yet small increase; in contrast to the behavior at rest, tension-time-index and rate-pressure-product remained unchanged during exercise, suggesting that overall oxygen consumption had remained unaltered. One may therefore assume that nifedipine leads to only mild coronary arteriolar dilatation, the arteriolar bed still being susceptible for beta-stimulation [4].

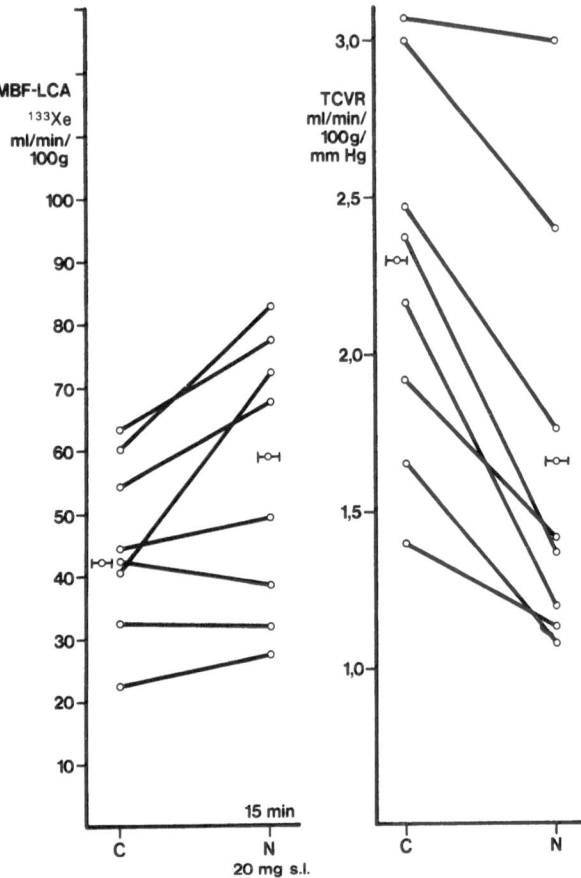

Fig. 7. Myocardial blood flow (MBF) and total coronary resistance (TCVR) at rest before and 15 min after administration of nifedipine (20 mg sublingually)

This point is further illustrated in Fig. 9 by combining the results of myocardial blood flow and coronary resistance at rest as well as during exercise, indicating single and average values. At rest, a 19% increase of myocardial blood flow, and a 21% drop of coronary resistance were observed; without the drug, exercise was followed by a 123% increase of flow and a 47% decrease of resistance. After nifedipine, average exercise flow and resistance reached identical levels. Most important, however: exercise flow values were significantly higher than resting values after nifedipine. Thus, in contrast to dipyridamole, the dilatory effect of nifedipine on the coronary arteriolar bed is obviously not a maximal one, the coronary arteriolar system still remaining susceptible to sympathetic stimulation and dilatation during exercise, i.e. to increased oxygen demand. It can therefore be assumed that nifedipine—like nitroglycerin—does not produce a change of collateral flow. Due to the uninhibited action of the beta-adrenergic system, there is, however, a significant increase in heart rate and dp/dt max mainly at rest, a phenomenon also observed with nitroglycerin.

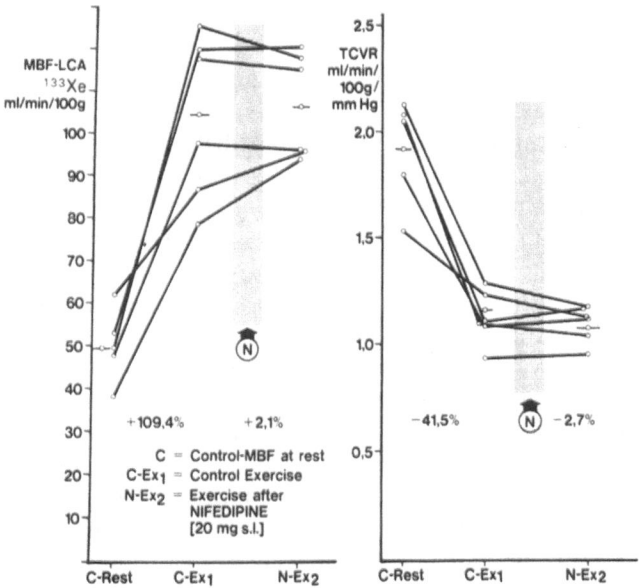

Fig. 8. Myocardial blood flow and coronary resistance during exercise before and after administration of nifedipine. Before nifedipine, there is a significant increase of flow and decrease of resistance from rest to exercise; under equal work loads, nifedipine did not change the control values during exercise

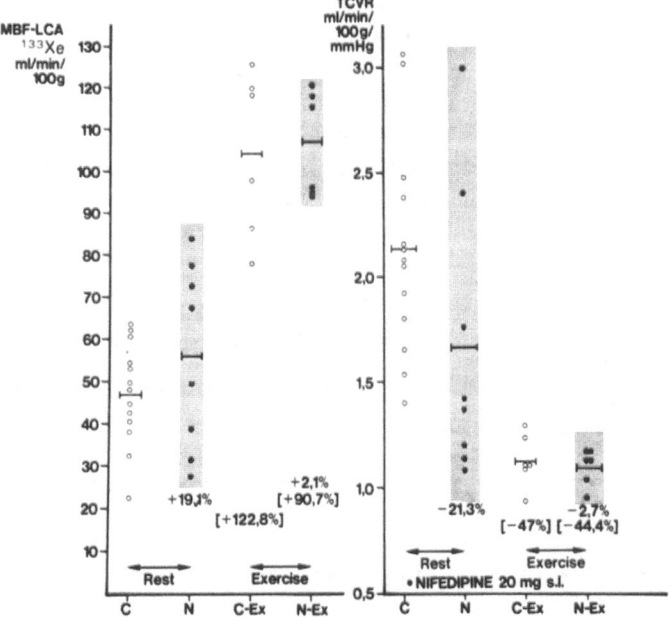

Fig. 9. Flow and resistance changes at rest and during exercise before and after nifedipine. C control at rest, N nifedipine values at rest, C_{ex} control value during exercise, N_{ex} nifedipine value during exercise (see text)

Conclusions (Table 1)

With regard to the coronary system, antianginal drugs can exhibit at least two effects:

1. They either lead to a decrease of myocardial blood flow, as in the case of nitroglycerin and beta-blocking agents, or 2. result in an increase of coronary flow, as observed mainly with dipyridamole and, to a lesser degree, with nifedipine. In the first group, a behavior difference is observed with regard to coronary resistance—it remains unchanged with nitroglycerin, yet increases considerably with beta-blocking agents. In the second group, a distinct difference in the amount and probably also in the type of coronary arteriolar dilatation is observed: Dipyridamole is followed by maximal coronary dilatation whereby the arteriolar tone is no longer susceptible to beta-stimulation. With nifedipine, coronary dilatation is only slight and arteriolar tone is preserved, i.e. beta-stimulation through exercise still produces a further increase in flow and a reduction of resistance. These observations lead to speculations on what is happening on the regional level, i.e. in the poststenotic, potentially ischemic zone of the myocardium where resistance vessels can, as a rule, be assumed to be maximally dilated due to hypoxia. Under nitroglycerin, where coronary resistance is unchanged, collateral flow is probably elevated, leading to a further rise of poststenotic flow [1, 3, 12]. The same is probably true for beta-blocking agents [1], leading to a higher resistance in the normal coronary bed and thereby obviously diverting blood to the ischemic area where resistance is suspected to remain low in spite of beta-blockade. Dipyridamole results in a maximal decrease of arteriolar tone in the normal area; in this way, flow might be diverted from the poststenotic area, thus producing a "steal phenomenon" [3, 10, 12] (Fig. 1). With nifedipine, coronary resistance is mildly decreased, indicating a minimal degree of arteriolar dilatation, probably enhancing collateral flow by collateral dilatation and increasing poststenotic regional flow. Thus, on the coronary level, nifedipine has an action on its own, differing both from the nitrates and dipyridamole as well as from beta-blockers. With regard to the hemodynamic changes [4], the similarity to the nitrates is obvious—both drugs lead to a decrease in left ventricular systolic and enddiastolic pressure,

Table 1

	Flow myocardium		Resistance myocardium		Arteriolar tone	Collateral flow	Hemodynamics				
							LV Pressure		HR	dp/dt max	MVO$_2$
	normal	post-stenotic	normal	post-stenotic			syst.	end-diast.			
NTG n = 47	↓	↑=	=	=	+	↑	↓	↓	↑	[↑]	[↓]=
BBL n = 32	↓	↑?	↑	?	[+]	↑?	↓	↑	↓	↓	↓
DIP n = 6	↑	↓=?	↓	=	−	↓steal	=	=	=	=	=
NIF n = 25	↑	↑=?	↓	?	+	↑	↓	↓	↑	↑	[↑]=

followed by a secondary increase in heart rate and dp/dt max, leaving average MVO_2 almost unchanged.

Based on these results, the calcium-antagonistic action of nifedipine represents a new pharmacological principle in treating angina pectoris; it produces a mild coronary arteriolar dilatation without interfering with the beta-adrenergic and metabolic vasomotor regulation and without causing any adverse changes of left ventricular function.

Abstract

Using the xenon-residue-detection-technique to record global myocardial blood flow, coronary dynamics were investigated at rest and, in some instances, under exercise after administration of various antianginal drugs in patients with angiographically proven coronary artery disease. The study included nifedipine, nitrates, beta-blocking agents (propranolol, pindolol, practolol) and dipyridamole.

Results: Nitrates and betablockers led to a significant decrease in coronary flow at rest; under nitrates, flow was also reduced at exercise when compared to control values obtained with identical work load (no exercise-flow-studies were done with betablockers). In contrast a marked increase in coronary flow after nifedipine and dipyridamole was observed already at rest; however, with these substances, flow remained unchanged under exercise and did not differ from exercise-flow without the drug or the resting values. With regard to coronary resistance, no changes were seen under nitrates at rest as well as under exercise; however, resistance decreased further with increasing work load, that is oxygen consumption (MVO_2) in spite of the nitrate; under betablockers, a significant increase in coronary resistance was found already at rest. On the other hand, nifedipine and dipyridamole led to a marked decrease in coronary resistance already at rest without further substantial decrease in coronary resistance under exercise.

Conclusions: It therefore seems that nifedipine leads to a considerable arteriolar dilatation in human beings, similar to the one observed after dipyridamole, although of a lesser magnitude. In contrast to dipyridamole, however, the increase in resting flow under nifedipine is associated with a significant rise of the rate-pressure-product, indicating a rise in MVO_2. This means that nifedipine leads, at least partially, to a secondary dilatory effect and that in contrast to dipyridamole, arteriolar tone is still maintained, at least to a certain extent, a situation similar to the one observed for nitrates. The various possible mechanisms for these flow changes will be discussed, especially also in relation to left ventricular hemodynamics.

References

1. BECKER, L., PITT, B.: Regional myocardial blood flow, ischemia and antianginal drugs. Ann. Clin. Res. **3**, 353 (1971).
2. BERNSTEIN, L. G., FRIESINGER, G. C., LICHTLEN, P. R., ROSS, R. S.: The effect of nitroglycerin on the systemic and coronary circulation in man and dogs. Myocardial blood flow measured with xenon 133. Circulation **33**, 107, 1966.

3. Fam,W.M., McGregor,M.: Effect of coronary vasodilator drugs on retrograde flow in areas of chronic myocardial ischemia. Circul. Res. **15**, 355 (1964).

4. Lichtlen,P.: The influence of Nifedipine on left ventricular and coronary dynamics at rest and under exercise in patients with coronary disease. "New Therapy of Ischemic Heart Disease", 1st Intern. Nifedipine "Adalat" Symposium, p.114. Tokyo: Univ. Tokyo Press 1975.

5. Lichtlen,P., Gattiker,K., Scholer,Y., Schibli,R.: Koronarfluß unter Arbeit bei Koronarsklerose, gemessen anhand der präkordialen Xenon-Clearance-Technik. Verhandl. Dtsch. Ges. Kreislaufforschung **39**, 301 (1973).

6. Lichtlen,P., Halter,J., Gattiker,K.: The effect of Isosorbidedinitrate on coronary flow, coronary resistance and left ventricular dynamics under exercise in patients with coronary artery disease. Basic Research in Cardiology **69**, 402 (1974).

7. Lichtlen,P., Moccetti,T., Halter,J.: Myocardial blood flow in man as shown by the precordial Xenon-Clearance-Technique. In: Maseri,A. (Ed.): "Myocardial Blood Flow in Man", Intern. Symp., Pisa 1971, p.309. Torino: Minerva Medica 1972.

8. Moccetti,T., Halter,J., Lichtlen,P.: Koronare und linksventrikuläre Dynamik dreier Substanzen mit unterschiedlicher beta-blockierender Wirkung: Propranolol, Prindolol, Practolol. Schweiz. Med. Wschr.**102**, 422 (1972).

9. Ross,R.S., Ueda,K., Lichtlen,P.R., Rees,R.J.: Measurements of myocardial blood flow in animals and man by selective injection of radioactive inert gas into the coronary arteries. Circul. Res. **15**, 28 (1964).

10. Schaper,W., Lewi,P., Flameng,W., Gijpen,L.: Myocardial steal produced by coronary vasodilatation in chronic coronary artery occlusion. Basic Res. Cardiol. **68**, 3 (1973).

11. Strauer,B.E., Tauchert,M., Heiss,H.W., Kochsiek,K., Bretschneider,H.J.: Relation between coronary blood flow, oxygen consumption and cardiac work in patients with and without angina pectoris. In: Maseri,A. (Ed.): "Myocardial Blood Flow in Man", Intern. Symp., p.465, Pisa 1971. Torino: Minerva Medica 1972.

12. Winbury,M.M., Howe,B.B., Weiss,H.R.: Effect of nitroglycerin and dipyridamole on epicardial and endocardial oxygen tension—further evidence for redistribution of myocardial blood flow. J. Pharmacol. Exper. Therap. **176**, 184 (1971).

Effect of Adalat (Nifedipine) on Left Ventricular Hemodynamics in Angina Pectoris (Comparative Study with Propranolol)

A. KURITA

Cedars Sinai Medical Center, Los Angeles, USA

M. KANAZAWA, H. HAMAMOTO, and G. MABUCHI

Nippon Medical School, Tokyo, Japan

Recently in Japan there have been several papers published concerning the mechanism of action of nifedipine in animal experiments [7, 8] and its efficacy in angina pectoris in clinical studies [11]. KIMURA et al. [10] studied its efficacy in treating angina pectoris by sequential analysis (Armitage); they concluded that it was almost as effective as isosorbide dinitrate and propranolol.

There are, however, no reports about the effects of nifedipine on left ventricular function during an attack of angina pectoris, so we decided to investigate its effect on left ventricular function. In this study we chose propranolol for the comparative agent, because the mode of action of propranolol is now considered to be more clearly defined than that of other antianginal agents.

Materials and Methods

Hemodynamic studies were performed in 17 patients with anginal pectoris (14 male and 3 female, 37–70 years). All patients had experienced typical anginal attacks, and their electrocardiograms did not demonstrate any remarkable changes in resting time other than ischemic ST, T wave changes, as determined by Master's double or treadmill test. To establish the minimal work load, exercise training was carried out with Ogawa's[1] bicycle ergometer at least 3–5 times prior to the experiment. Under local anesthesia, the right brachial artery and vein were isolated in the antecubital fossa. The tip of a No. 8 Cournand catheter was positioned in the right atrium, and a No. 8 Lehman catheter was advanced from the brachial artery to the left ventricle. Aortic pressure was measured by the same catheter. Pressures were measured with P 23 Db Statham strain gauges and cardiac output measurements made using a dye dilution technique. The V_5 of the electrocardiogram was monitored. Measurements were recorded on a Hewlett

---

[1] Institute of Tokyo Metropolitan Technology.

Packard 8890 A or Nihonkoden MR 2. Control pressure measurements were obtained, and supine leg exercise were carried out at the predetermined work load. Pressures were measured at the nearly maximum work load. Cardiac output was determined during the final 30 sec of this exercise period.

After the patients had rested for 15–20 min, control pressure, cardiac output and heart rate were again determined. In 9 patients, 0.02–0.03 mg/kg of nifedipine were given intravenously within 5 min, and in 8 patients 3–4 mg propranolol were given intravenously within 5 min. Approximately 5–10 min after administration of the medications, the patients performed a second series of supine leg exercises at the same work load as the initial exercise, and similar hemodynamic measurements were made. Calculation: Maximal rate of left ventricular systolic pressure (*dp/dt*) was obtained using a Hewlett Packard or Nihonkoden differentiating pressure amplifier. Vmax was obtained by the method of MASON [12], and the average of 3 items was used in this study. Tension-time index was determined using the formula:

TTI = LVm × HR × SEP

where LVm = mean left ventricular pressure in mm Hg, HR = heart rate in beats/min and SEP = systolic ejection period mm/sec. Left ventricular work was determined by the formula:

$$LVW = \frac{(LVSP - LVEDP) \times CI \times 13.6}{1000} \text{ (kg M/min/M}^2\text{)}.$$

Results

Effect of Exercise on Left Ventricular Hemodynamics

The hemodynamic changes after exercise are summarized in Table 1. Since we did not have a control group of normal subjects, we compared our results with those of other investigators. Our results of hemodynamic changes during exercise

Table 1. Effect of exercise on left ventricular hemodynamics (per cent change)

	Ischemic heart disease group				Normal subjects	
	KURITA et al. n = 17	PARKER et al. n = 13	WIENER et al. [17] n = 10	GAASH et al. [5] n = 5	PARKER et al. n = 7	GAASH et al. [5] n = 2
HR	49	60	47	22	69	
BPm	13	17		18	19	
LVEDP	103	302	180	69	12	no change
CI	52	55	38		101	
SI	0	−5	−10		15	
dp/dt	46	27	47	16	83	22
LVW	54	89	29		179	
TTI	66	88	79		128	
Vmax	42			no change 3 cases −18 to 20 2 cases		38

from ischemic heart disease patients showed tendencies that were similar to those reported by other investigators.

The most remarkable change in the ischemic group was the elevation of left ventricular enddiastolic pressure which increased by 103% ($p < 0.01$). PARKER et al. [9, 15] and WIENER et al. [17] reported that left ventricular enddiastolic pressure rose by 180% and 302% ($p < 0.01$). Max dp/dt, heart rate, cardiac index and tension-time index changed between 46 and 66% ($p < 0.01$).

In normal subjects, cardiac index, max dp/dt, LVW and tension-time index were more remarkably changed than in the ischemic group, but the change in left ventricular enddiastolic pressure was less.

Vmax in our group increased by 42%, but in 2 patients it decreased somewhat. GAASCH et al. [5] reported no change in 3 patients and on 18–20% decrease in 2 patients who had developed angina pectoris.

Effects of Nifedipine During Exercise

Table 2 is a summary of the hemodynamic response to nifedipine observed during exercise-induced angina. After medication but before exercise, left ventricular enddiastolic pressure was not significantly changed. During exercise after nifedipine, it increased to 19 ± 3 mm Hg; the difference between pre- and postmedication values was statistically significant ($p < 0.01$). There were no significant changes noted in heart rate, stroke index, max dp/dt, tension-time index and LVW before and during exercise after medication. Vmax increased from 1.8 ± 0.6 to 2.5 ± 0.8 muscle length/sec before medication.

Postmedication, Vmax rose only from 1.9 ± 0.8 to 2.0 ± 0.8 muscle length/sec; the difference during exercise between pre- and postmedication values was significant ($p < 0.01$).

Table 2. Hemodynamic effects of nifedipine at rest and during exercise-induced angina

	HR	BAm	LVEDP	dp/dt	TTI	CI	LVW	Vmax
Rest (m)	69	105	13	1376	1613	2.2	3.6	1.8
(SD)	9	9	3	203	403	0.5	1.1	0.6
Ex.	102	116	27	1908	2342	3.1	5.7	2.5
	20	7	7	351	508	1.6	1.3	0.8
Rest (N)	69	105	15	1396	1634	2.1	3.8	1.9
	10	8	3	213	547	0.6	1.8	0.8
Ex. (N)	98	111	19	1857	2291	2.7	6.4	2.0
	17	11	3	366	426	0.4	3	0.8
No. of subjects	9	9	9	9	9	6	6	9
P value	N.S.	N.S.	< 0.01	N.S.	N.S.	N.S.	N.S.	<0.01

m = mean, SD = standard deviation.
Ex. = final 30 sec of first exercise period.
Rest (N) = rest period after nifedipine.
Ex. (N) = final 30 sec of second exercise period after nifedipine.

Table 3. Hemodynamic effects of propranolol at rest and during exercise-induced angina

	HR	BAm	LVEDP	dp/dt	TTI	CI	LVW	Vmax
Rest (m)	81	104	11	1726	1300	3.1	5.8	2.0
(SD)	4	12	3	625	321	1	3	0.9
Ex.	112	119	23	2503	2187	4.5	9.2	2.8
	13	14	7	974	445	2	5	1.6
Rest (P)	75	97	12	1641	1205	3.1	5.6	1.7
	9	11	4	608	267	2	4	0.5
Ex. (P)	96	107	23	1857	1739	4.1	7.8	1.9
	9	13	5	815	313	2	5	0.5
No. of subjects	8	8	8	8	8	7	7	8
P value	<0.05	N.S.	N.S.	< 0.05	< 0.05	N.S.	N.S.	<0.05

m = mean, SD = standard deviation.
Ex. = final 30 sec of first exercise period.
Rest (P) = rest period after propranolol.
Ex. (P) = final 30 sec of second exercise period after propranolol.

Effects of Propranolol During Exercise

Table 3 contains a summary of the hemodynamic changes in response to propranolol observed during exercise-induced angina. Before exercise, heart rate, mean brachial pressure, max dp/dt, tension time index and Vmax were slightly suppressed, but the left ventricular enddiastolic pressure was not changed after propranolol.

During exercise after propranolol, however, heart rate, max dp/dt tension-time index and Vmax were suppressed; statistically significant ($p < 0.05$). Mean brachial pressure, cardiac index and left ventricular work tended to be suppressed, but the differences were not statistically significant.

Left ventricular enddiastolic pressure was not changed before and during exercise by propranolol.

Discussion

Our results of hemodynamic changes after exercise were similar to those previously reported by other investigators [9, 15]. PARKER and co-workers [9] reported that the most remarkable change elicited during a 7-minute exercise period by a predetermined work load was the elevation of left ventricular enddiastolic pressure by 302%.

On the other hand, WIENER et al. [17] reported a change of 180%, and GAASCH et al. [5] reported a change of 69%.

GAASCH et al. [5] reported that Vmax did not change after exercise in the nonanginal group, and that it was depressed in the anginal group.

Depressed Vmax in angina pectoris was also observed in a pacing study. CONTI et al. [3] reported that the peak Vce and Vmax fell in those patients who developed typical angina pectoris during pacing. In the 8 patients who did not develop angina pectoris, peak *Vce* and *V*max continued to rise or remained constant with an increasing rate. The authors concluded that peak *Vce* and *V*max normally increase with increasing heart rate, but decrease when myocardial ischemia is produced. Although there is some controversy about *V*max [1], it is still considered that *V*max may reflect a facet of contractility. QUINONES and co-workers [16] analyzed the left ventricular response to isometric exercise, using *V*max as one factor of a contractility index.

Our results showed an increase in *V*max of 42%, despite a decrease in 2 cases who had typical angina pectoris; this decrease was to be due primarily to minimal work loads. However, our hemodynamic data taken during exercise (Table 1) showed enough work load that developed an impaired left ventricular function and that could observe the mode of action of medication.

In this study, some of the hemodynamic responses to nifedipine confirmed the data (Table 2). The decreases in left ventricular enddiastolic pressure and *V*max were the primary results from our study. The decrease in left ventricular enddiastolic pressure was also observed after nitroglycerin. Although the mechanism of action of nitroglycerin is uncertain, it has been suggested that it may act by reducing myocardial oxygen needs through reduction of left ventricular volume or through an increase in coronary blood flow to ischemic areas or both [2, 13, 14].

Following intravenous administration of propranolol during exercise, the suppression of heart rate, tension time index, left ventricular work and max dp/dt was observed in this study. After propranolol, left ventricular enddiastolic pressure was higher at rest and during exercise in most patients in the presence of decreased or unchanged left ventricular stroke work. During exercise after propranolol, tension-time index, systolic ejection rate and left ventricular work were significantly lower than during the initial exercise period; such changes would be expected to reduce the myocardial oxygen requirement [15].

DWYER and co-workers [4] also reported that propranolol at rest and during exercise caused a decrease in heart rate, cardiac output, mean systolic ejection rate, stroke volume, left ventricular systolic pressure, first derivative and work. Left ventricular enddiastolic pressure did not change significantly.

They concluded that the improvement caused by propranolol was derived primarily from suppression of positive chronotropic and inotropic responses, which are major determinants of myocardial oxygen consumption.

Comparing these typical antianginal agents (Table 4), the suppression of elevation of left ventricular enddiastolic pressure is a common action with nitroglycerin and suppression of *V*max is the common action with propranolol.

HASHIMOTO et al. [7] reported in animal studies that the principal effect of nifedipine was the dilatation of coronary vasculature with increase of total cardiac output. Venous return was simultaneously increased, pulse pressure was increased due to reduction of blood pressure in diastole, and thus mean systemic pressure was slightly reduced. Nifedipine also caused negative chronotropic, dromotropic and inotropic effects. Although our data had no significant effect on left ventricular functions at rest, our results during exercise after medication were similar to these results.

GRÜN and FLECKENSTEIN [6] reported that nifedipine can completely block excitation-contraction coupling in potassium-depolarized coronary smooth mus-

Table 4. Effects of antiangial agents on left ventricular functions during exercise

	Effect of exercise $n=17$	Nifedipine $n=9$	Propranolol $n=8$
HR	↑	→	↓
BAm	↑	→	→
LVEDP	↑	↓	→
dp/dt	↑	→	↓
TTI	↑	→	↓
CI	↑	→	→
LVW	↑	→	→
Vmax	↑	↓	↓

cle preparations so that the contractile responses disappear. They reported that nitroglycerin proved to be an extremely strong and specific Ca-antagonistic coronary vasodilator, and it is expected that nifedipine will have similar pharmacological effects similar to those of nitroglycerin. The present study suggested that a decrease in left ventricular enddiastolic pressure would be effective in the treatment of angina pectoris, because, according to Laplace's law, a decrease in left ventricular enddiastolic pressure and dimension contributes toward diminished myocardial wall tension and thus to a decline in oxygen demand of the heart, which may reflect the suppression of Vmax.

We therefore concluded that the mode of action of nifedipine may be different from that of nitroglycerin and propranolol.

Abstract

The hemodynamic response to Adalat was compared with propranolol in 17 anginal patients induced by bicycle ergometer during left heart catheterization. During the procedures, anginal pain was occured in five among of these patients. After excercise left ventricular enddiastolic pressure was increased to 26.6 mmHg (103%), while other parameters such as heart rate, CI, dp/dt max Vmax and TTI were increased to 42 to 66% and there was no change in SI. Adalat (0.02 to 0.03 mg/kg) was intravenously given in 9 patients and the hemodynamic response to exercise was suppressed. The elevation of left ventricular enddiastolic pressure and Vmax was statistically significant.

Hemodynamic response after propranolol (3 to 4 mg, i.v.) was studied in 8 patients and the elevation of heart rate, mean blood pressure, dp/dt max, V max and TTI were statistically significant suppressed.

The common action of Adalat with propranolol suppressed the elevation of Vmax. Refering to the literature, the suppression of elevation of left ventricular enddiastolic pressure is the common action to nitroglycerin.

References

1. BENZING, G., STOCKERT, J., NAVE, E., et al.: Evaluation of canine left ventricular contractility. Cardiovasc. Dis. **8**, 313 (1974).
2. BRUCE, L., ROBINSON, P. H.: Medical management of angina pectoris. Circulation **41**, 1132 (1972).

3. CONTI, C. R., GRABER, J. D., GUNDEL, W. D., *et al.*: Effect of pacing induced tachycardia on myocardial force-velocity relationships in man. Circulation (Abstr.) **46**, 47 (Suppl. 111) (1970).
4. DWYER, E. M., WIENER, L., COX, J. W.: Effects of beta-adrenergic blockade (propranolol) on left ventricular hemodynamics and the electrocardiogram during exercise-induced angina pectoris. Circulation **38**, 250 (1968).
5. GAASCH, W. A., QUINONES, M. A., WAISSER, E., *et al.*: Alterations in the left ventricular contractile state during isometric exercise in patients with coronary artery disease. Amer. J. Cardiol. (Abstr.) **29**, 264 (1972).
6. GRÜN, G., FLECKENSTEIN, A.: Die elektromechanische Entkoppelung der glatten Gefäß-muskulatur als Grundprinzip der Coronardilatation durch 4-(2'-nitrophenyl)-2,6-dime-thyl-1,4-dihydropyridin-3,5-dicarbonsäure-dimethylester (BAY a 1040, Nifedipine). Arz-neim.-Forsch. (Drug Res.) **22**, 334 (1972).
7. HASHOMOTO, K., TAIRA, N., CHIBA, S., *et al.*: Cardiohemodynamic effects of BAY a 1040 in the dog. Arzneim.-Forsch. (Drug Res.) **22**, 15 (1972).
8. HAYASE, S., HIRAKAWA, S., HOSOKAWA, S., *et al.*: Basic and clinical studies on BAY a 1040 with special reference to its influence on the coronary systemic resistance and capacitance blood vessels. Jap. Heart J. **35**, 903 (1971).
9. KHAJA, P., PARKER, J. O., LEDWICH, J. J.: Assessment of ventricular function in coronary artery disease by means of atrial pacing and exercise. Amer. J. Cardiol. **26**, 107 (1970).
10. KIMURA, E., MABUCHI, G., KIKUCHI, H.: The clinical effect of 4-(2'-nitrophenyl)-2,6-dime-thyl-3,5-dicarbomethoxy-1,4-diphydropyridine (BAY a 1040) on angina pectoris eval-uated by sequential analysis. Arzneim.-Forsch. (Drug Res.) **22**, 365 (1972).
11. KOBAYASHI, T., ITO, Y., TAWARA, I.: Clinical experience with a new coronary-active sub-stance (BAY a 1040). Arzneim.-Forsch. (Drug Res.) **22**, 380 (1972).
12. MASON, D. T.: Usefulness and limitation of the rate of rise of intraventricular pressure (dp/dt) in the evaluation of myocardial contractility in man. Amer. J. Cardiol. **23**, 516 (1969).
13. PARKER, J. O., GIORGI, S. D., WEST, R. O.: A hemodynamic study of acute coronary insuffi-ciency precipitated by exercise. With observations on the effects of nitroglycerin. Amer. J. Cardiol. **17**, 470 (1966).
14. PARKER, J. O., WEST, R. O., GIORGI, S. D.: The hemodynamic response to exercise in pa-tients with healed myocardial infarction without angina. With observations on the effects of nitroglycerin. Circulation **36**, 734 (1967).
15. PARKER, J. O., WEST, R. O., GIORGI, S. D.: Hemodynamic effects of propranolol in coro-nary heart disease. Amer. J. Cardiol. **21**, 11 (1968).
16. QUINONES, M. A., GAASCH, W. H., WAISSER, E., *et al.*: An analysis of left ventricular re-sponse to isometric exercise. Amer. Heart J. **88**, 29 (1974).
17. WIENER, C., DWYER, E. M., JR., COX, J. W.: Left ventricular hemodynamics in exercise-induced angina pectoris. Circulation **38**, 240 (1969).

Discussion Remarks

to contributions LICHTLEN and KURITA *et al.*

HILGER: Dr. LICHTLEN, you made at the beginning of your paper a very important statement: that you did your examinations 40 min after performance of coronary angiography. You saw a drop of end-diastolic pressure from 18 to 7 mm Hg in the left ventricle after isosorbide dinitrate and a lesser drop after nifedipine. Did you see great changes in the left ventricular end-diastolic pressure before and after angiography and did you interpret this to the state of the myocar-dium?

Secondly, you said that you saw a great increase of coronary flow under dipyridamole and a smaller increase after nifedipine. We did a dose-effect relationship after nifedipine, 4 years ago, and we started with 3 μg/kg i.v. up to 30 μg/kg body weight and we saw that there is a maximum vasodilating effect of nifedipine when 20–30 μg/kg are given. Is the sublingual dose of 20 μg with fewer side effects, I know, the best dose for testing the coronary reserve?

LICHTLEN: In all these patients as a reference, we measured the left ventricular hemodynamics before coronary angiography; after angiography we waited until the end-diastolic pressure and the cardiac output returned to normal, that is, to the preangiographic level. Of course, we see quite significant changes in end-diastolic pressure during coronary angiography as does everybody else.

To the second question: We used the 20-mg dose because we were told that this would be a dose which should be given to the patients. We wondered whether if we had gone to higher doses, we would not have seen a greater dilatory effect on the coronary system. I think just from this data it is probably worthwhile not to go to higher doses—not to block completely the coronary system but to leave the arteriolar reaction of the coronary system intact.

HOCHREIN: I would like to comment on the behavior of the pulmonary and pulmonary capillary pressures as parameters of left ventricular function after oral application of 10 mg Adalat. We made calculations together with my co-workers, WITT and WOLF, in patients with coronary heart disease. In a compensated state with normal pressures, that is, without left ventricular heart failure, there are no significant changes in systolic, diastolic, mean pulmonary, and pulmonary capillary pressure within 90 min after administration. But in patients with elevated pressures, in a state of resting left heart failure, there is a marked drop of the pressures in the pulmonary circulation—best seen 60 min after administration. The systolic pulmonary pressure decreases from 48 to 30 mm Hg, the diastolic pressure from 21 to 15, the mean pressure from 35 to 24 and the pulmonary capillary pressure from 26 to 20 mm Hg. That means that Adalat has an important load-decreasing effect on the heart by the way of peripheral vasodilation and a decreasing venous return as we know it from nitroglycerin. The question still exists; can a drug with a calcium-antagonistic effect on the myocardium influence heart failure in coronary heart disease in such a beneficial way?

LYDTIN: I think we have difficulties here because whereas one finds a reduction in venous return, the other finds an increase in venous return.

I think we have to say that there is evidence for both and it seems that the basal status under which measurements and investigations are carried out, is very important for this. It is also important what kind of patients you are studying, in which body positions you do your studies, and at which time after ingestion of the drug you do your measuring; if you measure early you probably get much more sympathetic overdrive. If you measure later it might change and the increase in venous return seen by some might disappear after 20–30 min. This is just a suggestion.

Does anybody want to comment on these findings about venous return and end-diastolic pressure which went up in some and down in other studies?

LICHTLEN: I would like to ask Dr. KURITA how much work load he gave to these patients because I saw that the end-diastolic pressure did not increase under propranolol either and this is in contrast to most observers who exercise patients under propranolol. If you go to very low work loads of 20 watts, or even less, then of course you do not see much change, not in heart rate nor in venous return.

KURITA: If we had so-called anginal pain, we tested patients 3–5 times before catheterization. We applied the patients to a so-called minimal work load which provokes ST-segment depression and chest pains. I think that approximately 3–5 min under work load of 40–50 watts can cause ischemic ST-segment and elevation of end-diastolic pressure to the same extent as the so-called maximal exercise. My work loads were enough to see the change of left ventricular functions shown in the literature. The change of left ventricular end-diastolic pressure under propranolol during exercise did not suppress its elevation and almost the same grade of elevation before medication which Dr. JOHN O. PARKER and others published. Our results tended to be similar.

LOCHNER: Dr. LICHTLEN, you showed that coronary flow decreases 8% after nitroglycerin. What is your feeling with regard to the accuracy of the method you have used? Eight percent is a very small decrease. Another remark: There is very little evidence that there are alpha-receptors in the coronary vascular tree.

LICHTLEN: In the literature there are different opinions about alpha-receptors. American literature mainly believes in alpha-receptors in the coronary system. The decrease in flow under nitroglycerin was also shown by other groups. I had shown single figures and you could see that there was a decrease in almost all patients—in some up to 30% or even 40%—but there was a wide variation and this was also true at rest. So I think the statistics were correct.

KURITA: Dr. LICHTLEN, you saw no significant change after nitroglycerin in coronary flow. At Cedars Sinai Medical Center in Los Angeles Dr. GANZ and I are injecting nitroglycerin locally into the left coronary artery. We were able to see that the flow goes up. I think we should separate the local effects of nitroglycerin from the systemic effects.

LICHTLEN: BERNSTEIN, FRIESINGER, and I have published a paper in 1965 on the intracoronary effects of nitroglycerin and we were the first to demonstrate an increase of coronary flow after intracoronary injection and a decrease after sublingual administration.

The Effect of Adalat on Coronary Circulation after Sublingual Administration

J. A. KÖHLER

Medizinische Klinik der Städt. Krankenanstalten Landshut, Fed. Rep. Germany

The effect of 20 mg Adalat on the coronary circulation after sublingual or buccal administration was studied in 6 patients.

Method

During diagnostic right heart catheterization in 6 patients—25–44 years of age—with rather mild mitral stenosis still in normal sinus rhythm, the coronary sinus was catheterized. Simultaneous measurements of oxygen saturation (Sa O_2), of pressure in the coronary sinus and in the femoral artery and of O_2 consumption were made before and 5–40 min after sublingual or buccal administration of 20 mg Adalat.

Coronary flow and cardiac output were calculated using the Fick method and partly from dye dilution curves. The pulmonary pressure and the systemic pressure were in the normal range, i.e. neither pulmonary nor systemic hypertension was present.

Results

The rate of change of the coronary flow and of the blood pressure after administration of 20 mg Adalat is shown in Fig. 1. 100% represents the basic value of coronary flow before medication. Five minutes after administration of the drug, no change at all could be seen. About 6–10 min after administration, all patients exhibited a relatively prevalent flush and/or a warm feeling in their faces. After 10 min, a slight decrease of the blood pressure (systolic, − 10 mm Hg, diastolic, − 5 mm Hg), a slight decrease of heart rate and an increase of pulmonary flow of 25% was seen. After 15 min, the calculated coronary flow rose to 140% of the base value, whereas the blood pressure, heart rate, femoral arterial oxygen saturation and O_2 consumption remained unchanged. After 30 min the maximum rate of change of all diameters occurred. The coronary sinus oxygen saturation increased from 28% basic value to 56%, hence, an increased coronary flow of 70%, i.e. 170% of the basic value.

Only a small decrease in blood pressure from the basic value of 135/75 mm Hg to 125/68 mm Hg was recorded, whereas no demonstrable change of heart rate was observed.

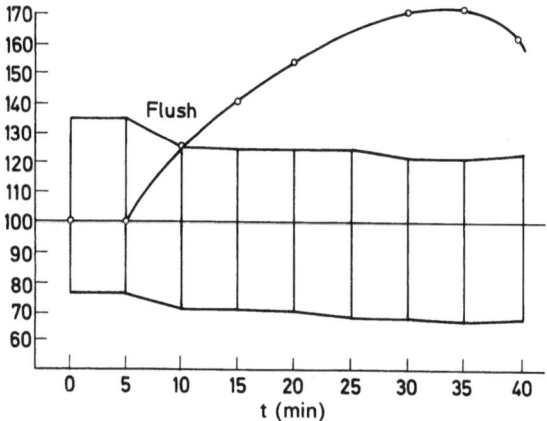

Fig. 1. Rate of change of coronary flow (o) and blood pressure (| |) after application of 20 mg Adalat

No side effects except the more or less pronounced flush appeared in the 6 patients studied.

Abstract

In 6 patients with mild mitral stenosis without any clinical signs of coronary artery disease or of systemic or pulmonary hypertension, a remarkable increase of coronary flow could be proved after sublingual or buccal administration of 20 mg Adalat.

At the same time only a small decrease of systemic blood pressure and of the heart rate appeared; however all patients were digitalized.

Also in the meantime, the anticoronary pain effect was confirmed in many clinical patients and outpatients, using the number of angina pectoris attacks and/ or the consumption of nitroglycerin as a measurement.

With a dosis of one capsule three times daily a very good result was observed in most of the patients.

Loading Tolerance after Adalat and Duration of Effect in Postmyocardial Infarction Studied in a Double-Blind Trial

G. STEIN

Curschmann Klinik, Timmendorfer Strand, Fed. Rep. Germany

During the first trial we studied the duration of effect of 10 mg Adalat given to postmyocardial infarction patients under stress. Thirty minutes after Adalat was given, an improvement in the stress tolerance and a statistically significant reduction of the ST depression were recorded. In contrast, 150 min after Adalat, an effect on the blood pressure, pulse and ST segment could not be statistically confirmed. During another trial we studied the efficacy and duration of effect of 20 mg of Adalat under the same conditions.

Materials and Methods

In 40 patients who had suffered myocardial infarctions 1–10 months previously, we studied the heart rate, blood pressure and ST segment of the ECG at rest, under increased loading and during the recovery phase. The study was carried out as a double-blind and cross-over study against placebo. A preliminary blank test (placebo) was carried out to exclude any effect which might have been induced by the test conditions. At the same time this test also served to establish (determine) the individual loading limits. The loading was stopped according to internationally laid down criteria. Increased loading of 50, 75, and 100 watts was carried out on a bicycle ergometer in the sitting position. Each stress stage lasted 3 min. The blood pressure was determined and recorded graphically (Tensiomat, Wilcken). An ECG was recorded after each minute using the Wilson leads V_2, V_4, and V_6.

The first loading test was carried out on the first day, 30 min and 150 min after administering 20 mg Adalat sublingually. At the same time, and at the same intervals of time, the test was repeated the following day. Determination of ST changes was carried out for each patient using that lead which showed the most pronounced changes. The value used for the calculation was the arithmetic mean (in mm) of the ST depressions and ST elevations from 5 QRS complexes. Only horizontally depressed or descending ST segments were measured. The ST elevations and depressions were measured 0.02 seconds after completion of the QRS wave.

Depending on the behavior of the ST segment during the first loading test the 40 patients were divided into 2 groups: 20 patients had an ST depression, 20 patients had an ST elevation. Table 1 shows the number of patients, sex, age, body weight, time after infarction and location of infarction.

Table 1. Nifedipine (20 mg sublingual). Double-blind cross-over study against placebo in patients with post myocardial infarction

No. of patients	Sex	Age (years)	Body-weight
40	39 males 1 female	54.9 ± 8.6	73.3 ± 7.8 kg

Time from infarction	No. of patients
1—4 months	21
4—5 months	7
5—6 months	4
6—7 months	2
> 10 months	6
Total	40

Localisation of myocardial infarction	No. of patients
anterior	28
diaphragmatic	10
antero-septal	2

Coronary agents and digitalis were discontinued 10 days before the trial to exclude digitalis-induced ST changes.

Results

1. Heart Rate (Fig. 1, Table 2)

After Adalat, the mean values at rest under and after loading were higher than after placebo. After 150 min the difference between Adalat and placebo decreases under loading. The ST elevation group behaved differently from that of the ST depression group.

The direct effect of Adalat under loading could only be detected in the 20 patients with ST depressions. In the case of the patients with ST elevations the difference, compared with placebo, was not statistically significant.

2. Blood Pressure (Table 3)

After Adalat, the systolic and diastolic blood pressures at rest, under and after loading were markedly lower than those after placebo. The differences at rest, 30 and 150 min under loading, and 3 min after loading are highly significant. The difference between Adalat and placebo increases under loading. The ST elevation group had lower initial values: Under Adalat or placebo the blood pressure increase was smaller than in the case of the patients with ST depressions.

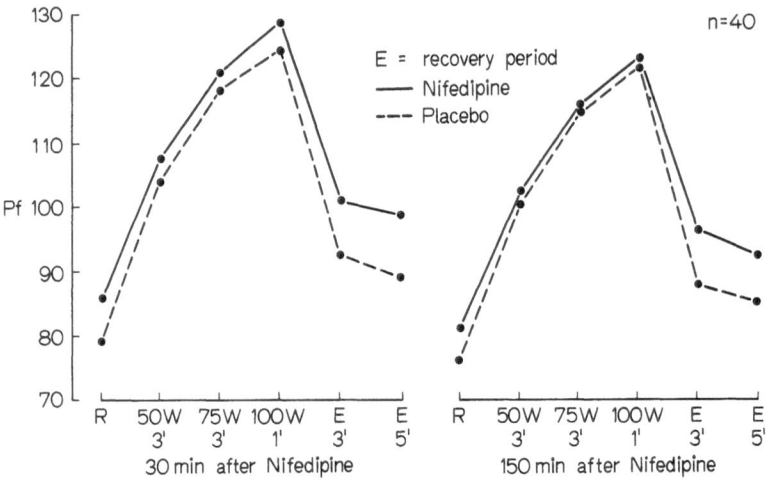

Fig. 1. Changes of heart rate (mean values). 30 and 150 min after nifedipine (20 mg sublingual) and placebo under standardized loading (50–75–100 watt = 300–450–600 kpm/min)

Table 2. Heart rate (mean values). 30 and 50 min after nifedipine (20 mg sublingual) and placebo under standardized loading (resting — 75 watt — recovery period)

		Nifedipine	Placebo	Difference	$p \leqq$
R	d	84.0	78.3	+ 5.7	0.0001
R	e	86.2	80.3	+ 5.9	0.0001
75 W 30'	d	121.5	117.0	+ 4.5	0.008
75 W 30'	e	120.0	119.1	+ 0.9	0.20
E 3'	d	100.8	90.2	+10.6	0.0001
E 3'	e	104.3	95.3	+ 9.0	0.0003
R	d	79.0	75.4	+ 3.6	0.0001
R	e	82.6	76.8	+ 5.8	0.0001
75 W 150'	d	117.0	114.5	+ 2.5	0.02
75 W 150'	e	116.0	115.4	+ 0.6	0.44
E 3'	e	96.2	86.1	+10.1	0.0001
E 3'	e	97.0	89.4	+ 7.6	0.0002

3. Loading Tolerance

In the 20 patients with ST depressions 30 min after Adalat, a statistically noticeable, but not significant improvement of the loading tolerance ($p < 0.09$) occurred. No significant or noticeable therapeutic effect was detectable 150 min after Adalat. The 20 patients with ST elevations did not reveal an increased loading tolerance after 30 min or 150 min.

4. ST Depressions (Fig. 2)

Compared with placebo, the ST segment 30 min after Adalat at 75 watts was 10% less and at 100 watts it was 15% less than that after placebo (not significant,

Table 3. Systolic and diastolic blood pressure (mean values). 30 and 150 min after nifedipine (20 mg sublingual) and placebo under standardized loading (resting — 75 watt — recovery period)

		Nifedipine		Placebo		Difference		$p \leqq$	
		syst.	diast.	syst.	diast.	syst.	diast.	syst.	diast.
R	d	115.8	81.5	124.5	89.2	− 8.7	− 7.7	0.0001	0.0001
R	e	114.5	84.0	124.2	91.8	− 9.7	− 7.8	0.0001	0.0001
75 W 30′	d	162.5	86.8	172.0	95.2	− 9.5	− 8.4	0.0001	0.0001
75 W 30′	e	147.2	85.2	159.0	94.2	−11.8	− 9.0	0.002	0.0003
E 3′	d	128.2	77.8	143.2	89.5	−15.0	−11.7	0.0002	0.0001
E 3′	e	125.5	83.0	139.2	92.8	−13.7	− 9.8	0.003	0.0001
R	d	112.5	82.8	121.5	90.2	− 9.0	− 7.4	0.0001	0.0001
R	e	113.5	85.0	124.2	95.5	−10.7	−10.5	0.0001	0.0001
75 W 150′	d	166.8	92.5	174.0	99.5	− 7.2	− 7.0	0.005	0.0002
75 W 150′	e	146.2	87.0	156.8	94.2	−10.6	− 7.2	0.0001	0.0001
E 3′	d	128.8	81.0	142.2	91.0	−13.4	−10.0	0.0001	0.0001
E 3′	e	124.8	83.8	143.8	96.2	−19.0	−12.4	0.0001	0.0001

d = ST depression ($n = 20$)
e = ST elevation ($n = 20$)
R = resting
E = recovery period.

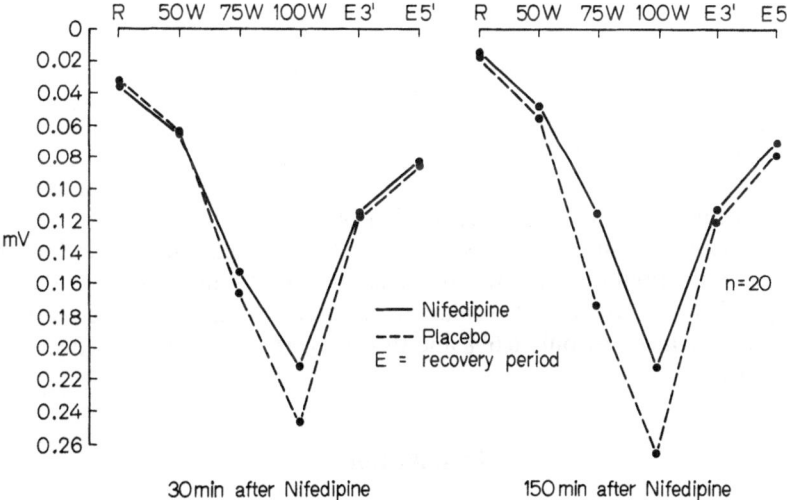

75 watt - 10.59% (non significant)   75 watt - 32.35% P ≤ 0.02 (significant)
100 watt - 15.60% (non significant)   100 watt - 21.48% P ≤ 0.02 (significant)

Fig. 2. ST depression (mean values). 30 and 150 min after nifedipine (20 mg sublingual) and placebo under standardized loading (50–75–100 watt = 300–450–600 kpm/min)

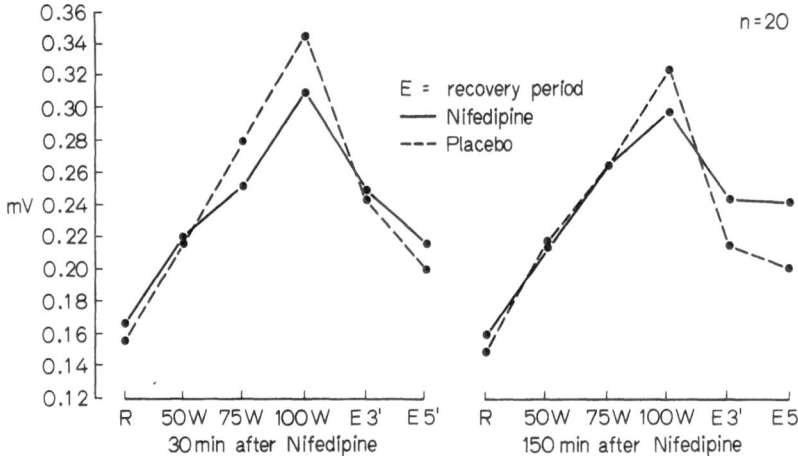

Fig. 3. ST elevation (mean values). 30 and 150 min after nifedipine (20 mg sublingual) and placebo under standardized loading (50–75–100 watt = 300–450–600 kpm/min)

but statistically noticeable). In contrast, 150 min after Adalat a statistically significant reduction of the ST depression occurred at 75 watts and 100 watts ($p < 0.02$). In 3 patients the ST depression 30 min after the administration of Adalat was greater than that under placebo. After 150 min, in only one of these 3 patients was the ST depression greater than after placebo. An indirect effect of Adalat was detectable 150 min after medication. This was expressed by the significant reciprocity between the treatment and the treatment times ($p < 0.007$). This means, as seen from the mean values, that with higher loading the ST depression is reduced by Adalat.

5. ST Elevations (Fig. 3)

At rest and under loading, 20 patients with anterior wall infarctions showed an increasing elevation of the ST segment. Thirty minutes after Adalat the ST elevation at 75 and 100 watts was reduced by 10%. Whereas the resting value for the ST segment under Adalat was above that of the placebo 30 min after Adalat, the ST segments at 75 and 100 watts were less elevated than under placebo. After correlation of the preliminary value, the difference of 0.04 millivolts is significant ($p < 0.05$) and shows an indirect Adalat effect. After 150 min, the ST elevation at 100 watts was reduced by only 6.6% and thus no certain therapeutic effect could be established.

Discussion

Ref. 1: Heart rate

Under 20 mg Adalat, the pulse rate at rest, under and after loading was higher than under placebo. After 10 mg Adalat a small decrease in the heart rate compared with the initial value was found. In the case of the ST elevation group, however, 20 mg Adalat had no direct influence on the pulse. At the same time, the blood pressure increase of this group was markedly reduced under loading when compared with the ST depression group. Thus the reflectory pulse increase resulting from the arterial blood pressure drop plays a subordinate role only and should not significantly reduce the effect of the increased loading tolerance induced by Adalat. Since, after Adalat under stress, the difference in pulse, compared with placebo, does not change significantly, this change should be of less importance than the central and peripheral pressures and resistances. This is also confirmed by the fact that after 150 min under loading, practically no difference is detectable when compared with placebo. On the other hand the blood pressure and ECG show marked changes at this particular time.

Ref. 2: Blood pressure

In the case of a drop in blood pressure there is a marked dose dependency as far as efficacy and duration of effect are concerned. According to our studies the drop is substantially greater after 20 mg Adalat than after 10 mg under the same conditions. Whereas, in our study with 10 mg practically no effect could be detected after 150 min, a constant and highly significant decrease at rest, under and after loading, was detectable 30 and 150 min after 20 mg. Under the prerequisite that the directions of other hemodynamic parameters during the same period of time also remain unchanged, it can be assumed that a protracted effect occurs.

Ref. 3: Loading tolerance

Under loading, the reduced blood pressure increase in patients with extensive myocardial infarctions caused premature exhaustion, but no angina pectoris. The insufficient blood pressure increase and exhaustion in postmyocardial infarcted patients are valid criteria for terminating the loading test. The absence of an increase in the loading tolerance after Adalat was probably due to the fact that in the majority of the patients (32 out of 40) the myocardial infarction was less than 6 months old and that the loading test did not have to be terminated because of angina pectoris, but because of other criteria. Thus the decrease in the ST segment was included as the main criterion.

Ref. 4: ST depressions

Here also a marked dose dependency was detectable as far as efficacy and duration of effect are concerned. Thirty minutes after 10 mg Adalat, a 33% reduction in the ST depression was established ($p < 0.024$). In contrast, after 150 min only a slight reduction in the ST depression was found ($p < 0.15$). However, after 20 mg Adalat a significant reduction in the ST depression still existed after 150 min. Whereas, 30 and 150 min after Adalat the absolute reductions of the ST depressions are the same (0.21 millivolts), under placebo a marked increase in the ST depression from 0.25 millivolts after 30 min to 0.27 millivolts after 150 min is detectable. These findings permit an indirect conclusion that an increasing and prolonged Adalat effect occurs, i.e. the heart is relieved (pre- and afterload) and the myocardium tolerates much better 2 loadings within 2 h.

Because after 30 min, no reduction of the ST depression was detectable in some patients, but after 150 min a pronounced reduction was detectable, it can be assumed that in the case of these patients a retarded absorption occurred and an effective concentration was first present after 1–2 h.

In stressed patients with an anterior wall infarction, very often no ST depression was observed, rather an ST elevation. As an explanation it is assumed that, under loading, a zone around the site of the infarction became anoxemic and as a result an ST elevation developed which in many ways reminds one of the curves of an acute myocardial infarction. In some cases these ECG changes do, with increasing intervals of time, return to normal and later even develop to an ST depression. From this, it was concluded that a reduced ST elevation should be seen as an expression of improved collateral circulation and as regeneration of hypoxemic cells. There was a very strong suspicion that several of the 20 patients with ST elevations under loading had an aneurysm of the heart wall. In the case of these patients the group proved to be inhomogeneous as some, for instance, had an anterior wall infarction. In such patients it was not statistically possible to establish a reduced ST elevation under loading after 20 mg Adalat.

Abstract

Investigations have shown that 20 mg compared with 10 mg Adalat markedly increases the intensity of the effect and duration of effect, particularly in association with a highly significant blood pressure drop and a significant reduction of the ST depression. In contrast to earlier investigations with 10 mg Adalat, the constant effect of 20 mg after 150 min is particularly noticeable. None of these patients reported subjective side-effects after this dose. Under the prerequisite that also after repeated daily doses a constant effect is maintained, a more favorable therapeutic effect can be expected in patients with myocardial infarctions after 20 mg than after 10 mg.

The Cardiopulmonary Loading Capacity
in Healthy Persons and Patients
with Coronary Heart Disease after Application of Adalat

W. HOLLMANN, R. ROST, H. LIESEN, and O. EMIRKANIAN

Department of Cardiovascular Research, German Sports College, Cologne, Fed. Rep. Germany

Materials and Methods

The purpose of these experiments was to test the effect of Adalat on the cardiopulmonary system under exercise conditions. The importance of physical activity in the realm of rehabilitation of coronary patients is increasing. Therefore it is necessary in particular to explore the effects of coronary active drugs under exercise conditions, since many coronary patients receive such drugs.

The effect of 10 mg Adalat administered sublingually on the cardiopulmonary system was investigated in the following experiments:

1. The influence on respiration was tested spiroergometrically in ten healthy physically trained students. Ventilation and oxygen uptake were measured with the subjects exercising in a sitting position on a bicycle ergometer. The load was increased by 4 mkp/sec every three minutes until exhaustion occurred, as determined by our standardized test. These experiments were carried out on two consecutive days, once after giving 10 mg Adalat, and once after giving a placebo. To eliminate the possible effect of better coordination, placebo and the drug were given in an alternating sequence.

2. The effects on circulation were tested in five physical-education students by the determination of cardiac output, stroke volume, heart rate and arterial pressure. The investigations were carried out at rest and during exercise on a bicycle ergometer in the supine position. Cardiac output was determined by the dye dilution technique; arterial pressure was measured directly in the brachial artery. The load level was 10 mkp/sec and lasted five minutes. To minimize the effects of previous exercise on the hemodynamics of a second exercise, the load level was made comparatively low. This test was repeated 40 min after giving Adalat.

3. The effect of Adalat on patients with coronary artery disease was explored in twelve cases. The severity of disease differed widely—from patients who experienced slight pain during exercise to patients who had suffered from myocardial infarction. All patients had a pathologic ECG under loading conditions. In these patients we studied exercise ECG's in a bicycle test as described in the first experiment before and after giving Adalat.

Results and Comments

Figure 1 shows the results of spiroergometrical investigations. In nine patients, the performance capacity was not decreased; one patient complained of feeling hot, which prevented him from achieving the same exercise level as in the placebo experiment. Since the subjects were trained to different degrees, they achieved different maximal performance levels between 19 and 35 mkp/sec, documented by the decreasing number of persons that were tested at the highest exercise levels.

The results indicate, that the respiratory parameters (ventilatory volume, oxygen uptake, respiration rate) are not significantly influenced at rest, at submaximal and maximal levels of exercise. This agrees with previous results that arterial oxygen saturation is not effected even under exercise.

In contrast, the oxygen pulse is diminished by the drug at rest and at submaximal level. This is the result of an increased heart rate, since the oxygen uptake did

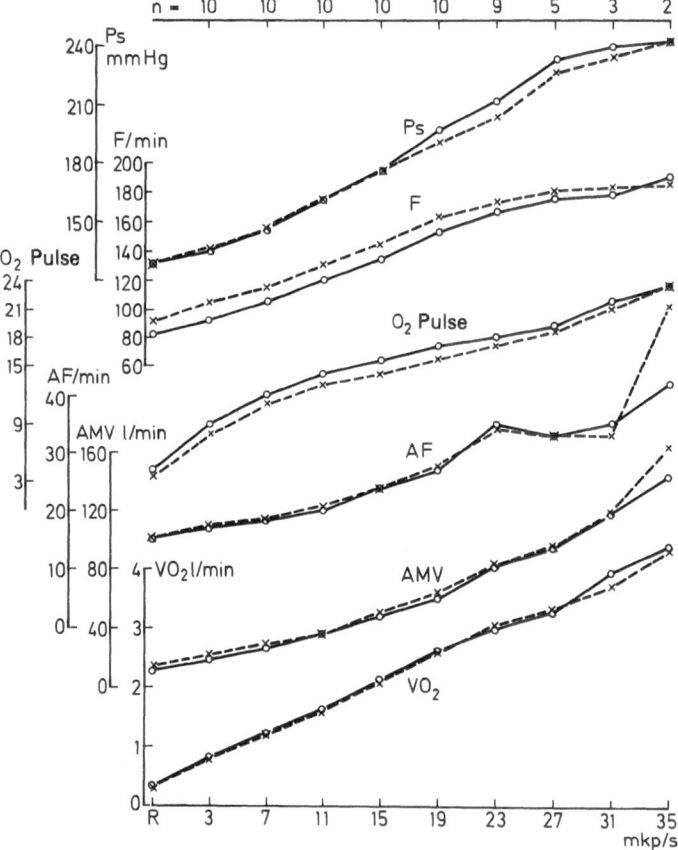

Fig. 1. Effects of Adalat in a spiroergometrical test. Values after giving Adalat are connected by a broken line. Abbreviations: P_s, systolic pressure; F, heart rate; O_2-pulse, oxygen uptake/heart rate; AF, respiration rate; AMV, ventilatory volume; VO_2, oxygen uptake

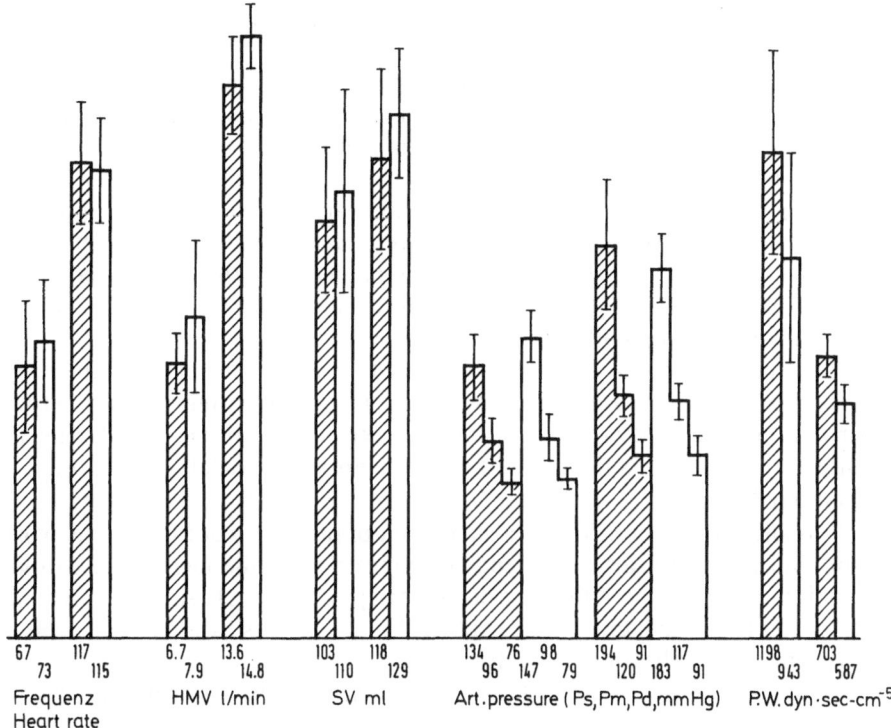

67		117	6.7		13.6	103		118	134	76	98	194	91	117	1198		703
	73	115		7.9	14.8		110	129		96	147	79	120	183	91	943	587
Frequenz			HMV l/min			SV ml			Art.pressure (Ps,Pm,Pd,mmHg)						P.W. dyn·sec-cm⁻⁵		
Heart rate																	

Fig. 2. Results of hemodynamic experiments. Mean values of heart rate, cardiac output (*HMV*), stroke volume (*SV*), arterial pressure (systolic, *P_s*), mean (*Pm*) and diastolic pressure (*Pd*) and peripheral resistance (*PW*) are dokumentated in the following sequence: resting before, resting after Adalat, exercising before, exercising after giving Adalat

not change. At the maximal level, the oxygen pulse and the heart rate again approach the control values.

The oxygen uptake per heart beat can be considered a measure of the efficiency of circulation. It corresponds to the product of stroke volume and oxygen arteriovenous difference. Because stroke volume does not decrease under Adalat, decreasing oxygen uptake per heart beat must be the consequence of a decrease in utilization. This can be considered to be a hyperkinetic state. The systolic pressure is slightly influenced; only at the higher levels of exercise can a diminution be seen. Due to the well-known methodologic difficulties, we disregarded the measurement of the diastolic pressure according to the indirect principle of RIVA ROCCI.

Figure 2 shows the result of further hemodynamic investigations. The heart rate during exercise was not increased in these tests. This fact suggests that the increase of heart rate in the sitting position could be a result of an orthostatic mechanism, i.e. a decrease of the venous tone. A considerable orthostatic effect of the drug could not be found during the Schellong-Test. Moreover, a venous pooling was not observed by previous investigators. It is possible to offer hypotheses to explain these different findings, but additional investigations, such as exact measurement of venous tone and cardiac output in the standing position, should be carried out.

Previous results concerning cardiac output are not unanimous. Our results show a significant increase of cardiac output after giving only 10 mg of the drug sublingually. The amount of increase is 1.2 l/min at rest and under exercise conditions. In the supine position, this increase is due to an enlargement of stroke volume; in the sitting position, the increase of heart rate may be important.

Arterial pressure was not decreased at rest; under loading conditions there was a slight decrease of systolic pressure, the influence on the mean arterial and diastolic pressures was negligible. Peripheral resistance decreased significantly at rest and under loading conditions.

In a general survey of our results we noted a vasodilating effect of the drug. The decrease of peripheral resistance results in an increasing cardiac output. Peripheral utilization decreases, so that hyperkinetic conditions result. The influence on arterial pressure is slight when a dosis of Adalat such as ours is administered.

Therefore it could be said that a slight shift of pressure work to volume work occurs. But external heart work tends to increase since the increase of cardiac output is more pronounced than the decrease of pressure work. As far as previous results differ from ours, this can be explained in most cases by a different type of experiment or of application of the drug.

The question is now, in view of our experiments, in what way can this drug be of benefit to coronary patients.

Two different possibilities are discussed. The first suggests a direct effect on the myocard or the coronary arteries. According to the second thesis, the only benefit lies in lowering the peripheral resistance and therefore the pressure work, because a sclerotic vessel cannot be dilated by any drug more than by myocardial ischemia.

Our findings do not confirm the latter suggestion. Decrease of peripheral resistance results primarily in an increase of volume work and only to a small degree in a decrease of pressure work.

These effects of the drug contrast remarkably with the general findings in sports medicine, which suggest that coronary patients would benefit from physical training, thereby effecting a more hypodynamic state. These findings are analogous to the effects of β-receptor blocking agents.

To an even greater degree, the findings in coronary patients indicate that the usefulness of the drug is due primarily to its cardiac effects. Our results varied considerably from patient to patient. In some patients, no effect could be observed. In others, there was a significant improvement of exercise tolerance and ECG (in our experiments, in only 3 of 12 patients).

These individual differences can be better explained by differences in the pathologic morphology of the coronary vessels, i.e. dissimilarities resulting in a different reaction to the drug, than by a general lowering of peripheral resistance.

Further, some patients under the influence of Adalat did tolerate a higher exercise level than during the control test without chest pain, despite an arterial pressure that exceeded the control value. This improvement cannot be explained by a lowering of pressure work.

Abstract

Investigations were carried out concerning the effect of the new drug Adalat on circulation and respiration during exercise. After oral intake of 10 mg of this drug we could find no deterioration in exercise performance, except for one person who complained of hot feeling. There was no effect on oxygen uptake; however, the increase of heart rate there was combined with a decreased oxygen pulse, i.e. oxygen uptake per heart beat. This could not be a consequence of a decreased stroke volume since the stroke volume increased to the same extent as the cardiac output at rest and during exercise. That means that the AVD O_2 decreased. Arterial pressure decreased only slightly, this being more important in the case of peripheral resistance. Heart work was not diminished, but there was a shift from pressure work to volume work for the cardiac muscle.

In patients with coronary heart disease, some noticable improvements in endurance were observed, but the effect was individually different. With the results of our findings we can not explain the effect of this new substance via peripheral mechanisms; e.g. through a decrease of peripheral resistance. There must therefore be an improvement of the myocardial oxygen supply, which depends on the individual pattern of coronary heart disease.

Remarks on Changes
of ST Segment Depression during the Day

U. Henkels and G. Blümchen

Klinik Roderbirken, Leichlingen, Fed. Rep. Germany

The effect on ST segment depression of drug therapy is often taken as an indicator of coronary insufficiency.

The following is a report on the reproducibility of ST segment changes during the day.

Figure 1 shows the wide range of ST segment depressions in the same patient on two consecutive days with no medication. Exercise tests were performed at 8 a.m., 11 a.m., 2 p.m. and 5 p.m. ST segment depression of more than 1 mV occurs at quite different work loads, ranging from 20 watts, 3 min to 60 watts, 2 min. Looking at comparable times each day, a wide range of ST segment depressions is evident.

Figure 2 shows an example of the increase in exercise tolerance during the period from 8 a.m. to 11 a.m., as judged by the ST segment values. If this patient had taken a drug, a false positive test would have resulted.

In this short report, we would like to emphasize the wide range of exercise tolerance, even when electrocardiograms are taken at the same time of day. This fact should be borne in mind if one uses ST segment changes in testing the effect of drug therapy.

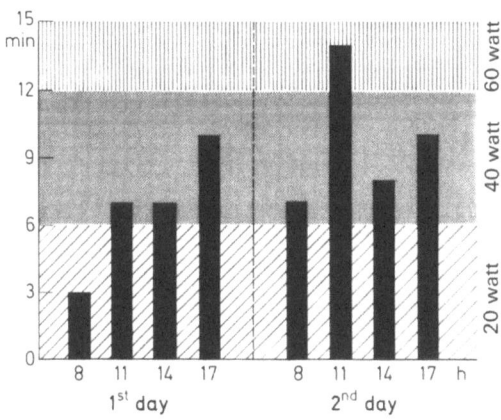

Fig. 1. The difference of exercise tolerance proofed by ST segment depression (>0.1 mV) shown in the same patient on two consecutive days at 8 a.m., 11 a.m., 2 p.m., and 5 p.m. The patient received no medication

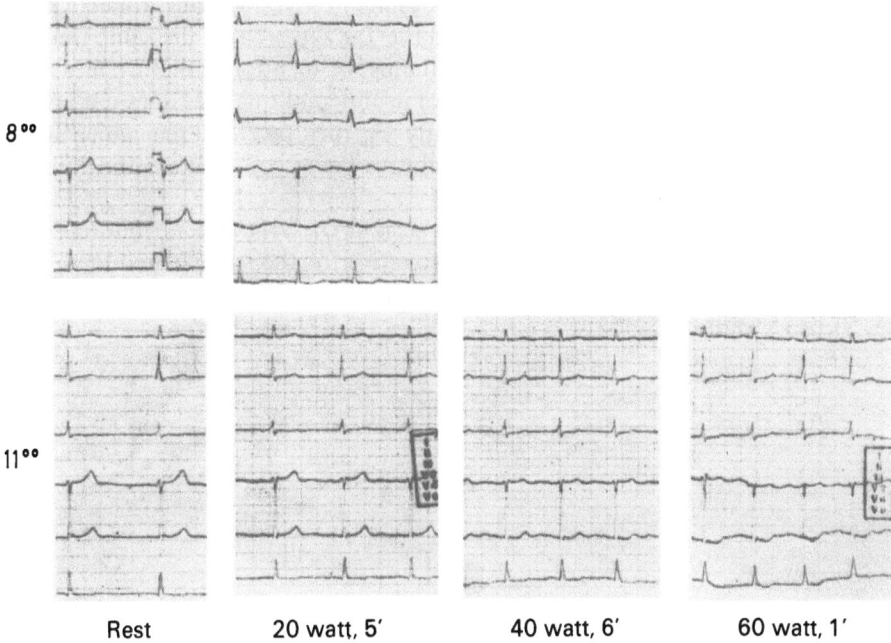

Fig. 2. Exercise electrocardiograms of a 48-year-old male patient with coronary heart disease (proofed by coronary angiography). Electrocardiograms were taken without medication. Exercise tolerance changed markedly from 8 a.m. to 11 a.m. on the same day

Abstract

As a basis for a double-blind trial with BAY a 1040 (nifedipine, Adalat) which is not yet finished, we investigated the daily variations of the coronary insufficiency in patients with previous myocardial infarction, which can be seen in the ECG under loading conditions.

Before administering BAY a 1040, loading tests were carried out on two consecutive days at 8 and 11 a.m. and at 2 and 5 p.m. with no other medication, if possible. In a few of these patients we saw that during the day the loading capacity varied considerably. This daily variation in the degree of coronary insufficiency is well known the treatment of angina pectoris patients.

The problems concerning these variations, which can be seen in the ECG under loading conditions, will be discussed with special regard to the objectification of therapeutical efficacy.

Discussion Remarks

to contributions STEIN, HOLLMANN *et al.*, and HENKELS and BLÜMCHEN

SCHÄCKE: With regard to the investigations of Dr. HENKELS and Dr. BLÜM-CHEN I would like to say that as I saw the diagram I thought of circadian rhythms. There was a maximum in the area of high performance and a minimum in the area of low performance. We had similar results in investigations from 6 a.m. to 6 p.m. When we measured the R-peak and the T-wave, we saw the same trend in both waves. As a further disturbing factor it must be mentioned that we measured the potentials on the skin, which because of its different qualities does not always let the myocardial potentials through equally. Further, one must remember that in precise measurement new electrodes are always being constructed, and thus we get artificial differences in potentials.

On the subject of load I would say—as seen in Dr. Stein's contribution—that in testing drugs it is, above all, necessary to strive for the submaximal load. One will first see effects clearly with 100 watts. I believe that there will be no effect with 25, 50, or 75 watts.

Hemodynamic Study of Nifedipine Using Doppler Flowmetry

B. Angelsen, A. O. Brubakk, and R. Rokseth

Section of Cardiology, Regional Hospital and Division of Engineering Cybernetics, Technical University of Norway, Trondheim, Norway

Introduction

To study the effect of drugs on the cardiovascular system, pressure and flow must be measured simultaneously. Flow measurement usually requires venous and arterial puncture (for dye dilution) or use of costly equipment (isotope techniques). This study was initiated in order to introduce the use of a pulsed Doppler velocity meter for recording changes in aortic flow. The method was used for studying changes in hemodynamic parameters in resting, normal man after sublingual administration of 10 mg of Adalat.

Materials and Methods

Eleven men and two women aged 30–49 years were studied in the supine, resting position. All persons were healthy and had no history or clinical signs of cardiovascular disease.

ECG was measured from chest electrodes, placed in a position giving a large R-wave. The blood pressure was measured using the occlusive cuff technique and recording the Korotkov sounds in the brachial artery with a stethoscope [3].

The velocity of flow in the ascending aorta was determined using a pulsed Doppler velocity meter, developed in this laboratory and described in detail elsewhere [1]. This instrument is capable of decoding the frequency shift in an ultrasonic beam reflected from the moving blood particles. Because the instrument uses pulsed ultrasound, it is possible both to record the direction of flow and the depth at which the flow is sampled. In this study a transducer with a diameter of 2 cm was used, utilizing an ultrasonic frequency of 2 MHz and a repetition frequency of 6.5 kHz.

As can be seen from Fig. 1, the transducer was positioned in the suprasternal notch and angled downwards, so that the velocity in the ascending aorta was recorded. The velocity was recorded at a depth which gave a normal velocity profile together with the highest velocity values. By angling the transducer, a position could be found that gave neither a positive nor a negative velocity signal, indicating the beam to be normal to the aorta. In this position the reflections from

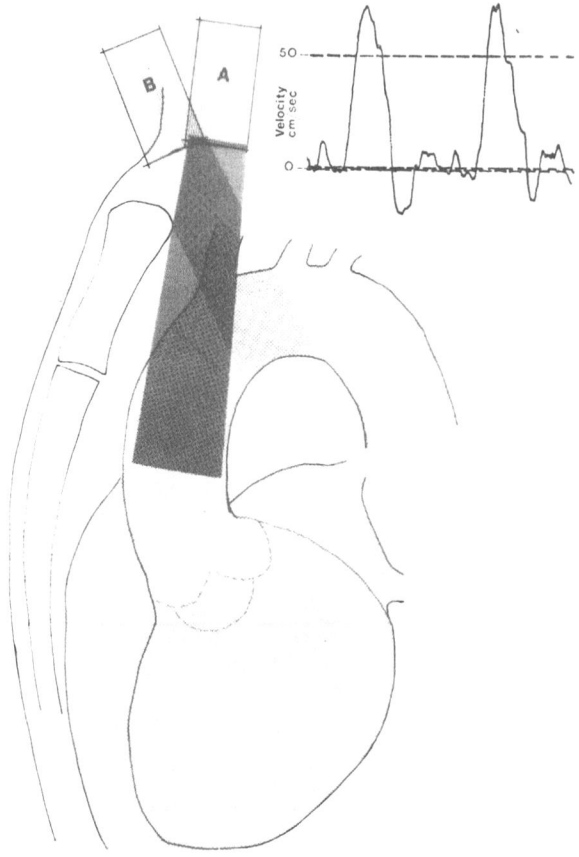

Fig. 1. The ultrasonic transducer positioned in the suprasternal notch. *A* shows the position for measuring velocities in the ascending aorta. *B* shows the position for measuring aortic diameter

the posterior and anterior wall of the aorta could be recorded and the diameter of the vessel calculated. An example of this can be seen in Fig. 2.

From these data it was possible to calculate the aortic flow and the stroke volume. Due to the fact that it is not possible to align the ultrasonic beam along the course of the ascending aorta, the absolute values of flow and stroke volume will be higher than those calculated by our method by a factor of the cosine of the angle between the ultrasonic beam and the ascending aorta. Because this factor changes from person to person, only relative values can be measured.

The mean arterial pressure was calculated as 2/3 of the pulse pressure + the diastolic pressure, and the total peripheral resistance was calculated by dividing the mean arterial pressure by the cardiac output.

The persons were tested in a semidarkened, quiet room after 5 min of rest and 20 min after sublingual administration of 10 mg of Adalat.

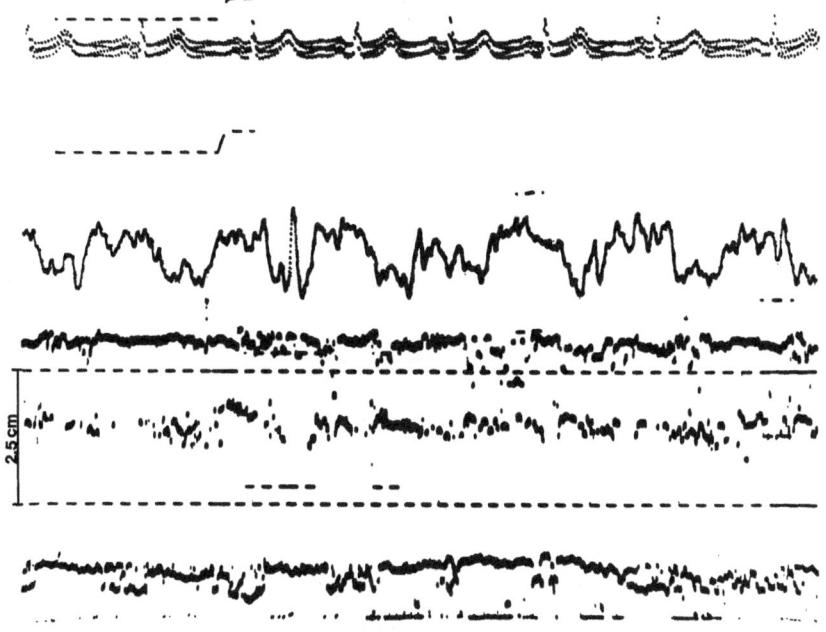

Fig. 2. A–T scan of aorta. ECG and velocity signal on top. Lower echoes represent the lumen of the aorta as measured from position B in Fig. 1 and as described in the text. The upper lumen is probably the brachiocephalic artery

Table 1. Subject data and percent change in measured variables 20 min after 10 mg Adalat

Subject	Sex	Age yrs.	Ao. diam cm.	MAP	HR	Peak Ao. flow	SV	CO	TPR
B.L.	M	49	2.6	−12	+13	+15	+12	+ 29	−33
A.G.	M	43	2.9	− 8	+14	+10	+16	+ 31	−30
J.M.	M	39	2.5	−13	+15	+23	+57	+ 74	−50
N.O.	M	43	2.9	+10	+10	+ 8	+ 6	+ 15	− 5
A.B.	M	33	2.4	+10	0	+24	+33	+ 32	−16
J.F.D.	M	38	2.4	+ 6	0	+ 8	+13	+ 9	− 3
B.A.	M	30	2.9	− 3	+ 9	+ 5	+22	+ 48	−35
T.T.	M	44	2.7	+ 8	+20	+25	+19	+ 41	−23
E.O.	M	36	2.4	− 5	+31	+28	+87	+190	−60
O.E.	M	38	2.5	− 9	+17	+14	0	+ 14	−20
T.J.	M	33	2.5	− 6	− 5	+10	+62	+ 54	−39
J.E.	F	40	2.2	− 5	+18	0	0	+ 18	−19
S.T.	F	37	2.2	− 6	+20	+ 5	+37	+ 50	−37
Mean		39	2.5	− 3	+12	+13	+28	+ 46	−28

Results

The results are compiled in Table 1. In this study the aortic diameter varied between 2.2 and 2.9 cm.

The changes in the various parameters are given as percentages of the resting values. As can be seen from the table, all persons examined showed an increase in

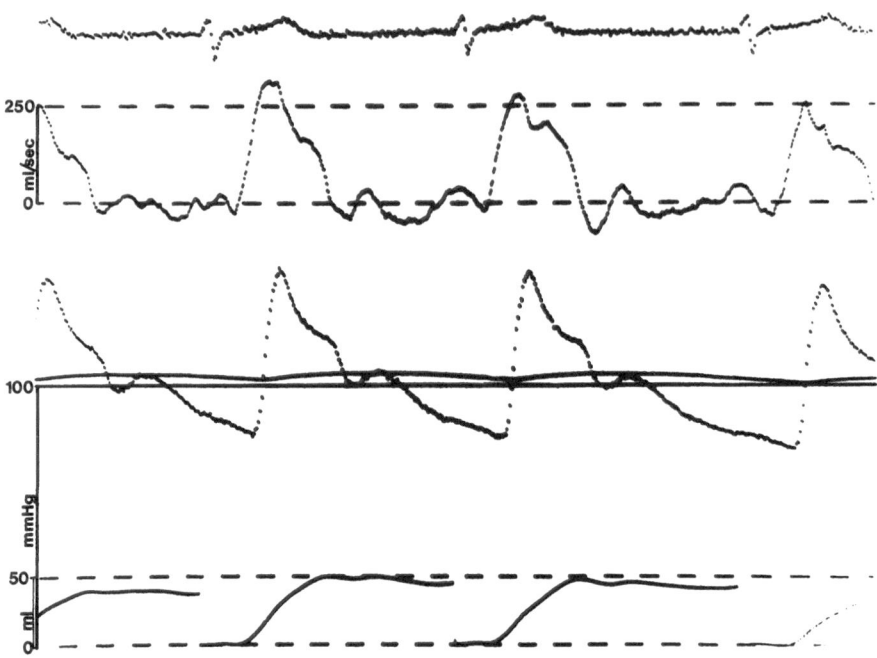

Fig. 3. Resting values. From top to bottom is shown ECG, aortic flow, arterial pulse pressure and mean pressure (radial artery) and stroke volume

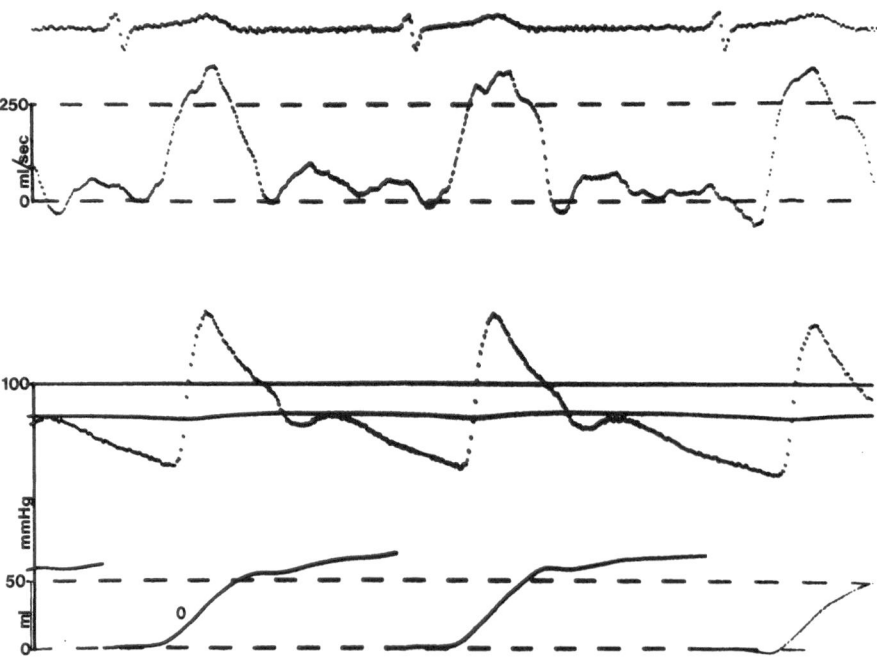

Fig. 4. The same measurements as in Fig. 3, 20 min after 10 mg Adalat sublingually

cardiac output and a decrease in peripheral resistance. Peak aortic flow and heart rate showed varying responses.

An example of the resting values are shown in Fig. 3 and the values 20 min after 10 mg of Adalat in Fig. 4. For purposes of illustration, the blood pressure was measured in the brachial artery in this subject. As in most of the subjects studied, the drug resulted in an increase in peak aortic flow and stroke volume and a decrease in arterial pressure.

Discussion

Adalat is a Ca-antagonist, which decreases the tone of arteriolar smooth muscle [5]. The hemodynamic effect, investigated by several authors, generally consists of a decrease in arterial pressure and an increase in cardiac output and heart rate [8]. In isolated myocardial muscle, the drug decreases contractility [4], but this effect seems to be compensated by a general increase in sympathetic tone, so that no inhibition of cardiac function is recorded.

There seems to be some disagreement on the effect on venous return and left ventricular enddiastolic pressure.

Some authors claim an increase in venous return and a rise in enddiastolic pressure [2, 6] while others claim that the enddiastolic pressure decreases [7]. This controversy is of some importance, because an increase in venous return and the decrease in peripheral resistance would indicate a different action on arterioles and veins. It is also of practical importance, since the well-known side-effects of nitroglycerin, notably the orthostatic phenomena, will not occur in the presence of increased venous return.

Nine of the persons investigated in this study showed a response similar to that reported by others. Surprisingly, 4 persons showed an increase in mean arterial pressure of +6–+10%. These 4 persons were all men in good physical shape. They all showed an increase in peak aortic flow, stroke volume and cardiac output and a decrease in total peripheral resistance. An increase in peak aortic flow in the face of rising pressure can either be the result of increased cardiac contractility or increased venous return. It is not possible from our data to conclude which of these mechanisms is responsible. It seems unlikely, however, that an increase in cardiac contractility should be caused by a Ca-antagonistic drug. Our results would therefore seem to indicate an increase in venous return.

As far as we know, no others have reported a rise in blood pressure after Adalat. Further work is needed to confirm these results, but we suggest that Adalat augments venous return and that this effect overrides the decrease in peripheral resistance in younger, well-trained subjects. This explanation is in agreement with the increase in left ventricular enddiastolic pressure reported by others.

If this theory is correct, no orthostatic symptom should be experienced by persons taking a larger dose of Adalat. This was tested in subject A, B, as can be seen from Fig. 5. 10 mg of Adalat were taken every 20 min, and after 80 min the subject suddenly changed from the supine to the standing position. The subject experienced a tachycardia with heart rate increasing from 95 to 110 beats per minute. No feeling of dizziness was experienced and as can be seen from the

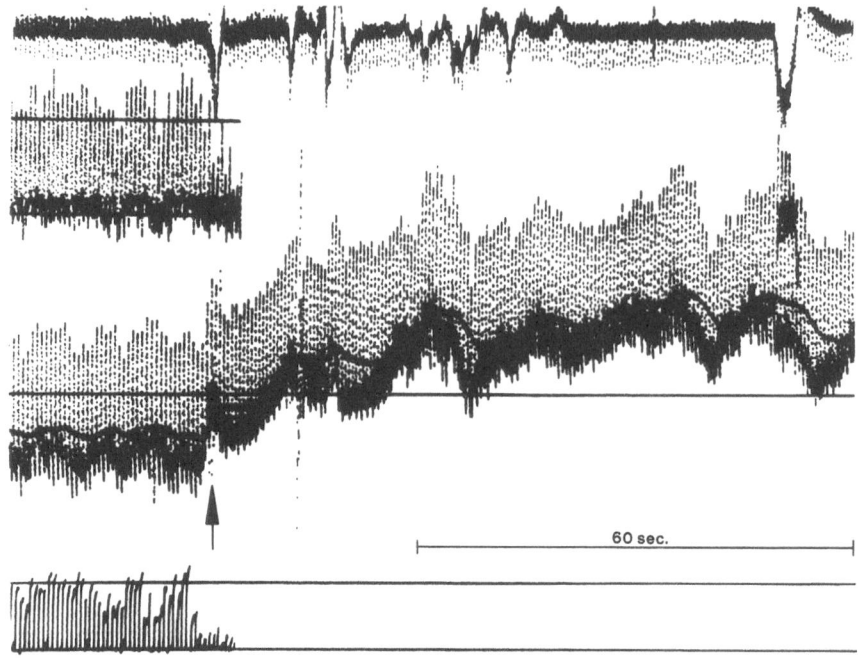

Fig. 5. The effect of changing from the supine to the standing position after 30 mg Adalat sublingually. Arrow indicates time of standing up. The measurements are the same as in Fig. 3 and 4

recording, the blood pressure showed a distinct rise. The results seem to confirm that no decrease in tone in the venous system could have occurred, as this would have resulted in a sharp decrease in pressure. The reason why the pressure rises, is not self-evident and further work is needed to clarify this point.

Abstract

This study was initiated in order to study the effect of Adalat (generic nifedipine) in normal, resting man. As most studies on the acute effect of this drug have been done with invasive methods, a study using non-invasive methods for measuring pressure and flow could be of interest.

Eleven men and two women aged 30–49 were studied in the supine position. All were healthy and none used any other drug.

Pressure was measured using the Riva-Rocci method. Heart rate was calculated from the ECG. Using a pulsed Doppler velocity meter developed in this laboratory the velocity in the ascending aorta was measured. Using an echo-technique, the diameter of the aortic arch was measured and used for calculating peak flow and stroke volume. From this data cardiac output and total peripheral resistance could be calculated.

These measurements were performed at rest and 20 min after 10 mg Adalat sublingually. It was then possible to study the change in hemodynamics caused by the drug. All patients had a fall in calculated total peripheral resistance and an increase in stroke volume, cardiac output and peak aortic flow. Rather surprisingly, 4 of the 13 persons investigated had a rise in mean aortic pressure. As this rise in pressure was accompanied by a rise in aortic flow, this finding can be explained either by an increase in myocardial contractility or by an increase in venous inflow. Both, the pharmacological properties of the drug and measurement of ventricular diameter, indicate that the drug augments venous return.

These findings indicate that Adalat decreases peripheral resistance while increasing venous tone. This effect, if confirmed by others, could make this drug preferable to nitroglycerin, particulary in patients with myocardial infarction.

References

1. ANGELSEN, B. A. J., AASLID, R., BRUBAKK, A. O.: Transcutaneous aortic blood velocity measurement by pulsed Doppler meter. Proc. III Nordic Meet. Med. and Biol. Eng., Tampere 1975.
2. VAN DEN BRAND, M., MEESTER, G. T., TIGGELAAR-DE-WIDT, L., DE RUITER, R., HUGEN-HOLTZ, P. G.: Hemodynamic effect of nifedipine (Adalat) in patients catheterized for coronary artery disease. [Proc. II. International Adalat-symposium, Amsterdam, 1974.]
3. BORDLEY, J., III., CONNOR, C. A. R., HAMILTON, W. F., KERR, W. J., WIGGERS, C. J.: Recommendation for human blood pressure determinations by sphygmomanometers. Circulation **4**, 503–509 (1951).
4. FLECKENSTEIN, A., TRITTHART, H., DÖRING, H. J., BYON, K. Y.: BAY a 1040 — ein hochaktiver Ca^{++}-antagonistischer Inhibitor der elektro-mechanischen Koppelungsprozesse im Warmblütermyokard. Arzneim.-Forsch. **22**, 22–33 (1972).
5. GRÜN, G., FLECKENSTEIN, A.: Die elektromechanische Entkoppelung der glatten Gefäßmuskulatur als Grundprinzip der Coronardilatation durch BAY a 1040, Nifedipine. Arzneim.-Forsch. (Drug Res.) **22**, 334–344 (1972).
6. HASHIMOTO, K., TAIRA, N., CHIBA, S., HASHIMOTO, K., JR., ENDOH, M., KOKUBUN, M., KOKUBUN, H., IIJIMA, T., KIMURA, T., KUBOTA, K., OGURO, K.: Cardiohemodynamic effects of BAY a 1040 in the dog. Arzneim.-Forsch. **22**, 15–21 (1972).
7. KALTENBACH, M., BECKER, H. K., KOBER, G., LOOS, A.: Veränderungen der Hämodynamik des linken Herzen unter der Wirkung von Nifedipin (BAY a 1040) im Vergleich mit Nitroglycerin. Arzneim.-Forsch. **22**, 362–365 (1972).
8. KOCHSIEK, K., NEUBAUM, J.: Die Wirkung von Nifedipin auf den Myokardstoffwechsel, die Hämodynamik, die Blutgase und den allgemeinen Stoffwechsel des Menschen. Arzneim.-Forsch. **22**, 352–358 (1972).

Session VI

Clinical Aspects: Special Studies

Chairmen: F. Camerini (Triest), F. Hagemeijer (Rotterdam)

Clinical-Therapeutic and Hemodynamic Studies with Adalat, a New Coronary Active Substance

K. Kodama, N. Ohgitani, and T. Minamino

Sakurabashi Watanabe Hospital, Osaka, Japan

Introduction

Adalat (generic nifedipine), a dihydropyridine derivative, was recently developed by Bayer AG, West Germany. The substance represents a new type of drug with a remarkable antianginal effect when administered orally or sublingually even in small doses. The antianginal efficacy of Adalat is well documented by numerous reports.

We investigated changes of circulatory parameters during exercise tolerance tests and caluclated the double product (calculated from blood pressure and pulse rate) in patients with angina on effort. Our results, comparing propranolol with nitroglycerin, have been reported elsewhere.

Subjects and Methods

In our present study, Adalat was included, using the same materials and methods. The same results of the exercise tolerance tests could be reproduced by maintaining well-controlled conditions.

Eleven ward patients with angina on effort, 7 males and 4 females, aged 42–75 years, took part in the study.

Figure 1 shows maximum exercise tests, which were performed with patients in supine position with a 30° elevation of the upper body using bicycle ergometer according to the modified method of Bruce and his co-workers.

Heart rate, blood pressure and electrocardiogram were monitored continuously from the start of the tests up to 10 min after completion of the series. The double product was calculated from data of heart rate and systolic blood pressure.

For each patient a series of 4 tests was carried out. The first with no medication served as control. Subsequent tests were done with nitroglycerin (0.3 mg) and nifedipine (10.0 mg) sublingually, with exercise always starting 3 min after administration. Propranolol (30 mg) was given orally for three days. The time of exercise, room temperature and humidity were kept as constant as possible. A series of 4 tests was planned to be completed within a period of 10–14 days.

Results

Figure 2 shows the changes in both exercise tolerance and double product at onset of anginal pain with nitroglycerin, nifedipine and propranolol compared to those with no medication as control. Exercise tolerance and double product

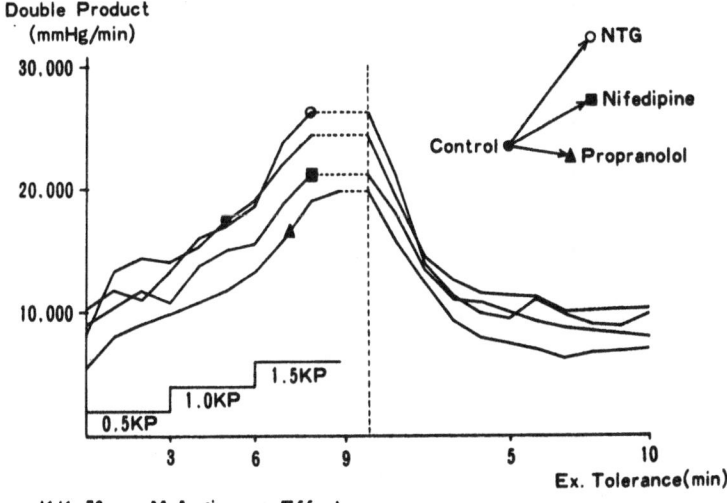

K.K. 76 yrs M. Angina on Effort

Fig. 1. Changes in exercise tolerance and double product in ergometric exercise test

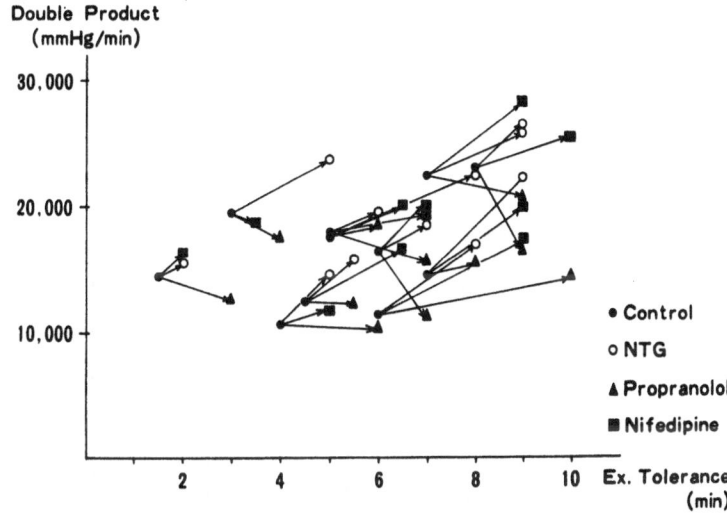

Fig. 2. Changes in exercise tolerance and double product in ergometric exercise test

increased with nitroglycerin and nifedipine. In contrast, with propranolol, exercise tolerance increased in all patients but double product increased only in some patients and decreased in others. The degree of change varied with individuals.

Some patients showed only a slight change, and others showed a comparatively great change.

Figure 3 shows the change in exercise tolerance in the short-term test using nifedipine, nitroglycerin and propranolol.

The results of further calculations of these groups were significantly superior to that of control, based on overall statistics.

But there were not significant differences observed in values obtained with these three drugs.

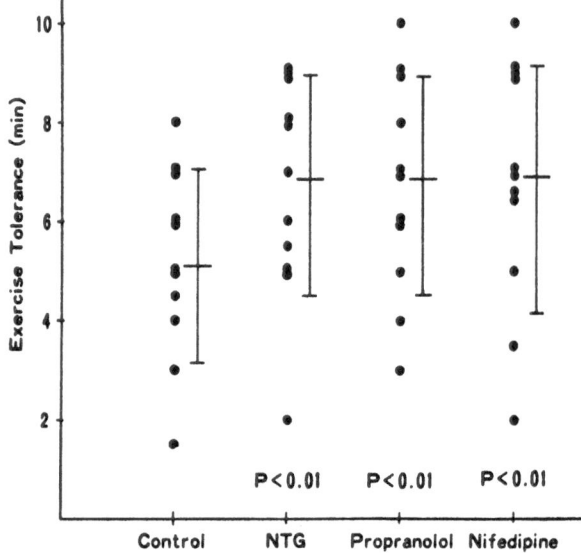

Fig. 3. Exercise tolerance in ergometric exercise test ($n = 11$)

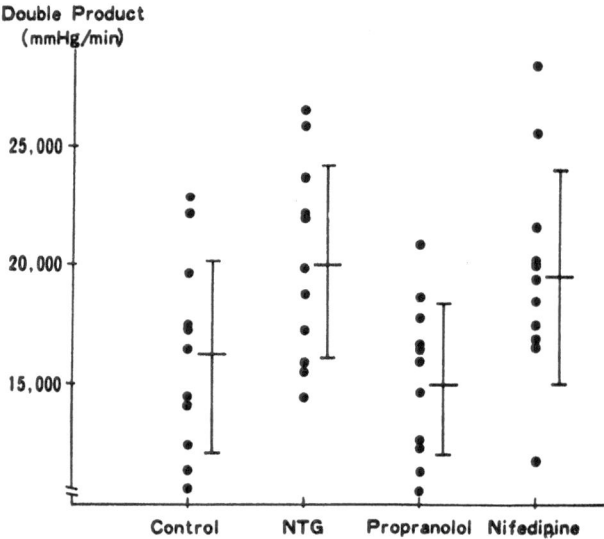

Fig. 4. Double product at onset of pain induced by ergometric exercise test ($n = 11$)

Figure 4 shows that the double product at onset of pain increased with nifedipine compared to control, but only slightly in comparison to nitroglycerin. Propranolol, on the other hand, showed a distinct tendency to decrease it.

The systolic blood pressure at onset of pain was elevated with nifedipine and nitroglycerin which is shown in Fig. 5, with propranolol, however, it was slightly decreased.

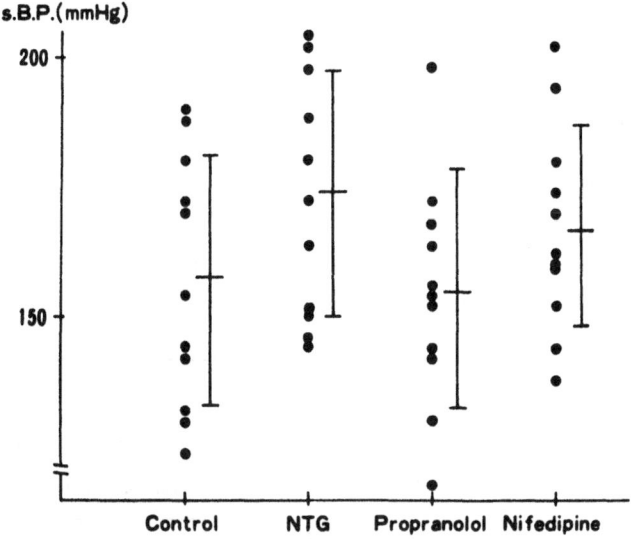

Fig. 5. Systolic blood pressure at onset of pain induced by ergometric exercise test ($n=11$)

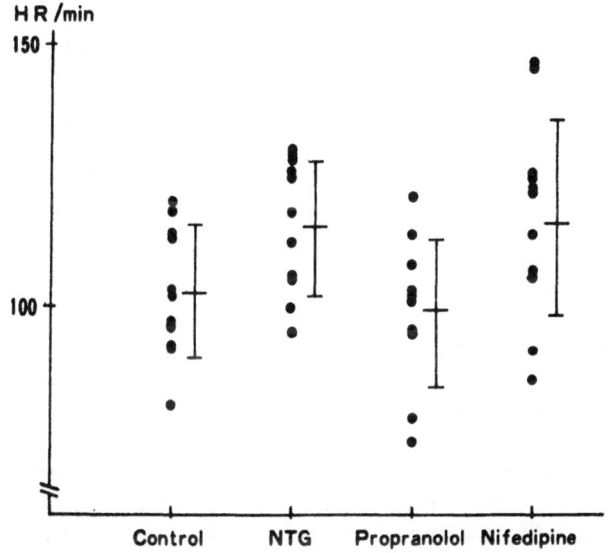

Fig. 6. Heart rate at onset of pain induced by ergometric exercise test ($n=11$)

The heart rate at onset of pain was increased with nifedipine and nitroglycerin (Fig. 6), but with propranolol, the decrease was minimal.

Figure 7 summarizes our principal results. Compared to control, the values of exercise tolerance and double product at onset of pain significantly increased with nifedipine and nitroglycerin.

Propranolol, on the other hand, produced a significant increase in exercise tolerance but a slight decrease in double product. On the basis of available

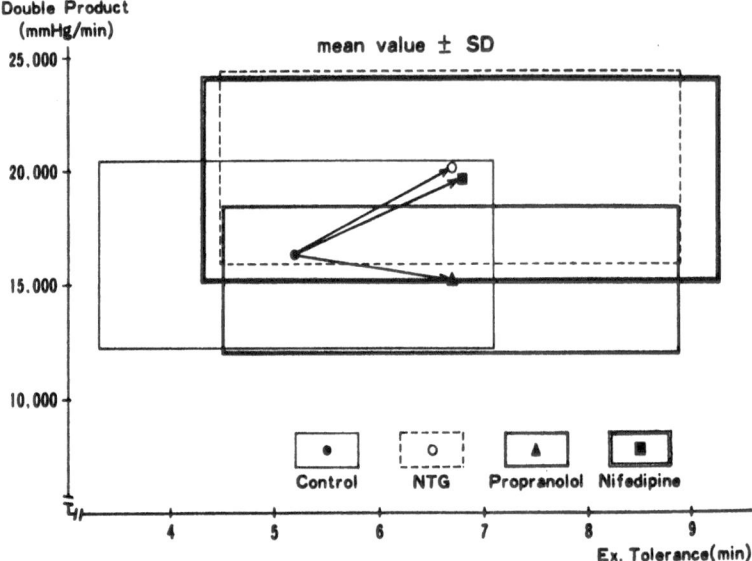

Fig. 7. Mean changes in exercise tolerance and double product in ergometric exercise test
(n = 11)

Table 1. Patients examined in a long-term therapeutic trial with nifedipine

Angina on Effort	16 Cases
Angina on Effort and at Rest	9 Cases
Angina at Rest	3 Cases
Variant Form of Angina	7 Cases
Total	35 Cases

evidence, it seems likely that the mechanism of action of nifedipine is similar to
that of nitroglycerin.

Thirty-five in- and outpatients were admitted to a subsequent long-term therapeutic study with nifedipine (Table 1).

The case-load consisted of 27 males and 8 females, aged 46–76 years. The
patients were either resistant to or poorly responding to therapy with other
antianginal drugs and had typical ischemic ECG changes during attacks.

They received 30 or 40 mg of nifedipine daily, taken orally in 3 or 4 single
doses for up to 12 weeks.

The main parameters for evaluating therapeutic results included reduction of
frequency of anginal attacks and decrease of nitroglycerin consumption. When
the number of anginal attacks and/or consumption of nitroglycerin was reduced
to less than 1/2 the original number, the therapeutic results were graded as
"Good". The other cases were graded as "Poor". Comparison of initial and final
ECG's was used as supplementary evidence.

Nifedipine therapy was judged "Good" in 11 out of 16 patients with angina on
effort, in 7 out of 9 patients with angina on effort and at rest, and in 2 out of
3 patients with angina at rest (Table 2).

Table 2. Effect of nifedipine on subjective symptoms in a long-term therapeutic trial with nifedipine

Angina on Effort	$^{11}/_{16}$	(68.8%)
Angina on Effort and at Rest	$^{7}/_{9}$	(77.8%)
Angina at Rest	$^{2}/_{3}$	(66.7%)
Variant Form of Angina	$^{7}/_{7}$	(100.0%)
Total	$^{27}/_{35}$	(77.1%)

Seven patients with variant forms of angina, whose blood pressures, ECGs, etc. were monitored continuously in our Coronary Care Unit, responded particularly well. In all 7 patients nifedipine was judged "Good".

Discussion and Conclusions

In previous ergometric tests, we investigated changes of exercise tolerance and double product of patients with angina on effort, who were medicated with nitroglycerin and propranolol. At that time we concluded that nitroglycerin resulted in an increase in the double product that was proportional to that of exercise tolerance. Propranolol improved exercise tolerance but the value of the double product either remained the same or decreased slightly. The double product levels for nitroglycerin and propranolol during attacks were significantly different. Assuming that the work threshold of anginal pain did not change during exercise, patients under the effects of nitroglycerin could tolerate a higher double product, i.e., a higher oxygen demand of the myocardium.

In the present study the same method was used as in the previous one, but with the addition of the new drug, nifedipine.

The use of all 3 drugs increased exercise tolerance in all patients. The double product was also increased with nifedipine and nitroglycerin, whereas with propranolol it did not change in some cases, and was even lowered in others. In view of these results, we believe that the therapeutic profile of nifedipine exhibits combined features of both nitroglycerin and propranolol. In a long-term study of the oral administration of nifedipine to patients with various types of angina pectoris, the drug was found to be effective in 68.8% of patients with angina on effort, in 77.8% of patients with angina on effort and at rest, in 66.7% of patients with angina at rest and in 100% of patients with variant forms of angina.

During nifedipine therapy for up to 12 weeks, neither side-effects nor changes of liver function and of other clinical laboratory tests for pathological values were observed.

Abstract

Ergometric exercise tolerance tests were carried out in 11 patients with stable angina, reproducible by physical effort, after medication with nifedipine, nitroglycerin and propranolol. Physical capacity and double product (calculated from blood pressure and pulse rate) were measured. Nifedipine and nitroglycerin, both taken sublingually, increased physical capacity and double product. Propranolol, taken orally, increased exercise tolerance in some patients, but double product values either remained unchanged or decreased.

Admitted to a subsequent therapeutical trial, were 35 in- and outpatients of Sakurabashi Watanabe Hospital with typical anginal attacks and ischemic ST-changes during attacks or exercise tests. Nifedipine in a daily dosage of 30–40 mg administered for up to 12 weeks proved to be remarkably effective. It was found to be effective in 68.8% of patients with angina on effort, in 77.8% of patients with angina on effort and at rest, in 66.7% of patients with angina at rest and in 100% of patients with variant forms of angina. No adverse reactions were recorded. Clinical laboratory tests such as GOT, GPT, alkaline phosphatase remained within normal range throughout the investigation.

Influence of Different Doses of Adalat on Angina Pectoris Induced by Exercise

A. PREMPREE and B. TABATZNIK

North Charles General Hospital, Baltimore, USA

Introduction

The purpose of this study was to examine the effect of different doses of Adalat on exercise performance in patients with chronic stable angina pectoris.

Materials and Methods

Twenty-one male patients were initially recruited according to the following criteria:

All patients had had classical angina of effort for at least 4 months and there had been no recent increase in the frequency or severity of attacks. A treadmill exercise test had resulted in the development of typical ischemic chest pain and typical ischemic changes in the ST segment. All patients were able to complete at least the first stage of the Bruce treadmill test, namely 3 min of exercise at 1.7 miles per hour at a gradient of 10%, equivalent to 5 mets of energy expenditure.

The following study protocol was used:

1. All medications with the exception of nitroglycerin were discontinued 48 h prior to the study.

2. No food or cigarettes were used for at least 3 h prior to the study.

3. Three consecutive exercise periods were performed with the patient in the upright position on a motor-driven treadmill. The work load was increased every 3 min until either the onset of angina or fatigue.

Exercise period I was performed without premedication.

Exercise period II was carried out 10 min after premedication with known placebo.

Exercise period III was performed 30 min after administration of either unknown placebo (Group I), 10 mg of Adalat (Group II) or 20 mg of Adalat (Group III), according to random allocation.

The assigned medication was given in the form of 2 capsules such that absorption took place from the buccal mucosa. Parameters for evaluation, namely heart rate, blood pressure, ST segment depression, exercise capacity and presence or absence of chest pain were determined before, during and after each exercise period.

Table 1. Influence of different doses of Adalat on angina pectoris induced by exercise

Patient profile	
Age range	41—67 (mean 54)
Prior MI	2
Normal resting ECG	19
Exclusions	
< 5 mets	2
Side effects	1
Mean duration of exercise	
Group I	3.68 min
Group II	5.72 min
Group III	3.62 min

The relevant characteristics of the recruited patients are shown in Table 1. The age range was between 41 and 67 with a mean of 54. Two patients had sustained a prior myocardial infarction. The remaining 19 had normal resting electrocardiograms. Two patients could not complete 3 min of exercise at an energy expenditure of 5 mets and were excluded from the subsequent analysis. A third patient was also excluded from analysis because he developed severe side-effects after administration of 20 mg Adalat and could not perform the third exercise period.

Satisfactory randomization into the 3 groups was probably not achieved because of the small number of patients studied. Thus, the mean duration of exercise achieved in Group II (10 mg Adalat) was significantly greater than that achieved in Groups I (placebo) and III (20 mg Adalat). In the first exercise period the mean duration of exercise in Group I patients was 3.86 min, in Group II patients 5.72 min, and in Group III patients 3.62 min. This implies a less severe degree of angina in Group II patients compared with the other groups.

The only other significant difference between the groups was in height— Group II patients were significantly taller than Groups I and III patients. Nine patients, almost equally distributed among the groups, underwent coronary cineangiographic studies.

Results

1. Onset of Angina

The onset of exercise-induced angina pectoris was delayed in both Group II and Group III patients (Table 2). All patients developed chest pain either during or immediately after the first exercise period; one patient in Group I and two patients in Group II did not have pain at an equivalent work load during the second exercise period, presumably due to a training effect. During the third exercise period, the same patient pretreated with placebo who did not have pain during the second exercise period again had no pain. None of the patients pretreated with 10 mg of Adalat had pain at a generally increased work load, and only 1 patient pretreated with 20 mg Adalat had pain, again at an increased work load. These results are statistically significant at $p \leq 0.005$ comparing placebo with the 10 mg dose and $p \leq 0.080$ comparing placebo with the 20 mg dose.

Table 2. Influence of different doses of Adalat on angina pectoris induced by exercise

Exercise induced chest pain Angina	Placebo (n = 6)	10 mg (n = 7)	20 mg (n = 6)
Exercise I			
Yes	6	7	6
No	0	0	0
Exercise II (known placebo)			
Yes	5	5	6
No	1	2	0
Exercise III (active drug)			
Yes	5	0[a]	1[b]
No	1	7	4

[a] Placebo VS 10 mg nifedipine — $p \leq 0.005$.
[b] Placebo VS 20 mg nifedipine — $p \leq 0.080$.

2. Duration of Exercise

The mean duration of exercise was increased in patients who received active drug as compared with placebo. A very slight training effect was observed in patients in each of the three groups. Thus, patients in all 3 groups increased their exercise duration between the first and second exercise periods (Fig. 1). However, a greater increase was observed in both treatment groups between the second and third exercise periods. Patients on 10 mg Adalat were able to exercise by an

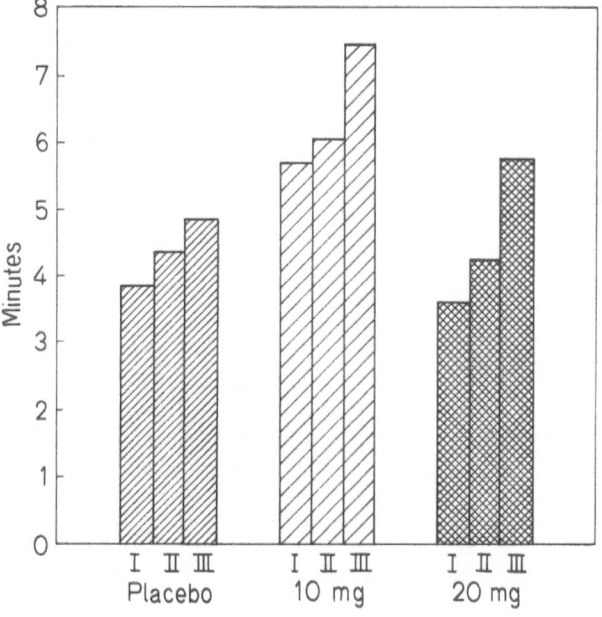

Fig. 1. Influence of different doses of Adalat on angina pectoris induced by exercise

additional mean time duration of 1.44 min at either the same or an increased work load, whereas patients on 20 mg Adalat increased their exercise performance by a mean duration of 1.65 min, generally at the same work load. These increments in exercise duration show a clear trend of superiority of Adalat over placebo.

3. Effect on ST Segment Depression

Although exercise performance was improved and angina did not occur under the influence of Adalat, ischemic changes appeared on the electrocardiogram at an increased work load in all instances.

4. Alterations in Heart Rate and Blood Pressure

Alterations in heart rate and blood pressure occurred much as anticipated from the peripheral vasodilator action of Adalat. The resting heart rate rose by a mean value of 33 beats per minute, 24 min after administration of 20 mg Adalat and 10 beats per minute on the 10 mg dose (Fig. 2). The systolic blood pressure dropped by a mean value of 8 mm Hg on the 10 mg dose and 17 mm Hg on the 20 mg dose, 20 min after ingestion of the drug (Fig. 2). Only modest drops in diastolic pressure occurred.

Significantly greater heart rates were achieved at the end of exercise under the influence of active drug, commensurate with the improvement in exercise performance (Fig. 3). Blood pressure levels achieved at the end of the third exercise period were consistently lower on active drug compared with the first two exercise periods (Fig. 3), but these alterations were not statistically significant.

5. Side-Effects

Significant side-effects occurred in 8 patients, all on active drug (Table 3). Four of seven patients had side-effects at both doses of active drug. These included flushing, headache, dizziness, postural hypotension, nausea and weakness. One

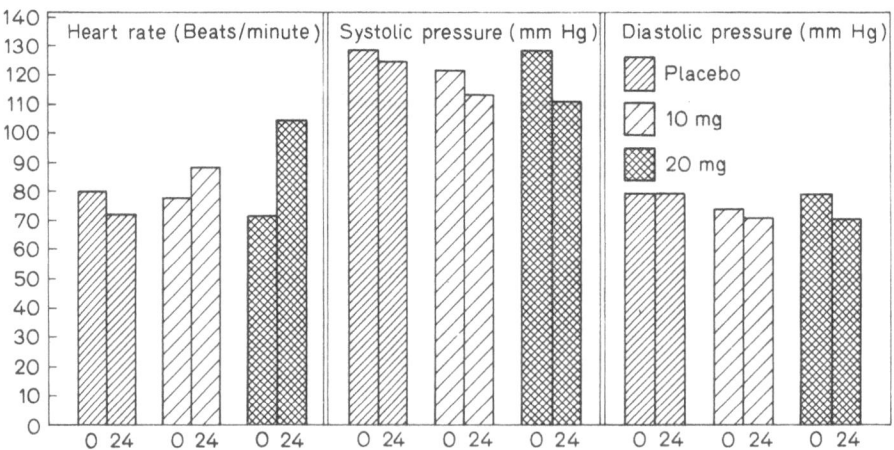

Fig. 2. Influence of different doses of Adalat on angina pectoris induced by exercise

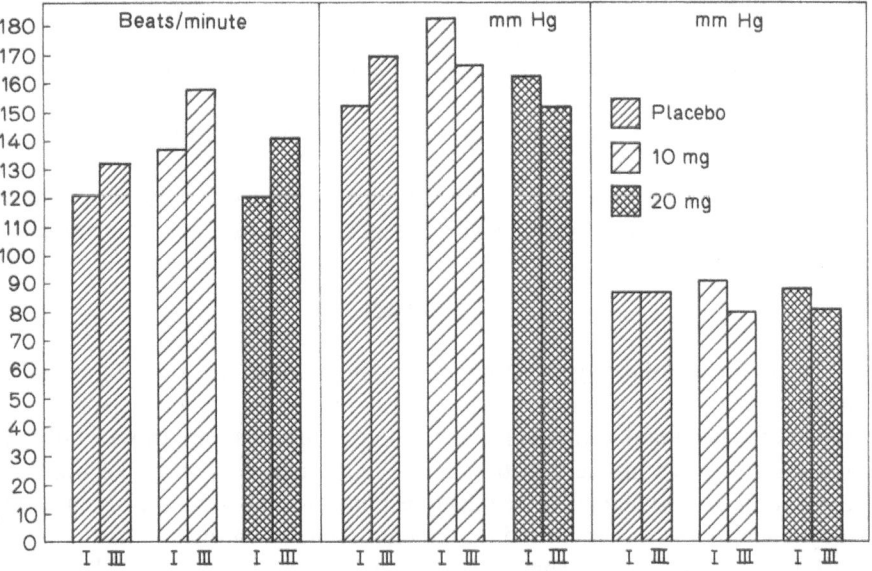

Fig. 3. Influence of different doses of Adalat on angina pectoris induced by exercise

Table 3. Influence of different doses of Adalat on angina pectoris induced by exercise

Number of patients reporting side effects			
Side effect	Placebo	10 mg	20 mg
Postural hypotension			2
Junctional rhythm			1
PVC's		1	
Chest discomfort		1	2
Dizziness		1	2
Headache		4	1
Blurring of vision			1
Flushing		1	2
Nausea			1
Weakness			1
Total	0/7	4/7	4/7

patient had very frequent ventricular extrasystoles accompanied by flushing and pounding in the head; another patient developed postural hypotension and dizziness associated with sinoatrial depression and a junctional escape rhythm at 43 per minute, and a third patient had marked dizziness associated with hypotension, flushing and chest and arm pain.

Conclusions

1. Adalat at both 10 and 20 mg doses significantly delays the onset of chest pain in patients with stable angina pectoris tested on a motor-driven treadmill at graded work loads.

2. It increases the duration of exercise in these patients, although in this small series, not in sufficient magnitude to be statistically significant.

3. It does not abolish the ischemic response of the ST segments at increased work loads.

4. There does not appear to be a clear-cut advantage of the 20 mg dose over the 10 mg dose.

5. Side-effects, particularly flushing, dizziness, nausea, and postural hypotension, and rhythm disturbances in some instances, are common, particularly at the 20 mg dose.

Abstract

The effect of Adalat (generic nifedipine) in a single oral dose of 10 mg and 20 mg on exercise performance was studied in a group of male patients with moderately severe stable angina pectoris. Eligible subjects were those whose maximal exercise performance was between 5 and 8 mets and who had both chest pain and typical ischemic ST segment response as end points in their control study. Each patient was exercised to maximal capacity on the treadmill at graded work loads according to Bruce's protocol in 3 successive periods. The first two exercise periods were performed without premedication, and the third exercise period was performed 30 min after treatment with a single tablet containing either placebo (Group I), 10 mg of Adalat (Group II) or 20 mg of Adalat (Group III), administered in a double-blind fashion.

Of the 19 patients studied, 1 was unable to perform the third exercise period because of postural hypotension and nausea following administration of 20 mg of Adalat. Six patients were randomly allocated to each of Groups I, II, and III. In the third exercise period as compared with the second exercise period, the duration of exercise (in minutes) was increased by 12% in Group I (presumed training effect), 23% in Group II and 32% in Group III. Whereas all 18 patients developed chest pain as a clearcut end point in the first exercise period, none of the patients in Group II and only 2 of 6 patients in Group III developed chest pain in the third exercise period in spite of significantly higher heart rates; only 1 patient pretreated with placebo failed to develop angina in both the second and third exercise periods. Maximal effects of Adalat on pulse rate and blood pressure were noted from 20 to 30 min after ingestion of the drug. The systolic pressure fell significantly (mean fall 16.3 mm Hg) and the heart rate rose significantly (mean rise 33.3 beats per minute) with the 20 mg dose prior to the third exercise period.

It is concluded that Adalat increases exercise performance in patients with moderately severe angina pectoris and delays the onset of exercise induced chest pain. This effect occurs with a dose of 10 mg as well as 20 mg. There seems little advantage in the 20 mg dose over the 10 mg dose, particularly since the larger dose may induce hypotension, nausea and flushing.

Discussion Remarks

Kober: You found an increase in exercise tolerance and the subsequent appearance of chest pain after administration of nifedipine, but you also said that there was no influence on ST depression in the ECG. Did you mean that this ST-segment depression was not altered when you compared the control exercise test with that under nifedipine during a higher work load, or did you compare the ST-segment during and after nifedipine on the same work load?

TABATZNIK: This was at the higher work load. I think had we compared the ST-segment at the same work load we might have come to the same conclusion that, although the angina disappeared and exercise performance was improved under nifedipine, the ischemic ST changes did occur at the point at which exercise was terminated usually by fatigue.

MCARTHUR: Dr. TABATZNIK, you mentioned that you had more side effects with the 20-mg dose than with the 10-mg dose and yet on your slide you noted four out of seven patients had side-effects in both the 10-mg and 20-mg doses. Do I take this to mean that the severity of the side effects was different under the two doses schedules?

TABATZNIK: That is correct; we had two patients on the 20-mg dose; one patient could not be exercised following administration of the drug because of partial hypotension and the second patient was the patient who developed very striking sinorhythm depression with a junctional rhythm at 42/min on the 20-mg dose. So the differences were quantitative.

Nifedipine in the Treatment of Ischemic Heart Disease

S. YASUI, Y. MIZUNO, I. SOTOHATA, and Y. WATANABE

First Department of Internal Medicine, Nagoya University School of Medicine and
Department of Internal Medicine, Fujita Gakuen University, School of Medicine,
Nagoya, Japan

Introduction

Clinical trials with Adalat (generic nifedipine) in patients with ischemic heart disease have been performed continuously by many investigators for several years.

Basic investigations concerning the mechanism of its pharmacologic action have been made at the same time. According to FLECKENSTEIN [1], nifedipine restricts the transmembrane Ca influx during excitation. In reducing the Ca supply to the contractile system, nifedipine interferes with the activation of the Ca-dependent myofibrillar ATPase. The production of mechanical tension and oxygen consumption decrease, and the tone of vascular smooth muscle fibers, particularly in the coronary arteries, is also diminished.

HASHIMOTO [2] showed that nifedipine produced a marked coronary dilatation in dogs. The principal cardiodynamic effect was dilatation of the coronary vascular bed with increased total cardiac output, while an overdose of nifedipine produced negative chronotropic, dromotropic and inotropic effects.

Taking these basic studies into consideration, we have given nifedipine, with excellent results, to patients with angina pectoris. At this symposium, we will report on our experience with nifedipine treatment.

Materials and Methods

1. Patients

Thirty-eight patients with ischemic heart disease were admitted to the study. Thirty cases had angina pectoris on effort, two, angina pectoris both on effort and at rest, one, angina pectoris at rest, and five, angina pectoris with obsolete or acute myocardial infarction (Table 1).

The patients, 18 men and 20 women, ranged in age from 36 to 78 years.

2. Administration of Nifedipine

Three placebo capsules per day were first administered for one or two weeks to observe the frequency of anginal attacks. Thereafter, daily doses of 3–6 capsules, each containing 10 mg of nifedipine, were given after meals. Nifedipine

Table 1. Subjects receiving nifedipine

Subjects (36—78 years)	
1. Angina pectoris on effort	30
2. Angina pectoris on effort and at rest	2
3. Angina pectoris at rest	1
4. Angina pectoris with obsolete or acute myocardial infarction	5
Total	38 cases

was administered over a period ranging from 2 weeks to 3 years, except for 6 cases in whom the drug was discontinued because of side-effects.

Nine out of 13 cases with systemic hypertension received concomitantly anti-hypertensive agents, and one received digitalis for prevention of paroxysmal atrial tachycardia. Three were continuously on coronary dilators, which they had taken previously.

3. Clinical and Laboratory Examination

Measurement of blood pressure, physical examination and ECG examination with double Master's exercise test were usually performed every week or every two weeks. The patients had a daily card on which they described the medicine they took and their subjective symptoms, especially concerning anginal attacks.

At every outpatient visit, deficiencies of the records were filled in through a questionnaire.

"Excellent" was used to denote the patients whose anginal attacks disappeared during administration of nifedipine. "Good" refers to those with diminished complaint of angina after nifedipine treatment.

The ECG findings were also classified according to the degree of beneficial response. The efficiency of the drug was graded as "excellent" in patients in whom ST-T changes became normalized or in whom a previously positive Master's exercise test became negative with nifedipine. It was classified as "fairly good" in patients whose resting and postexercise ECG's were improved but not normalized.

Results

Several cases in whom there was improvement in ECG findings as well as in subjective symptoms after nifedipine will be presented first.

Case 1 H.K., 48 years old, female

Angina pectoris on effort and at rest

This patient complained of a sense of tightness in her chest during exertion and occasionally at rest and came to the hospital in September, 1970. At the first visit, her resting ECG showed slight ST depression of horizontal type in leads V_3 through V_6. Master's two-step test was diagnosed as positive with the ST segment more depressed than in the control.

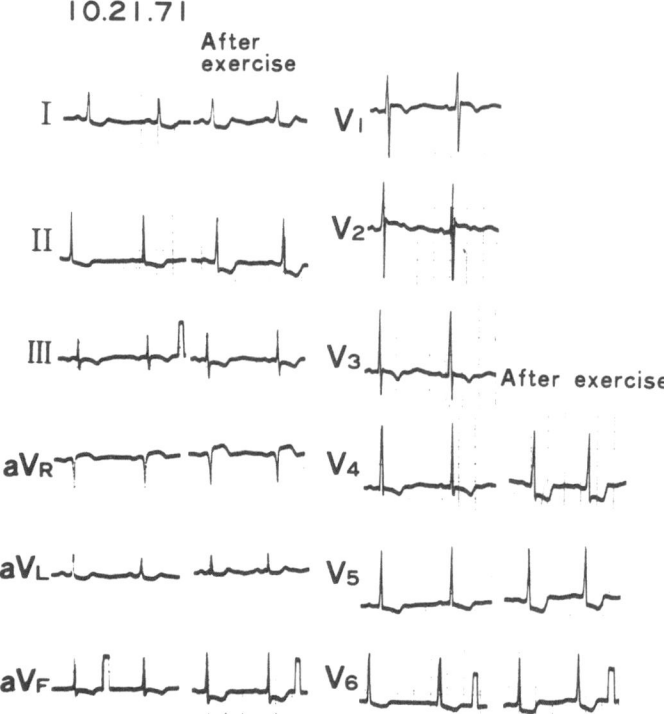

Fig. 1. Case 2. (H.S., 61 years, female). ECG was obtained before treatment with nifedipine

With a daily dose of nifedipine of 30 mg for one week, her anginal attacks disappeared. One month later, the patient could go on a trip free from anginal pain. A remarkable improvement in ECG occurred in November (just 4 weeks after starting the treatment with nifedipine). The resting and exercise ECG's became normalized.

At the beginning of the treatment, she complained of transient headache, which was presumably a side-effect of nifedipine, but did not require interruption of the treatment.

Case 2 H.S., 61 years old, female

Angina pectoris on effort and diabetes mellitus

She suffered from substernal pain when walking up a slight incline. Her substernal pain and dyspnea were relieved by the administration of isosorbide dinitrate. The brachial blood pressure was 162/82 mm Hg. Her resting ECG in October 21, 1971 showed ischemic ST-T changes in left precordial leads. With Master's exercise test, a sagging type of ST depression became more distinct in leads V_4 through V_6 (Fig. 1).

With 30 mg of nifedipine daily, her complaints diminished within two months. In January 13, 1972, ischemic ST changes became less marked as compared with the previous ECG. Furthermore, the grade of ST depression in leads V_4 through V_6 was decreased in Master's exercise test (Fig. 2). Then, a type of dinitrate was administered in place of nifedipine, but dyspnea and angina on exertion reap-

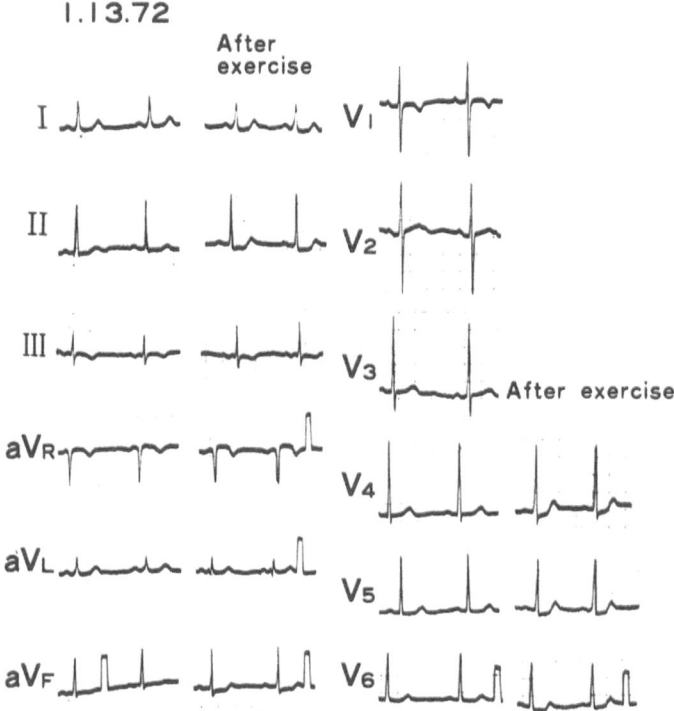

I. I 3.72

Fig. 2. Case 2 (H.S., 62 years, female). ECG was recorded on Jan. 13, 1972, during nifedipine treatment

peared. After January 27, 1972, nifedipine was resumed in the same way as before, and subjective symptoms again were relieved. During the three-year-period of treatment, her course was satisfactory, both in subjective symptoms and ECG findings (Fig. 3).

During the observation period, liver function and blood cell examination revelated no abnormalities.

Case 3 T.Y., 61 years old, male

Angina pectoris on effort and at rest

At the beginning of October, 1969, he came to the hospital, complaining of precordial pain during walking. In the ECG dated October 16, 1969, there was a slight ischemic ST change in V_6, and Master's double two-step test induced more marked ST depression of the horizontal type in leads 11, 111, aVF and V_{4-6}.

On October 30, 1969, treatment with 30 mg of nifedipine per day was begun, no recognized improvement of subjective symptoms was noted in four weeks. At this point, exercise ECG showed slight improvement. Therefore, nifedipine was changed for verapamil with a daily dose of 6 tablets, and subjective symptoms disappeared.

In August, 1970, he again complained of precordial pain during walking and also at rest early in the morning. Master's exercise test induced 1 mm ST depression of the sagging type in V_6. Nifedipine was administered again.

1.24.74   8.15.74

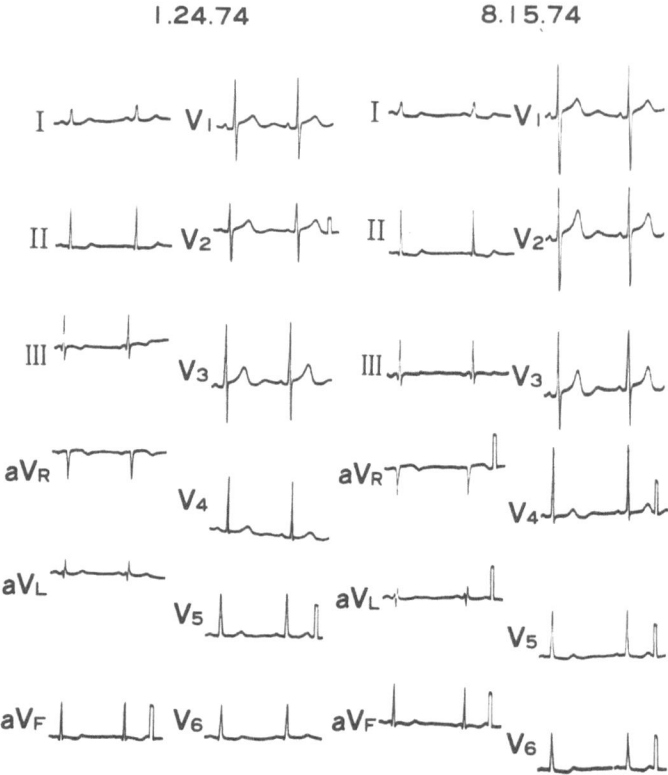

Fig. 3. Case 2. (H.S., 64 years, female). ECG recorded after three-year-period of treatment with nifedipine

Two months later, the ECG findings were slightly improved, while subjective symptoms remained unchanged.

Nifedipine was replaced by Inderal. Two months later, he had severe anginal pain lasting longer than thirty minutes and died of acute myocardial infarction.

Case 4 T.S., 58 years old, female

Angina pectoris and essential hypertension

She came to the hospital with complaints of precordial pain during walking. Her brachial blood pressure was 184/60 mm Hg. She began to take 30 mg of nifedipine daily on October 23, 1969, and the daily dose was increased to 60 mg on November 6.

The ECG recorded on October 23, 1969, indicated left ventricular hypertrophy and strain. Master's exercise test showed 4 mm depression in V_5. With nifedipine treatment for six weeks, subjective complaints were remarkably relieved so that she could take a bath.

At this time, the resting ECG showed a normal pattern, while the exercise test revealed 2.5 mm ST depression in V_5.

Ankle edema and liver swelling were observed, liver function remaining normal.

In this case, nifedipine was administered for a 3- to 4-month period three times, separated by a time interval of 2 months.

Significant improvement in ECG findings and subjective symptoms occurred invariably upon resumption of nifedipine.

Ankle edema and liver swelling were observed only during the first trial.

Summary

The effects of nifedipine on 38 patients with coronary heart disease have been investigated.

In regard to the complaints, 9 cases exhibited excellent responses with disappearance of anginal pain or chest pain, and 19 cases, fairly good response, making a total of 28 effective cases (74%) (Table 2).

The effects on ischemic ST-T changes and the response to Master's exercise test were remarkably good in 6 cases and fairly good in 12 cases, totalling 18 cases with a good response (48%) (Table 3).

The effect of nifedipine on the subjective complaints appeared within the first week and on ECG findings, after one week.

Concerning the side-effects, hot flushes appeared in three cases, throbbing headache in four, itching in one, epigastric discomfort in one, and ankle edema in one. Six cases discontinued treatment due to these side effects, particularly flushing and headache (Table 4).

In the course of the treatment, remarkable changes in blood pressure and heart rate were not observed.

There were also no significant changes in the values of serum electrolytes such as Na, K, and Cl, which were measured before and after medication at an interval of 4 weeks.

As to liver function disturbances, no abnormal values could be seen in GOT, GPT and alkaline-phosphatase during treatment with nifedipine.

Table 2. Effect of nifedipine on subjective symptoms

Excellent	9 (24%)	28 (74%)
Good	19 (50%)	
Unchanged	10[a] (26%)	
Total	38 cases	

[a] Discontinued within 2 weeks due to flushing etc. in 6 cases.

Table 3. Effect of nifedipine on ECG changes

Excellently improved	6 (16%)	18 (48%)
Fairly good	12 (32%)	
Unchanged	20[a] (52%)	
Total	38 cases	

[a] Discontinued within 2 weeks due to flushing etc. in 6 cases.

Table 4. Side-effects of nifedipine

Flushing	3 (2)[a]
Headache	4 (3)[a]
Itching	1 (1)[a]
Epigastric discomfort	1
Ankle edema	1

[a] Discontinued within 2 weeks.

Abstract

A clinical trial with nifedipine was performed including 38 patients with ischemic heart desease.

It was recognized that nifedipine is an excellent drug for the treatment of angina pectoris, because it resulted in marked improvement in ECG findings as well as in subjective symptoms.

References

1. FLECKENSTEIN, A., TRITTHART, H., DÖRING, H.-J., BYON, K. Y.: BAY a 1040 — ein hochaktiver CA^{++}-antagonistischer Inhibitor der elektro-mechanischen Koppelungsprozesse im Warmblüter-Myokard. Arzneim.-Forsch. (Drug Res.) **22**, 22 (1972).
2. HASHIMOTO, K., TAIRA, N., CHIBA, S., HASHIMOTO, K., JR., ENDOH, M., KOKUBUN, M., KOKUBUN, H., IIJIMA, T., KIMURA, T., KUBOTA, K., OGURO, K.: Cardiohemodynamic effects of BAY a 1040 in the Dog. Arzneim.-Forsch. (Drug Res.) **22**, 15 (1972).

Clinical Observations on the Efficacy of Adalat Compared with a Pentaerythrityl Tetranitrate Preparation

G. C. Maggi and F. Piscitello

Department of Cardiology, Ospedale Bassini, Milan, Italy

Introduction

During the First International Nifedipine "Adalat"-Symposium, held in Tokyo in November 1973 we presented a preliminary paper on the clinical activity of this new coronary active drug (generic: nifedipine; Adalat).

As discussed in the pharmacology sections in Tokyo as well as here, the most important properties of Adalat are well known.

The only point I would like to emphasize concerns the pharmacokinetics of Adalat; taken orally 90% of the drug is absorbed and 55–65% is excreted in the urine.

The maximum pharmacological effect is reached between 10 and 30 min, but the drug is present in the blood in active concentrations up to 3 h after administration.

Thus Adalat acts almost immediately and is long-lasting. Consequently it is probably useful in prevention of angina pectoris attacks.

In Tokyo Professor Kimura and his colleagues discussed the clinical evaluation of the effects of Adalat on angina pectoris: sequential analysis indicates the significant efficacy of the drug. It is as effective as propranolol and isosorbide dinitrate, as was shown in comparative clinical trials of these drugs.

Good and satisfactory results are generally reported with the use of pentaerythrityl tetranitrate (PETN) preparations to prevent attacks of angina pectoris.

The effect of PETN has a relatively quick onset, the drug is well tolerated in a good percentage of patients and, finally, is very popular in therapy, as the sales figures indicate. For these reasons, we chose for this trial a PETN-preparation as a comparison drug for Adalat.

The purpose of our trial was to compare the clinical efficacy of Adalat with a timed-release form of PETN in a group of patients with typical attacks of angina pectoris. We ran this trial either double blind or open.

Materials and Methods

From a roster of ambulatory anginal patients at the Bassini Hospital in Milan, 50 were approved for admission to this study. The patients included 40 males and 10 females, ranging from 32.5 to 60.4 years of age.

Each met the criteria of Gazes and colleagues, who stated that "the diagnosis of angina pectoris is dependent upon the history and electrocardiographic changes".

Twelve patients were examined coronarographically.

The symptoms had been present for at least 6 months and did not alter during that time.

No one needed digitalis therapy. The primary disability was a typical anginal syndrome precipitated by effort and/or emotion and relieved by sublingual tablets of glyceryl trinitrate. None had been hospitalized before for myocardial infarction or intermediate syndrome.

A thorough physical examination was made in each case. An accurate history was taken separately by two different physicians with particular reference to the frequency, intensity and duration of anginal pain, exercise tolerance, and number of tablets of glyceryl trinitrate consumed daily. During the preliminary screening examination, characteristic ischemic ST segment displacements appeared in the rest or in the work loading electrocardiograms obtained following the classic criteria.

The nature of our investigation was explained to these patients, and they participated voluntarily in the trial.

Both gelatine capsules looked the same, but one contained PETN and the other, Adalat. The daily doses were 3×80 mg of PETN or 3×10 mg of Adalat given orally.

Neither the physcian nor the patient had any foreknowledge of the content of the capsules.

Each patient was given Adalat or the PETN preparation for a 2-week period.

The allocation was randomized, and the trial was designed as a double-blind cross-over comparison.

Patients were asked to take glyceryl trinitrate as usual for the attacks of pain, but not prophylactically and to keep a record of the attacks of pain and number of tablets of glyceryl trinitrate taken; they were given a record sheet for a week. The patients were asked to record the time of onset of any attack, the duration, to assess severity as mild, moderate, or severe, to note the number of glyceryl trinitrate tablets consumed, and to record any comment they desired. Patients were reexamined weekly; subjective impressions and any complaint of side-effects were noted.

Results

The results have been analyzed from three aspects:

1. number of attacks of pain from each patient during the trials when on Adalat or PETN preparation; each attack was scored as one, regardless of severity or duration;

2. number of glyceryl trinitrate tablets consumed and

3. subjective feeling of the patients, whether they felt generally better when taking the drug, apart from relief of pain.

Since the number of attacks and the number of glyceryl trinitrate tablets used were similar from week to week and from patient to patient, statistical analysis was carried out only on the number of attacks.

Of the 50 patients, 44 had fewer attacks when on Adalat than when on PETN preparation; this in itself is statistically significant ($p = 0.003$) and has the advantage over other analyses of being independent of subjective opinions.

The weekly subjective reports of the patients were expressed, according to Prichard and colleagues, as much better ($+2$), better ($+1$), same (0), worse (-1), and much worse (-2).

Examination of these results showed a consensus in favor of Adalat that was significant.

No significant side-effects were reported with either drug for the doses used in our trial.

Another group of 30 patients, a number of whom participated in the a.m. double-blind study, was treated with both drugs in an open trial.

In this trial about 80% of the patients claimed improvement. They consistently preferred Adalat and claimed fewer benefits on any occasion from PETN preparation.

In summary, a marked improvement in the typical anginal syndrome was observed during Adalat treatment, both in double-blind and open trials.

The results with Adalat were definitively superior to those obtained with PETN preparation.

Abstract

The aim of this clinical double-blind trial was to compare the efficacy of nifedipine versus pentaerythrityl tetranitrate preparation.

From a roster of ambulatory anginal patients, 50 were approved for admission to this study. The patients included 40 males and 10 females. The symptoms had been present for at least six months and did not alter appreciably during that time.

A thorough physical examination was made in each case: an accurate history was taken separately by two different physicians of our department with particular reference to the frequency, intensity and duration of anginal pain, exercise tolerance and number of tablets of glyceryl trinitrate consumed daily.

The results were analyzed from three aspects:

1. number of attacks of pain experienced by each patient during the trial, when on nifedipine and PETN preparation; each attack was scored as one, regardless of severity of duration;

2. number of glyceryl trinitrate tablets consumed and

3. subjective feeling of the patients.

Of the 50 patients 44 had significantly fewer attacks when on nifedipine than when on PETN preparation.

A marked improvement in anginal syndrome could be shown during nifedipine treatment; the results were definitely superior to those obtained with PETN preparation.

Discussion Remarks

Hagemeijer: Did you observe those side effects as often as Dr. Tabatznik has shown, and is it clinically worrisome?

Maggi: With doses used by us there are no side effects but with "single" doses of 30 mg headache may occur.

Tabatznik: With reference to the side effects, I think it should be emphasized that the side effects that I observed were under acute experimental conditions and may have had no bearing on the observations of other workers; that in chronic studies the same side effects may not be observed as in a third exercise period, when the patient had already been exercised twice, was peripherally dilated, and so on, and the conditions are different.

Clinical Studies on the Combined Effect of Various Antihypertensive Agents and Adalat

U. Laaser, K. A. Meurer, H. Krüger, and W. Kaufmann

Medizinische Universitäts-Poliklinik, Cologne, Fed. Rep. Germany

Introduction

According to BEGEMANN [1] one cannot postulate linear-causal relationships when evaluating synchronous drug effects. Since we usually do prescribe more than one drug to a patient, it is of high priority to analyze the interaction of drugs during the phase of their experimental and clinical testing.

Although this type of analysis seems to be most advanced in the study of anticoagulants [3], the problem applies also to the therapy of angina pectoris with its polypragmatic approach.

Because coronary heart disease is often a complication of hypertension [5], the combination of coronary with antihypertensive drugs is not a rare event.

In order to evaluate more precisely the possibility of interactions between Adalat and antihypertensive agents, a 6-week double-blind cross-over experiment was designed for the outpatient department of the University of Cologne.

As can be seen from Table 1, 30 patients completed the study. After a one-week pre-test period, they received Adalat and placebo in a double-blind technique. The dosage of Adalat was 10 mg, 3 times daily.

Table 1. Experimental design

Group	Antihypertensive	Diuretic	N
A	methyl-dopa 750 mg (Presinol)	triamteren 50 mg and hydrochlorothiazide 25 mg (Dytide H)[a]	10
B	reserpine 0.25 mg (Serpasil)	triamteren 50 mg and hydrochlorothiazide 25 mg (Dytide H)	7
C	*various* methyl-dopa reserpine dihydralazine clonidine alprenolole	*various* triamteren hydrochlorothiazide clompamide mefruside spironolactone	13

[a] 2 patients with mefruside, 10 and 25 mg.

In 7 other patients, we discontinued Adalat-intake because of adverse reactions. One patient was eliminated from the final analysis because he did not show up for check-ups regularly enough due to a common cold.

The 30 patients who completed the study received their test medication (Table 1) and:

either 750 mg methyl-dopa daily and a diuretic (group A) or 0.25 mg reserpine and the same diuretic (group B). A third group (C) received various but constant antihypertensive medications.

Any accompanying medication was stopped whenever possible except for nitroglycerin (Nitrolingual grün) sublingually for severe intermittent attacks of angina. But some patients took digitalis (usually Novodigal 2×0.2 mg).

Throughout the trial period the patients came in for check-ups on days 1, 8, 22, 29, and 43.

Blood pressure measurements were taken, with some exceptions, by an automatic registering device of Bosch AG in the supine and in the upright position, allowing the patient at least one minute to adapt his circulation to this position. In addition, at each check-up, we questioned the patients concerning side-effects, anginal attacks and nitroglycerin consumption and whether they took their tablets regularly.

Although some doubts have been raised with regard to an outpatient setting in the evaluation of drugs [2], most of the patients had only a few capsules left in their bottles at the end of each three-week period.

We could not arrange a certain time of day for check-ups nor could we assure a constant time interval between intake of medication and the performance of the check-up. In almost every case, the time lag was longer than 60 min.

Due to the specific character of our clinic as a highly specialized diagnostic unit, there is considerable selection and heterogeneity among patients. Usually we receive our hypertensive clientele only for diagnostic procedures or if they do not respond to routine treatment.

From Table 2 one can see that the three groups are roughly comparable, at least with regard to age, weight and sex.

Because of a lower mean weight, group B patients received a slightly higher dose, per kg of Adalat.

All but two patients showed mild degrees of angina pectoris according to the Rose-questionnaire with little or no hypoxic changes in the ECG at rest. Most patients showed mild retinopathies corresponding to degree I or II in a modified Keith-Wagner system.

Table 2. Description of population

Group	Mean age (years)	Mean weight (kg)	Male/female
A	49	81	6/4
B	47	73	5/2
C	49	79	8/5

Results

The results reported here are preliminary. For each patient we calculated the mean arterial pressures (MAP) according to the formula:

$$MAP = D + 1/3\,(S - D)$$

where D ist the distolic and S the systolic pressure.

Then we averaged all measurements taken in the supine or upright position during each phase of treatment. Thus, each patient is entered into the mean arterial pressures of the various groups (Table 3) with 4 measurements under Adalat (2 supine, 2 upright) and with 4 measurements under placebo. For orientation we also indicated the corresponding pre-test-values (2 measurements per patient, 1 supine, 1 upright).

Table 3 summarizes the results from patients who received Adalat first. Directed differences of pressure under Adalat minus pressure under placebo could not be detected. The same was found for patients who received placebo first (Table 4).

Comparing treatment groups A, B, and C, again the differences are not impressive.

Although the proper statistical analysis has not yet been performed, we believe that it is safe to say, as can be seen from the summary in Table 5, that no additional hypotensive effect of clinical importance can be ascribed to Adalat on the basis of these results.

This is strengthened by the impression that the sequence Adalat—placebo versus placebo—Adalat does not cause a different trend of any importance.

Table 3. Mean arterial blood pressures (mm Hg)

| Adalat given first | | | | | |
Group	N	Pre-test	I Adalat	II Placebo	Diff. I—II
A	5	119	124	123	+1
B	2	121	104	101	+3
C	6	114	108	113	−5
Sum	13	117	114	115	−1

Table 4. Mean arterial blood pressures (mm Hg)

| Placebo given first | | | | | |
Group	N	Pre-test	II Adalat	I Placebo	Diff. II—I
A	5	129	125	131	−6
B	5	112	105	105	0
C	7	129	121	127	−6
Sum	17	124	117	122	−5

Table 5. Mean arterial blood pressures (mm Hg)

Medication-sequence	N	Pre-test	Adalat	Placebo	Diff. Adalat — Placebo
Adalat I	13	117	114	115	−1
Placebo I	17	124	117	122	−5
Total	30	121	116	119	−3

Discussion

The hypotensive effect of nitroglycerin and its derivatives is well documented [9].

From the literature, we know that some hypotensive effects have also been observed after administration of the calcium-antagonistic drug Adalat.

After doses of about 10–20 mg orally or sublingually, pressures fell by 10–20% [4, 8, 10, 11] with a minimum after 20–30 min. The dose of 1 mg intravenously lowered the systemic pressure of hypertensive patients after 10 min by 20% [6].

KOBAYASHI [7] treated 47 patients with angina, among them 26 hypertensives. The average before-after difference was less than 10 mm Hg.

Our results are in perfect accordance with these findings described in the literature. Thus far, there is no indication from the data that Adalat given on a long-term basis in combination with antihypertensive agents lowers the systemic pressure more than during a monotherapy. The decrease of blood pressure seems rather to be smaller.

Some patients, however, might experience a short hypotensive phase immediately after the ingestion of Adalat, which is probably of the same sort as that known from nitroglycerin.

Thus, we would conclude from the results of our investigation that Adalat can be given to hypertensive patients without additional precautions in regard to associated antihypertensive medication.

Abstract

In a double-blind cross-over technique 38 hypertensive outpatients with various levels of blood pressure were given Adalat (generic name nifedipine) in an oral dose of 3×10 mg daily for 3 weeks followed by a three-week placebo treatment and vice versa. There was a one-week preparation period, so patients usually remained under observation for 7 weeks.

As a specific treatment, mainly reserpine, methyl-dopa and clonidine were used. Adalat did not seem to cause any clinically relevant additional lowering of blood pressure.

References

1. BEGEMANN, H.: Med. Klin. **68**, 569 (1973).
2. BOURNE, H.R.: Internist **13**, 345 (1972).
3. GUGLER, R., DENGLER, H.J.: Klin. Wschr. **51**, 1081 (1973).

 4. Hayase,S., Hirakawa,S., Hosokawa,S., Mori,N., Kanyama,S., Iwasa,M.: Arzneim.-Forsch. **22**/2, 370 (1972).
 5. Kannel,W.B., Gordon,T., Schwartz,M.J.: Amer. J. Cardiol. **27**, 335 (1971).
 6. Klütsch,K., Schmidt,P., Grosswendt,J.: Arzneim.-Forsch. **22**/2, 377 (1972).
 7. Kobayashi,T., Ito,Y., Tawara,I.: Arzneim.-Forsch. **22**/2, 380 (1972).
 8. Kochsiek,K., Neubaur,J.: Arzneim.-Forsch. **22**/2, 353 (1972).
 9. Robinson,B.F.: Brit. Heart J. **30**, 295 (1968).
10. Schneider,K.W., Jesse,R.: Arzneim.-Forsch. **22**/2, 373 (1972).
11. Weidemann,R., Klepzig,H., Woicke,S., Gellhorn,D.: Klinikarzt **2**/6, 13 (1973).

Discussion Remarks

Lydtin: Dr. Laaser, we learned yesterday that nifedipine has a strong effect on the larger arteries and less so on the peripheral ones. Why did you use mean arterial pressure instead of systolic pressure. Is it possible that the impedence to flow is much more influenced by nifedipine than the overall peripheral resistance you measured? I also wonder why a drug, which has a dilating action on the vessels even after prolonged treatment and also eventually a pooling effect, does not stimulate the renin-angiotensin-aldosteron system. Did you get any change in serum potassium hinting in that direction?

Laaser: We did not find any important differences in the blood pressure even when we separated or analyzed diastolic and systolic pressures separately and I gave the mean pressure just to simplify the impression. We will do a proper statistical analysis during the coming week and then perhaps we will have more to say about this problem.

With regard to the potassium and other laboratory findings, we analyzed the first 11 patients very intensively for various laboratory results and did not see any important differences, so for the other 26 or 27 we did not continue this detailed laboratory analysis.

Kaufmann: The fact that there is no reduction of the serum potassium concentration does not exclude a stimulatory action of nifedipine on the renin-angiotensin-aldosteron-system. It is certainly suggestible to set up a study on the influence of nifedipine on the discussed system.

Peschl: For investigating whether renin-angiotensin really has significance in the application of Adalat, measuring renal blood flow would be of interest, because this would provide checkpoints on whether the renin-angiotensin system was actually being stimulated or not.

Lydtin: We get β-adrenergic drive following nifedipine administration both in the acute experiment and after prolonged treatment; β-adrenergic drive should stimulate the renin secretion as far as we know. So this is just a theoretical argument. Any drug that causes chronic pooling should, in some way, do the same thing. I have no data but I would suggest that this is to be studied in the future.

Kaufmann: We have done those experiments with other drugs and we know for sure that isoprenaline is able to stimulate the β-adrenergic system.

Response of Intraocular Pressure in Normal Subjects and Glaucoma Patients to Single and Repeated Doses of the Coronary Drug Adalat

D. SCHNELL

Ophthalmologic University Clinic, Cologne, Fed. Rep. Germany

Introduction

The use of drugs that are intended to enhance coronary circulation plays an important role in modern medicine.

Frequently, however, necessary treatment with coronary drugs is omitted because of the presence of other diseases for which such drugs are believed to be contraindicated. For example, glaucoma is considered by many to be a contraindication to the administration of nitroglycerin.

We have been unable to find any reports in the literature on an observed increase in intraocular pressure due to nitroglycerin. Nevertheless, this drug is still described as being strictly contraindicated in glaucoma in recently published papers, e.g. by MATZKE [27], BACHMANN [1], DONAT [7], and KURZ [22]. In fact, nearly all the manufactures of nitroglycerin preparations cite glaucoma as a contraindication. Evidently, a false analogy has been drawn to amyl nitrite. In 1918, KÖLLNER [20] noted a 3 mm Hg pressure increase in a glaucoma patient.

BAILLART and BOLLOCK [2] also observed a pressure rise lasting about 2 min, followed by a pressure drop, in normal subjects and glaucoma patients who inhaled this substance. CHRISTINI and PAGLIARANI [5, 6] noted a small, brief increase of pressure in cases of congestive glaucoma.

GRANT [11] reported a small pressure rise not exceeding 3 mm Hg a few seconds after inhalation of amyl nitrite.

BECKER [3] unsuccessfully tried to provoke a glaucoma attack with amyl nitrite in patients with narrow-angle glaucoma who had responded with such an attack to a mydriasis provocation test. Although there is no indication in the literature that an attack of glaucoma has ever been induced by amyl nitrite, the drug should be used with caution in patients with narrow-angle glaucoma.

In the case of nitroglycerin the situation is different—the statement that this drug is contraindicated in glaucoma patients is not supported by any author known to us. On the contrary, BOTHMANN and COHEN [4] as early as 1927 observed a decrease of blood pressure and intraocular pressure in dogs and cats following intravenous administration of this more-than-a-century-old drug, which proves to be so effective against angina pectoris.

When ZAHN [32] administered 0.5 mg of nitroglycerin to twenty patients (average age 53) in 1957, he observed no changes in intraocular pressure.

In 1964, WHITWORTH et al. [31] administered 0.3–1.2 mg of glyceryl nitrate as well as 20 mg of pentaerythritol tetranitrate to 34 subjects, normal individuals and patients with open and narrow-angle glaucoma (some of whom had previously suffered a glaucoma attack) who were not receiving any specific glaucoma therapy. In none of the cases did they see a pressure rise; instead, they noted no change in intraocular pressure or a slight, transitory decrease.

Thus, it seemed to us appropriate to present this brief review because the new coronary drug Adalat, dimethyl-1,4-dihydro-2,6-dimethyl-4-(o-nitrophenyl)-3,5-pyridinecarboxylate (generic nifedipine), which we study with regard to its effect on intraocular pressure, has a mode of action similar to that of nitroglycerin [9, 12, 13, 16, 21, 24, 26, 28–30].

We will not discuss the structure, mechanism of action, and therapeutic use of this drug since these areas have been covered at length elsewhere.

Our purpose was to determine whether single and repeated doses of Adalat cause an increase of intraocular pressure in normal individuals or glaucoma patients, that is, whether or not this coronary drug is contraindicated in glaucoma.

Methods

a) Patients

We set up four groups:

Group A of eleven eyes of seven normal subjects, that is, subjects unsuspected of glaucoma, with an average age of 60 years, the youngest being 43 and the oldest 80.

Group B was composed of sixteen eyes of eight glaucoma patients ranging in age from 49 to 83 years, with an average age of 69. Ten eyes had chronic simple glaucoma, one eye secondary acute glaucoma, two primary acute glaucoma, and two had low-pressure glaucoma.

After tonometry, the foregoing two groups received a single dose of 20 mg Adalat.

Group C consisted of eleven eyes of seven subjects unsuspected of glaucoma who had an average age of 58 years. The youngest subject was 27 and the oldest 82 years old.

Group D numbered twenty glaucomatous eyes (10 subjects). The patients average age was 60, the youngest being 34 and the oldest 83 years old. Fourteen of the eyes had open-angle glaucoma, four narrow-angle (attack) glaucoma, and two low-pressure glaucoma.

Groups C and D received 20 mg Adalat 3 times a day for several days.

All the patients were hospitalized at the Ophthalmologic University Clinic in Cologne.

In four subjects we studied the pressure response both after single and repeated doses.

b) Procedure

In Groups A and B, applanation tonometry was performed at least 2 h prior to administration of 20 mg Adalat and at least 6 times thereafter.

All the patients in Group B were kept off glaucoma therapy for at least 2 days, but in most cases for much longer periods, preceding the study.

In Groups C and D, applanation tonometry was performed at least once before the first dose of Adalat. In most of the glaucoma patients of Group D, the intraocular pressure had been followed for some time prior to administration of the coronary agent.

As a rule, 20 mg Adalat was then given 3 times a day and the intraocular pressure was measured 4 times during the day. Administration of Adalat was generally continued for 4 days.

Intraocular pressure measurements were taken in two patients of Group D for 9 days, and in three further patients each for 7, 6 and even 13 days respectively. In some patients, we determined the intraocular pressure several more times after withdrawal of the coronary medication.

Whereas five eyes in Group D received no treatment whatever, the others on which measurements were made were on antiglaucoma drugs. In four eyes, glaucoma therapy was temporarily suspended.

The following antiglaucomatous drugs were employed: Diamox (LEDERLE), Epinal, Glaukostat, Isopto-carbachol (ROLAND), Isopto-pilocarpine (ROLAND), Ocusert, Piladren (THILO), Pilocarpol (Dr. WINZER), and Syncarpin (Dr. WINZER).

All measurements of intraocular tension were carried out with newly calibrated Goldmann applanation tonometers using Haag-Streit slit lamps.

Single doses of Adalat were given sublingually since the drug is more effective by this route than from swallowed capsules [15]. For repeated doses capsules were swallowed.

Results

a) Single Dose of Adalat (Groups A and B)

Table 1 presents the results obtained in Group A (normal), while Table 2 presents the results for Group B (glaucoma). Results are shown in Fig. 1 (right eyes) and Fig. 2 (left eyes).

In both groups a more or less pronounced decrease of intraocular pressure occurred within 15–45 min after the administration of Adalat, followed by a phase in which the intraocular tension increased again (at 30–60 min). From the 60th minute on, the pressure decreased again.

Understandably, the variance of the individual values as expressed by the standard deviation of the mean was considerably greater in the glaucoma patients (Group B) than in the normal subjects, but it remained approximately constant within the groups.

Whereas the pressure decrease following a single dose of Adalat (comparison between value before and at different intervals after administration) was not significant in the normal subjects (Group A), the reduction in intraocular pressure was significant—in fact, highly significant in some cases—in the glaucoma pa-

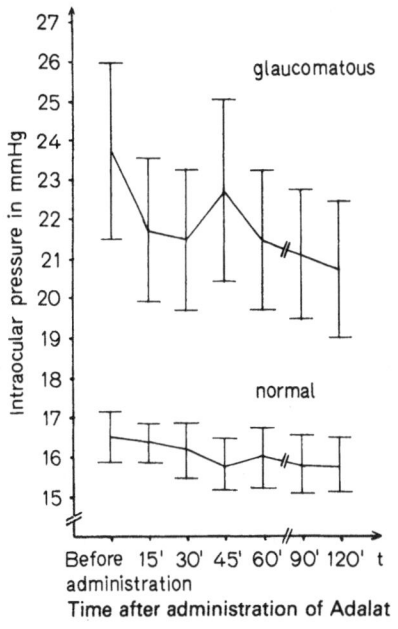

Fig. 1

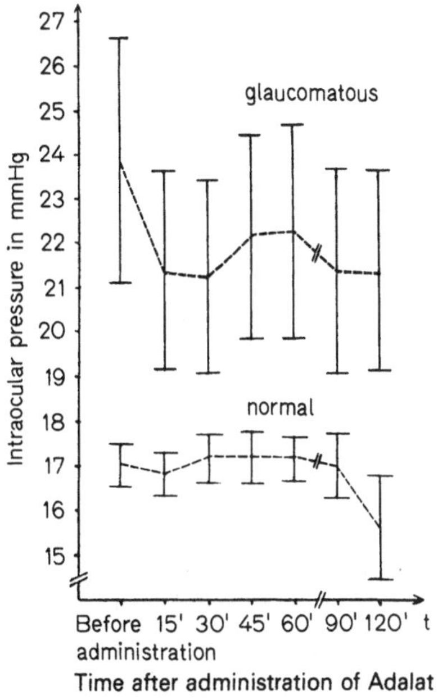

Fig. 2

Fig. 1. Average values and standard errors of mean values of intraocular pressure in right eyes of 7 normal and 8 glaucomatous patients before and after a single dose of 20 mg Adalat (BAY a 1040)

Fig. 2. Average values and standard errors of mean values of intraocular pressure in left eyes of 7 normal and 8 glaucomatous patients before and after a single dose of 20 mg Adalat (Bay a 1040)

tients (Group B) (except for the right eyes after 45 min). However, in view of the small number of subjects, less importance should be attached to the statistical analysis than to the individual responses.

Examining the curves of the normal subjects—Fig. 3 presents a typical example—we note that the average pressure decrease stems from just a few subjects, whereas no change in pressure occurred in the majority of cases.

In this group, all subjects, with the exception of one eye, showed a pressure decrease within the first 30 min after administration, followed by an increase back to the base line value or above it, with nearly all subjects exhibiting another pressure drop between the 45th and the 150th minute.

In a few patients the intraocular pressure fluctuated about the base line value.

In none of the subjects, however, did the intraocular pressure increase by more than 1 mm Hg.

Whereas the observed decrease in intraocular pressure was small in the normal subjects, reaching 3 mm Hg in a single case, two eyes of glaucoma patients showed a maximal decrease of 4 mm Hg, and in five other eyes the maximal decrease was 5 mm Hg, in two 6 mm Hg, and in one eye even 8 mm Hg.

Thus, the intraocular pressure was reduced by more than 3 mm Hg in ten out of sixteen eyes.

Table 1. Intraocular pressure values before and after a

Subject	Time after admin. of Adalat → Age ↓	before R	L	after 15 min R	L	after 30 min R	L	after 45 min R	L
A₁	60 yrs	18	17	17	16	18	18	16	16
A₂	80 yrs	16	16	15	16	14	16	14	16
A₃	58 yrs	17	—	17	—	17	—	17	—
A₄	51 yrs	14	—	16	—	15	—	14	—
A₅	43 yrs	—	18	—	18	—	18	—	18
A₆	70 yrs	16	16	15	16	15	16	16	17
A₇	57 yrs	18	18	18	18	18	18	18	19
Mean value	59.86 yrs	16.50	17.00	16.33	16.80	16.17	17.20	15.83	17.20
Standard deviation of the mean (standard error)		±0.62	±0.45	±0.49	±0.49	±0.70	±0.49	±0.65	±0.58
Significance of decrease of intraocular pressure after administration of 20 mg Adalat				No	No	No	No	No	No
Level of significance		—	—	—	—	—	—	—	—

Table 2. Intraocular pressure values before and after a

Subject	Time after admin. of Adalat → Age ↓	before R	L	after 15 min R	L	after 30 min R	L	after 45 min R	L
B₁	83 yrs	24	25	20	20	20	22	21	24
B₂	80 yrs	15	10	15	10	14	9	15	10
B₃	65 yrs	20	18	18	17	19	18	19	19
B₄	69 yrs	22	22	20	20	18	19	18	18
B₅	49 yrs	24	26	22	24	23	25	23	25
B₆	61 yrs	35	33	32	30	30	29	34	30
B₇	71 yrs	30	34	26	28	27	26	31	29
B₈	72 yrs	20	23	21	22	21	22	21	22
Mean value	68.75 yrs	23.75	23.87	21.75	21.38	21.50	21.25	22.75	22.13
Standard deviation of the mean (standard error)		±2.21	±2.75	±1.84	±2.23	±1.80	±2.17	±2.30	±2.29
Significance of decrease of intraocular pressure after administration of 20 mg Adalat				Yes	Yes	Yes	Yes	No	Yes
Level of significance				1,5%	1.1%	1.7%	2.3%	—	4.7%

b) Repeated Administration of 20 mg Adalat t.i.d. (Groups C and D)

The results in Groups C and D were not compared statistically because differences in glaucoma therapy, in measurement times after the administration of Adalat, and in the frequency of measurement precluded a comparison of the values.

single dose of 20 mg Adalat (Bay a 1040) in seven normal subjects

after 60 min		after 90 min		after 120 min		after 150 min		after 180 min	
R	L	R	L	R	L	R	L	R	L
17	16	17	17	17	12				
13	16	13	15	13	14				
17	—	15	—	16	—				
15	—	15	—	15	—				
—	18	—	19	—	18				
16	17	17	16	16	16	15	16	17	16
18	19	18	18	18	18	18	19	18	18
16.00	17.20	15.83	17.00	15.83	15.60	16.50	17.50	17.50	17.00
±0.73	±0.58	±0.75	±0.71	±0.70	±1.17				
No	No	No	No	No	No	No	No	No	No
—	—	—	—	—	—	—	—	—	—

single dose of 20 mg Adalat (Bay a 1040) in glaucoma patients

after 60 min		after 90 min		after 120 min		after 150 min		after 180 min	
R	L	R	L	R	L	R	L	R	L
22	25	22	24	21	24				
14	10	15	10	15	10			14	9
19	18	19	18	19	19				
18	18	18	16	17	17				
22	25	20	23	18	21				
30	31	30	30	30	30				
26	29	25	28	26	28				
21	22	20	22	20	22	21	22	21	23
21.50	22.25	21.13	21.38	20.75	21.38			17.50	16.00
±1.75	±2.40	±1.63	±2.31	±1.75	±2.24				
Yes	Yes	Yes	Yes	Yes	Yes				
1,5%	4,8%	1%	2,4%	0.9%	3%	—	—	—	—

Moreover, as in Groups A and B, which received single doses Adalat, it seems more appropriate, considering the small number of subjects, to review the individual cases rather than to discuss statistical data.

Figure 5 presents the typical pressure response of a normal subject.

The intraocular pressure values of the curves for Group A were all within normal limits.

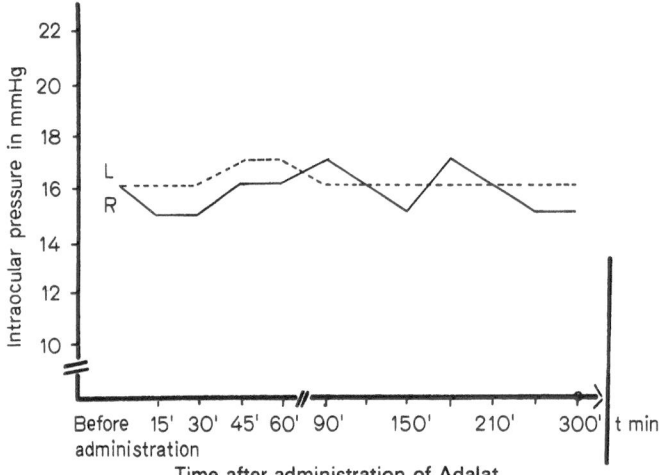

Fig. 3. Intraocular pressure in a normal subject (No. A_6) before and after a single dose of 20 mg Adalat (Bay a 1040)

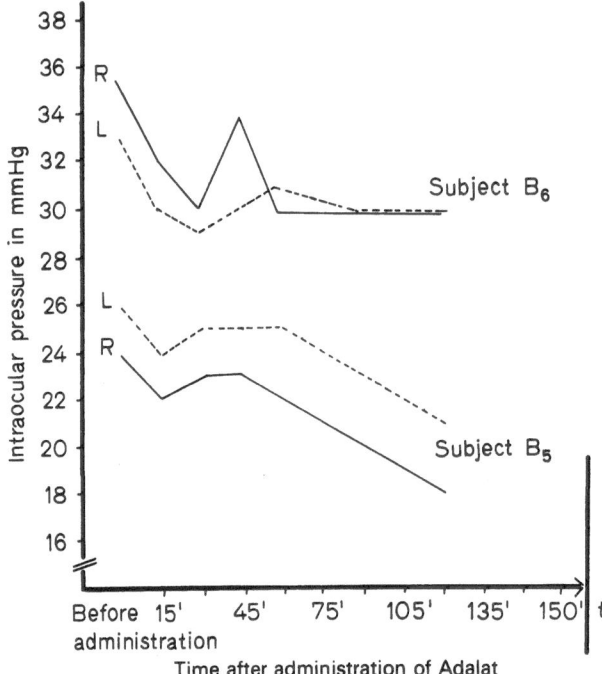

Fig. 4. Intraocular pressure in two glaucoma patients (Nos. B_5 and B_6) before and after a single dose of 20 mg Adalat (Bay a 1040)

In no case did the average pressure decrease or increase by more than 2–3 mm Hg. Individual deviations from the average pressure during administration of Adalat never exceeded 4 mm Hg.

Figure 6 presents the typical curve of a glaucoma patient who was receiving antiglaucoma medication in the right eye but none in the left.

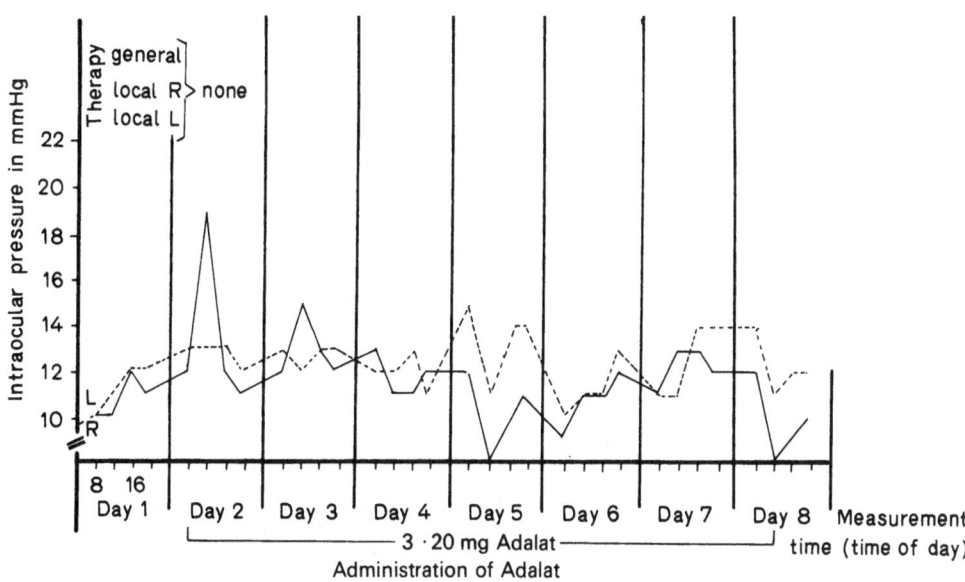

Fig. 5. Intraocular pressure in a normal subject (C_4) before and during 6 days of treatment with 20 mg Adalat (Bay a 1040) t.i.d.

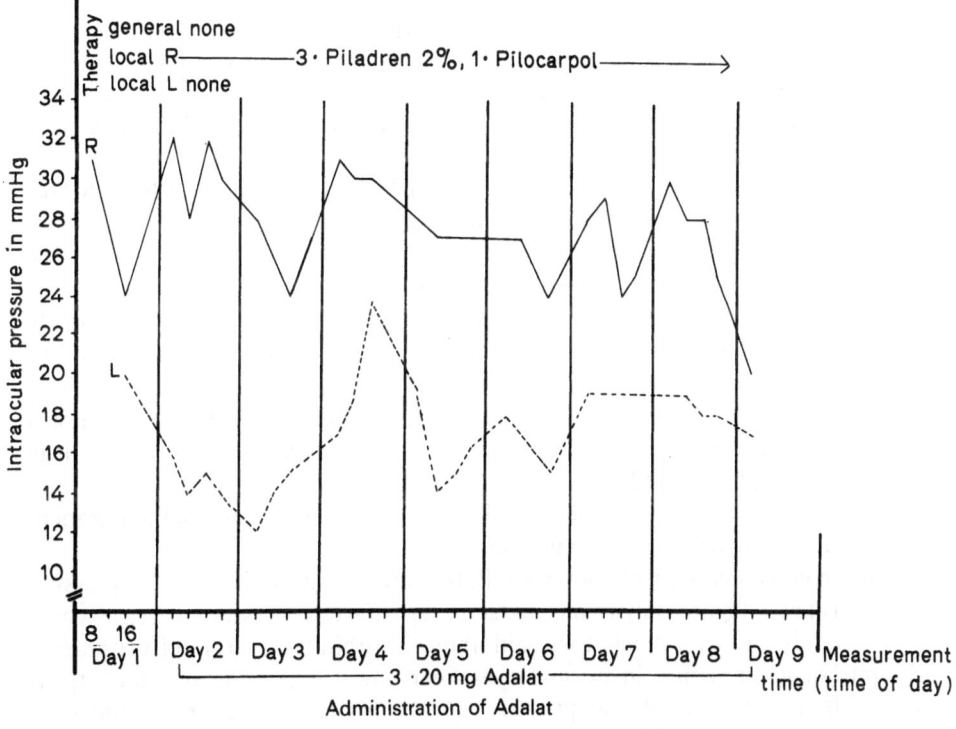

Fig. 6. Intraocular pressure curves of a glaucoma patient (D_2) before and during 7-day administration of 20 mg Adalat (Bay a 1040) t.i.d. (right eye receiving glaucoma therapy, left eye none)

Seven further glaucoma patients or 10 eyes received Adalat without concomitant glaucoma therapy.

In none of these eight subjects did the pressure rise above the base line level during Adalat treatment.

In five eyes the pressure decreased perceptibly during Adalat medication; in the remaining eyes it remained about the same.

It appears difficult if not impossible to ascertain the effect of Adalat on the intraocular pressure in patients concomitantly receiving antiglaucomatous medication because too many factors then act upon the eye.

Since our main concern in the present study was the detection of adverse pressure changes, we shall focus attention on this aspect.

In no case did we observe an increase of intraocular pressure attributable to Adalat. In particular, the patients with paroxysmal glaucoma who did or did not receive glaucoma therapy exhibited no rise in the pressure level.

Adalat was generally well tolerated. During repeated administration two patients (C_3, age 49; D_5, age 36) showed manifestations of intolerance in the form of severe headache.

Discussion

Our study centered on the question of whether the coronary drug Adalat causes an increase of intraocular pressure, that is, whether it can induce or exacerbate glaucoma. In the case of the normal subjects in Group A it was therefore necessary to know what possible fluctuations in intraocular tension may have occurred during the study period.

Unfortunately, the literature is of little help in this respect. While sharply divergent data may be found on the normal diurnal variation of intraocular pressure [8, 23], precise information is lacking about possible fluctuations within the relatively short test period of 2 h used in our study.

Taking as our premise the diurnal variations of at most 4–6 mm Hg (± 3 mm Hg) cited by LEYDHECKER [23], we find that none of the glaucoma-free eyes of Group A that we examined reached these limits.

Even though the mean pressure in Group A did show a decrease, if not a significant one (Figs. 1 and 2), a pressure-lowering effect of the coronary drug Adalat may not be inferred.

There is no evidence whatever that the drug causes an increase of the intraocular pressure in subjects free of glaucoma.

In the glaucoma patients of Group B, too, an increase in intraocular pressure may be ruled out since only two of sixteen eyes showed a pressure increase which was certainly—in view of what we said above—within the margin of variance of the intraocular pressure in normal eyes, reaching a maximum of 2 mm Hg. It should be borne in mind that pressure variations due to glaucoma could have reached several times this normal value during the test period [8]. It appears probable, however, that at least in some of the glaucoma patients Adalat caused a decrease of the intraocular pressure.

This is suggested not only by the high statistical significance of the findings but also by the fact that ten of sixteen eyes showed a maximum pressure decrease of 3–8 mm Hg during the test period.

The duration of the pressure drop induced by Adalat cannot be specified since in most of the eyes in which a decrease of intraocular pressure was observed the pressure remained below the base line value at the end of the measurement time.

The results obtained in Groups C and D, that is, in the patients who took Adalat over a longer period, argue against an increase of intraocular pressure by this coronary drug in normal subjects or in glaucoma patients with or without concomitant glaucoma therapy. Yet by the same token there is also no evidence that the drug benefits the pressure levels continuously, presumably because the pressure-lowering effect of Adalat does not last long enough, although in acute studies swallowed capsules had a longer-lasting effect, at least on the coronaries, than sublingual doses (due to slower absorption) [15].

Even those glaucoma patients who were tested in both the single-dose and the repeated-dose study, and who had shown a marked decrease of intraocular pressure after the single dose, exhibited no change in the pressure level following repeated administration of Adalat.

Thus, our results conform to results obtained by WHITWORTH et al. [31] and by ZAHN [32] with the similarly acting Nitrolingual. They, too, noted either no change in pressure levels or a decrease of the intraocular tension.

Adalat exercises its effect through withdrawal of Ca^{++}, which leads to relaxation of the smooth musculature and also of the vessel wall, hence to vasodilation and a small decrease of intravascular pressure; a similar effect has been discussed with regard to Nitrolingual but has not been proved beyond doubt [4, 9, 12–14, 16, 18, 19, 21].

According to current concepts, the therapeutic effect on the heart consists not in dilation of the coronaries, which are already maximally dilated as a result of the hypoxia, but in dilation of vessels close to the heart and peripheral vessels, that is, in a reduction of the peripheral resistance, as a consequence of which cardiac work is reduced and the oxygen demand is decreased.

It is not certain how the brief reduction of the intraocular pressure following administration of Adalat, to glaucoma patients comes about. Inasmuch as increases in intraocular pressure are caused by a disproportion between production and outflow of aqueous humor, the drug may theoretically improve outflow or reduce aqueous production. Less probable is a reduction in outflow resistance, although an improvement of outflow via iris vessels—dilated by Adalat—is also a possibility.

More likely, it is the output of aqueous humor that is decreased. Conceivably, the ciliary arteries are dilated and this leads to a pressure drop in these vessels, which in turn brings about a reduction of the pressure gradient and, consequently, decreased output.

A decrease of pressure in the small arteries and arterioles of the body periphery was noted by HAYASE et al. [14] in cardiac patients and by KLÜTSCH et al. [17] in patients with renal hypertension.

The renewed rise of the pressure observed in most of the glaucomatous (and several normal) eyes after 30 min could reflect a counterregulation.

The fact noted by KOCHSIEK and NEUBAUR [19] that the reduction of intra-arterial pressure (also in peripheral vessels) occurred only after a single dose of Adalat, not after repeated doses, may explain the absence of a decrease of intra-ocular pressure with repeated doses.

It seems of importance that no increases in intraocular pressure occurred in patients with narrow-angle glaucoma. It might be imagined that a dilation of the ciliary body and the iridic vessels would lead to a further narrowing of the chamber angle and, consequently, to pressure increases and possibly even to glaucoma attacks. However, no such adverse effect on acute glaucoma has been observed after administration of nitroglycerin or other vasodilators such as Priscol and Vasculat [31], except in a case described by GALLOIS [10] in which a glaucoma attack occurred after administration of Priscol, and this attack was probably unrelated to the vasodilator treatment. In fact, improvements in glaucoma were generally seen even with these vasodilators containing no nitrate or nitrite [31].

The fact that side-effects developed in only two (fairly young) of 28 subjects and led to interruption of the study in only one case attests to the safety of Adalat.

Abstract

The response of the intraocular pressure to administration of the new coronary drug Adalat was studied in fourteen subjects with no evidence of glaucoma (22 eyes) and in fourteen glaucoma patients (28 eyes).

Approximately one half of these two groups each received a single 20 mg dose (sublingual) or repeated doses of 20 mg t.i.d. (capsules).

In four of the glaucoma patients the intraocular pressure was measured both before and after single and repeated doses.

No indication of an increase in intraocular pressure was found in any of the subjects.

In the single-dose study, the glaucoma patients showed a significant decrease of the intraocular pressure; in ten of sixteen eyes the pressure decrease within the test period of 2 h exceeded 3 mm Hg.

A non-significant, small pressure decrease was noted in the glaucoma-free reference group.

No changes in the diurnal curve of pressure levels were observed during repeated Adalat doses in either the normal subjects or in the glaucoma patients (with or without glaucoma therapy).

The coronary agent Adalat was tolerated very well in the majority of cases.

References

1. BACHMANN, K.: Moderne Therapie der Koronarinsuffizienz, Zeitschrift für Allgemeinmedizin/Der Landarzt 24, 1200–1204 (1970).
2. BAILLART, P., BOLLOCK, J.: De l'action comparée de certaines substances medicamenteuses sur la tension intraoculaire et sur la pression artérielle. Ann. Oculist 158, 641–654 (1921).
3. BECKER, B.: In: Conference on Glaucoma Transactions, New York Josiah Macy Jr. Foundation, 32 (1955).

4. BOTHMANN, L., COHEN, S. J.: Studies in intraocular pressure. Arch. Ophthal. **56**, 110–115 (1927).
5. CHRISTINI, G., PAGLIARANI, N.: Amyl nitrite test in primary glaukoma. Brit. J. Ophthal. **37**, 741–745 (1953 a).
6. CHRISTINI, G., PAGLIARANI, N.: Esplorazione clinica della circolazione unveale anche a scopo prognostico, nel. glaucoma primario. Arch. Oftal B Air **28**, 145–149 (1953 b).
7. DONAT, K.: Differentialdiagnose und Differentialtherapie. Herz/Kreisl., 2. Jg., Nr. 19, 455–460 (1970).
8. DUKE-ELDER, S.: System of Ophthalmology, Vol. XI, 2nd ed., pp. 456–461. London: Henry Kimpton 1971.
9. FLECKENSTEIN, A. *et al.*: Bay a 1040 — ein hochaktiver Ca^{++}-antagonistischer Inhibitor der elektromechanischen Kopplungsprozesse im Warmblüter-Myocard. Arzneim.-Forsch. (Drug Res.) **22**, 22–33 (1972).
10. GALLOIS, J.: Glaucoma aigu aprés Pricol. Soc. Opththal Franc. **1951**, 131–132.
11. GRANT, W. M.: Physiological and pharmacological influences upon intraocular pressure. Pharmacol. Rev. **7**, 143–182 (1955).
12. GRÜN, G., FLECKENSTEIN, A.: Die elektromechanische Entkoppelung der glatten Gefäß-muskulatur als Grundprinzip der Coronardilatation durch 4-(2′-Nitrophenyl)-2,6-di-methyl-1,4-dihydropyridin-3,5-dicarbonsäure-dimethylester (Bay a 1040 Nifedipine). Arzneim.-Forsch. (Drug Res.) **22**, 2, 334–344 (1972).
13. HASHIMOTO, K., *et al.*: Cardiohemodynamic effects of Bay a 1040 in the dog. Arzneim.-Forsch. (Drug Res.) **22**, 1, 15–21 (1972).
14. HAYASE, S., *et al.*: Hemodynamic and therapeutic effect of Bay a 1040 on the patients with ischemic heart disease. Arzneim.-Forsch. (Drug Res.) **22**, 2, 370–373 (1972).
15. HORSTER, F. A., *et al.*: Klinische Untersuchungen zur Pharmakokinetik von radioaktiv markierten 4-(2′-Nitrophenyl)-2,6-dimethyl-1,4-dihydropyridin-3,5-dicarbonsäure-dime-thylester. Arzneim.-Forsch. (Drug Res.) **22**, 2, 330–334 (1972).
16. KALTENBACH, M., *et al.*: Veränderungen der Hämodynamik des linken Herzens unter der Wirkung von Nifedipine (Bay a 1040) im Vergleich mit Nitroglycerin. Arzneim.-Forsch. (Drug Res.) **22**, 2, 362–365 (1972).
17. KLÜTSCH, K., *et al.*: Der Einfluß von Bay a 1040 auf die Nierenfunktion des Hypertoni-kers. Arzneim.-Forsch. (Drug Res.) **22**, 2, 377–380 (1972).
18. KOBAYASHI, T., *et al.*: Clinical experience with a new coronary active substance (Bay a 1040). Arzneim.-Forsch. (Drug Res.) **22**, 2, 380–389 (1972).
19. KOCHSIEK, K., NEUBAUR, J.: Die Wirkung von 4-(2′-Nitrophenyl)-2,6-dimethyl-1,4-dihy-dropyridin-3,5-dicarbonsäure-dimethylester auf den Myocardstoffwechsel, die Hämody-namik, die Blutgase und den allgemeinen Stoffwechsel des Menschen. Arzneim.-Forsch. (Drug Res.) **22**, 2, 353–358 (1972).
20. KÖLLNER, H.: Über den Augendruck beim Glaukoma Simplex und seine Beziehungen zum Kreislauf. Arch. Augenheilk. **83**, 135–167 (1918).
21. KOSCHE, F., *et al.*: Zum Wirkungsmechanismus der Coronardilatation durch Nifedipine. Arzneim.-Forsch. (Drug Res.) **22**, 1, 39–42 (1972).
22. KURZ, J. F.: Die Behandlung der Koronarinsuffizienz mit Nitrolingual. Zeitschrift für Allgemeinmedizin/Der Landarzt, 46. Jg., **26**, 1319–1323 (1970).
23. LEYDHECKER, W.: Glaukom, ein Handbuch, p. 7. Berlin-Göttingen-Heidelberg: Springer-Verlag 1960.
24. LICHTLEN, P., *et al.*: Die Wirkung des Nitroglycerins auf die Koronardurchblutung am Menschen, unter Berücksichtigung der selektiven Koronarangiographie und Messung der Koronardurchblutung mit Xenon 133. Cardiologia **48**, 371–373 (1966).
25. LICHTLEN, P., BAUMANN, P. C.: Zur Therapie und Diagnose der Angina pectoris. Praxis **58**, 135–144 (1969).
26. LOOS, A., KALTENBACH, M.: Die Wirkung von Nifedipine (Bay a 1040) auf das Belastungs-Elektrocardiogramm von Angina pectoris-Kranken. Arzneim.-Forsch. (Drug Res.) **22**, 1, 358–362 (1972).
27. MATZKE, H.: Die Intervallbehandlung der Angina pectoris mit Nitrodurat. Münchner Med. Wochenschrift **104**, 2299–2301 (1962).

28. RAFF, W. K., *et al.*: Untersuchungen mit Nifedipine, einer coronargefäßerweiternden Substanz mit schneller sublingualer Wirkung. Arzneim.-Forsch. (Drug Res.) **22**, 1, 33–39 (1972).
29. ROSKAMM, H., *et al.*: Der Einfluß von Propranolol und Nitroglycerin auf das Elektrokardiogramm und die intrapulmonalen Drucke während körperlicher Belastung von Angina pectoris-Patienten. Deutsche Med. Wochenschrift, **95**, 2593–2599 (1970).
30. VATER, W., *et al.*: Zur Pharmakologie von 4-(2'-Nitrophenyl)-2,6-dimethyl-1,4-dihydropyridin-3,5-dicarbonsäure-dimethylester (Nifedipine; Bay a 1040). Arzneim.-Forsch. (Drug Res.) **22**, 1, 1–14 (1972).
31. WHITWORTH, C. G., *et al.*: Der Gebrauch von vasodilatierenden Nitraten und Nitriten bei Glaukom-Patienten. Archives of Ophthalmology **71** (April, 1964).
32. ZAHN, K.: The effect of nitroglycerin on the retinal circulation. Cesk Oftal **13**, 146–149 (1957); (abstr.) Zbl Ophthal. **72**, 235 (1957).

Extracardial Effects of Nifedipine (Adalat): Measurements of Liver Blood Flow in Animals and Humans and of Peripheral Circulation in the Lower Limbs

A. Mostbeck, H. Partsch, and L. Peschl

Isotopenstation des Wilhelminenspitals und Medizinische Abteilung des Kaiserin-Elisabeth-Spitals der Stadt Wien, Austria

Like other antianginal drugs, nifedipine has cardial and extracardial effects. We investigated the extracardial influence of nifedipine

1. on liver blood flow in dogs and healthy volunteers, recording simultaneously arterial blood pressure, heart rate and cardiac output;

2. on the resting blood flow of lower legs and feet, and ankle pressure measured over the dorsal artery of the foot;

3. on the venous distensibility of the forearm and lower leg (Table 1).

Table 1. Extracardial effects of nifedipine

Subjects	Parameters	Methods
I. 10 dogs	Liver blood flow	^{133}Xe-clearance flowmeter
	Cardiac output	Indicator-dilution (^{131}I-albumin)
	Blood pressure	Mercury manometer
	Heart rate	ECG
II. 15 healthy volunteers	Liver blood flow	^{198}Au-clearance
III. 15 healthy volunteers	Resting blood flow of lower leg and foot	Strain gauge plethysmography ^{133}Xe-clearance
	Venous distensib. of lower leg	Strain gauge plethysmography
	Systemic blood pressure	Brachial artery auscultation
	"Ankle pressure"	Doppler ultrasonic detector
	Heart rate	Strain gauge plethysmography
IV. 5 healthy volunteers	Venous distensib. of forearm and lower leg	Capacitance plethysmography

Influence of Nifedipine on Liver Blood Flow in Dogs

Method

Ten anesthetized mongrel dogs (10–20 kg) received 1 mg/kg nifedipine sublingually. Liver blood flow was recorded by liver washout of intraportally injected physically solubilized ^{133}Xe (100–300 µCi). The liver washout of ^{133}Xe is a function

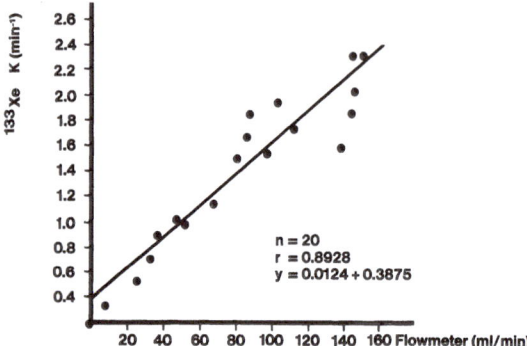

Fig. 1. Correlation between liver washout of ^{133}Xe and flowmeter values under changing circulatory conditions [11]

of liver blood flow. The quantification of liver blood flow with the aid of the tissue/blood partition coefficient of 0.7 as determined by CONN [2], seems to be unreliable because of the individual variations in liver fat content. On the other hand there is good correlation between the changes in portal blood flow measured by flowmeter and the changes of the disappearance constant of ^{133}Xe detected by scintillation counting over the liver, as could be shown by 20 simultaneous measurements in dogs with ligated liver arteries [9] (Fig. 1). Therefore in our investigations, only the disappearance constant k was calculated from the first slope of the activity curve registred on a logarithmic scale.

Cardiac output was calculated according to the method of STEWART-HAMILTON after injection of 10 µCi ^{131}I-albumin into a jugular vein [4, 6, 8].

Blood pressure in the femoral artery was measured directly by a mercury manometer.

Heart rate was detected by ECG.

Liver blood flow measurements were made after achieving constant circulatory conditions and at intervals between 5 and 15 min after sublingual administration of nifedipine (1 mg/kg). Cardiac output was determined before, and 30 min and 60 min after administration.

Results

After administration of nifedipine, heart rate increased from 126 to 140–150/min (statistically significant) and mean blood pressure decreased significantly from 131.8 ± 9.2 to 104.0 ± 2.6 mm Hg after 40 min (p<0.05).

Table 2. Disappearance constant $K(\bar{x} \pm s_{\bar{x}})$ of intraportally injected ^{133}Xe in 7 dogs before and after nifedipine

	Basic value	Minutes after nifedipine	
		11–30	31–50
$K(\min^{-1})$	2.0092 ± 0.2279	2.9363 ± 0.4017	2.6766 ± 0.3953
%	100%	146%	133%
p		< 0.025	< 0.1

Table 3. Cardiac output ($\bar{x} \pm s_{\bar{x}}$) in 7 dogs before and after nifedipine

	Basic value	Minutes after nifedipine	
		20–30	> 60
Cardiac output (ml/kg)	142.5 ± 26.6	232.0 ± 30.9	190.2 ± 17.0
%	100%	163%	134%
p		< 0.001	< 0.001

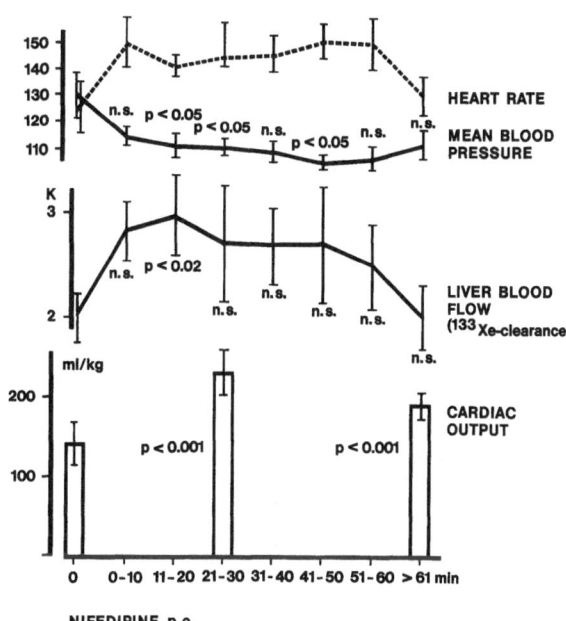

Fig. 2. Heart rate, mean blood pressure, liver blood flow and cardiac output in 7 dogs after nifedipine (1 mg/kg p.o.)

Liver blood flow increased and reached its maximum 11–30 min after nifedipine.

This maximal increase amounts to 146% of the base line value and is statistically significant (p < 0.025) (Table 2).

There was also a highly significant increase of cardiac output of 62.8% after 20–30 min and of 35.5% after 1 h (p < 0.001) (Table 3, Fig. 2).

Influence of Nifedipine on Liver Blood Flow in Man

Method

In a group of 15 healthy volunteers, aged 21–53 years, liver blood flow was determined by the disappearance rate of intravenously injected colloidal [198]Au (average diameter 300 Å) from the blood. In healthy persons the microparticles of [198]Au are removed from blood mainly by the reticuloendothelial cells of the liver. Changes in the disappearance rate of [198]radiogold in one subject are indicative of

changes of liver blood flow [3,10]. In the first 15 min after the injection of 20 μCi
^{198}Au, the values of plasma radioactivity follow a monoexponential function that
can be evaluated simply in terms of the disappearance half-time t/2. From this the
disappearance constant k, given by the formula $k = \ln 2/t/2$, was calculated before
and 15 min after sublingual application of 20 mg nifedipine.

Results

Table 4 and Fig. 3 show the influence of nifedipine on the ^{198}Au clearance in
15 healthy persons. The average disappearance constant k increased only moderately after sublingual application of 20 mg nifedipine. This increase is not statistically significant.

Table 4. Disappearance constant $K(\bar{x} \pm s_{\bar{x}})$ of ^{198}Au in 15 healthy volunteers before and
after nifedipine

	Before	15'after
	Nifedipine	
K(min^{-1})	0.1931 ± 0.0137	0.2076 ± 0.0124
%	100%	108%
p		< 0.1 n.s.

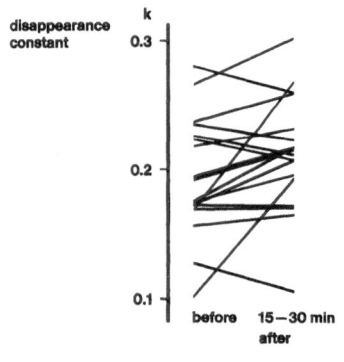

NIFEDIPINE p.o.

Fig. 3. ^{198}Au-clearance before and 15–30 min after 20 mg nifedipine p.o. in 15 healthy volunteers

Influence of Nifedipine on Resting Blood Flow of the Lower Leg

Method

In a group of 15 healthy volunteers (24–68 years old) the following parameters
were measured:
1. Resting blood flow of the lower leg and of the foot by strain gauge plethysmography (Periquant 102) [5].
2. ^{133}Xe clearance from depots in the anterior tibial muscle and in the skin of
the dorsum pedis [9].

3. Blood pressure of brachial artery by Riva-Rocci and

4. ankle pressure measured over the dorsal artery of the foot by ultrasonic Doppler Detector (Model 806, Parks Electronics) [1, 11].

The investigation was started after 30 min of rest in a recumbent position with slightly elevated legs. The room temperature during the investigation ranged between 22 and 25° C.

Measurements were done before and 30 and 60 min after sublingual administration of 20 mg nifedipine. After 1 h we placed lead shields over the previously injected Xe depots and reinjected new depots.

Results

The results of peripheral flow and pressure measurements in a group of 15 persons before, 30 and 60 min after sublingual administration of 20 mg nifedipine are shown in Table 5 and Fig. 4, respectively. Mean blood pressure and ankle pressure decreased by 6–8% ($p < 0.02$) and heart rate increased from 73 to 82/min ($p < 0.005$). In each case the ankle pressure was higher than or equal to the systolic brachial artery pressure, thus excluding arterial occlusions in the leg.

There was an increase of peripheral resting blood flow in the calf and in the foot region as observed by venous occlusion plethysmography and also by ^{133}Xe clearance technique. Blood flow into the calf segment increased by 67% after 30 min and by 54% after one hour ($p < 0.02$). Muscle blood flow measured by ^{133}Xe clearance showed an increase of 68% ($p < 0.025$) 1 h after nifedipine.

Resting blood flow in the foot increased by 11% after 30 min and by 87% after 1 h following drug administration ($p < 0.005$). ^{133}Xe clearance from the skin of the foot showed an average increase of 155%. This increase is statistically not significant because of the considerable scattering of the single values.

In our experience blood flow measurements by venous occlusion plethysmography seem to provide more reliable results for the assessment of circulatory drug effects than ^{133}Xe clearance. On the other hand, with venous occlusion plethysmography alone, it is not possible to distinguish between muscular and dermal circulation, although calf flow measurement in the foot is mainly referred to as muscle blood flow, and measurement in the foot, mainly referred to as skin flow. Therefore also Xenon clearance technique providing regional blood flow values was performed.

Influence of Nifedipine on Venous Distensibility

Method

In 15 healthy persons, venous distensibility of the lower leg was measured in a calf segment by strain gauge plethysmography (Periquant 102). 5 healthy volunteers were investigated by capacitance plethysmography. Venous distensibility was measured simultaneously on segments of the forearm and lower leg by inflating cuffs on the upper arm and on the distal thigh respectively to 20, 40, and 60 mm Hg and registering the volume increase of the limb segments. This procedure was performed three times before and three times after the application of 20 mg nifedipine, 0.8 mg nitroglycerin and placebo, respectively. The time of venous congestion was 2 min for each pressure increment, the intervals between the periods were 5 min.

Results

Venous distensibility of the lower leg measured by strain gauge plethysmograph decreased by 19% ($p<0.005$) (Fig.4, Table 5). Figure 5 shows the changes of venous distensibility of forearm and lower leg obtained during a congestion pressure of 60 mm Hg after placebo, nifedipine and nitroglycerin. There was an increase of venous distensibility after nifedipine and nitroglycerin in the forearm and a decrease of this parameter in the lower leg. This decrease was statistically significant for both drugs. The placebo group showed a non-significant decrease of venous distensibility in the forearm and in the lower leg.

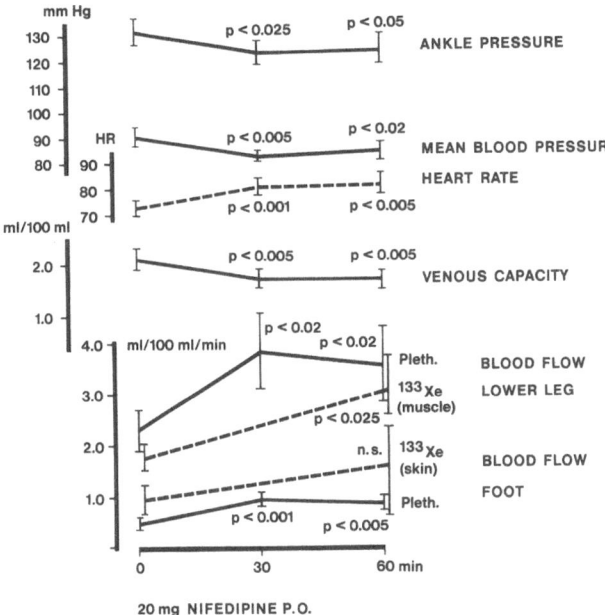

Fig.4. Peripheral circulation parameters after sublingual application of 20 mg nifedipine in 15 healthy volunteers

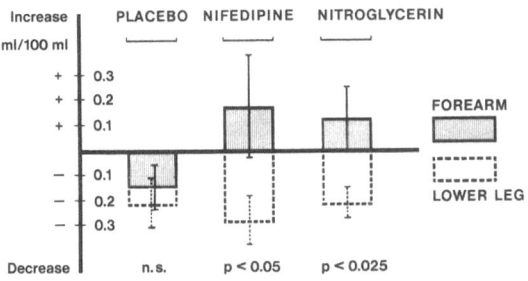

Fig. 5. Change of venous distensibility

Table 5. Peripheral circulation parameters in 15 healthy volunteers after nifedipine

	Basic value	Minutes after nifedipine	
		30	60
Heart rate (min^{-1})	72.5±3.1	81.5±3.2	82.3±3.5
%	100%	112%	113%
p		< 0.001	<0.005
Mean blood pressure (mmHg)	90.6±3.2	82.7±2.7	85.0±3.0
%	100%	91%	94%
p		< 0.005	< 0.02
Resting blood flow calf (Plethysmography) ml/100 ml/min	2.3±0.1	3.8±0.7	3.5±0.7
%	100%	165%	152%
p		< 0.02	< 0.02
Muscle blood flow (^{133}Xe-clearance) (ml/100 ml/min)	1.96±0.28		3.30±0.66
%	100%		168%
p			< 0.023
Resting blood flow, foot (Plethysmography) (ml/100 ml/min)	0.46±0.08	0.97±0.13	0.86±0.14
%	100%	211%	187%
p		< 0.001	<0.005
Skin blood flow (^{133}Xe-clearance) (ml/100 ml/min)	0.89±0.25		2.27±0.80
%	100%		255%
p			< 0.2
Venous distensibility (ml/100 ml)	2.15±0.22	1.74±0.18	1.72±0.16
%	100%	81%	80%
p		< 0.005	< 0.005

From these measurements it is suspected that the response to nifedipine and nitroglycerin in terms of the venous distensibility of lower leg and forearm is the same. The quantitative differences depend upon the time of measurement and perhaps upon the dosage and should be further evaluated with more experiments.

Abstract

Peripheral hemodynamic effects of nifedipine were investigated
A. in 10 anesthetized mongrel-dogs
B. in 3 groups of healthy volunteers.

In the animal experiments the following parameters were determined: pulse rate, blood pressure, liver blood flow (flowmeter and radioxenon-technique) and cardiac output (^{131}I-albumin).

In group 1 of healthy persons liver blood flow was assessed by ^{198}Au clearance method.

In group 2 blood flow of the lower leg and of the foot and venous capacity (strain gauge plethysmography), ^{133}Xenon clearance of muscle and skin, blood pressure of a. brachialis and distal a. tibialis anterior (Doppler ultrasonic detector) and pulse rate were determined.

In group 3 comparative studies of the venous distensibility simultaneously measured in a calf and in an arm segment by capacitance plethysmography after nitroglycerin and after nifedipine were carried out.

After nifedipine sublingually some hemodynamically relevant extracardial effects could be observed. Peripheral blood flow was increased (liver, muscle, skin) and changes of distribution of blood flow and of venous distensibility were found.

References

1. BOLLINGER, A., MAHLER, F., ZEHENDER, O.: Kombinierte Druck- und Durchflußmessungen zur Beurteilung arterieller Durchblutungsstörungen. Dtsch. med. Wschr. **95**, 1039 (1970).
2. CONN, H. L.: Equilibrium distribution of radioxenon in tissue: xenon-hemoglobin association curve. Dtsch. Wschr. **95**, 1039 (1970).
3. DOBSON, E. L., JONES, H. B.: The behavior of intravenously injected particulate material. Its rate of disappearence from the blood stream as a measure of liver blood flow. Acta med. Scand., Suppl. 273 (1952).
4. DONATO, L., GIUNTINI, C., LEWIS, L., DURAND, J., ROCHESTER, D. F., HARVEY, R. M., COURHAND, A.: Quantitative radiocardiography. I. Theoretical considerations. Circulation **26**, 174 (1962).
5. GUTTMANN, J., KRÖTZ, J.: Quantitative Messungen bei Durchblutungsstörungen. Diagnostik **3**, 205 (1970).
6. HUFF, R. L., FELLER, D. D., BOGARDUS, G.: Cardiac output by body surface counting of ^{131}I-human serum albumine. J. clin. Invest. **33**, 944 (1954).
7. LASSEN, N. A., LINDBJERG, I., MUNCK, O.: Measurement of blood through skeletal muscle by intramuscular injection of Xenon-133. Lancet **1964/I**, 686.
8. MOSTBECK, A.: Die Bestimmung des Plasma- und Blutvolumens sowie des Herzminutenvolumens mit ^{131}J-Albumin. Wien. klin. Wschr. **75**, 444 (1963).
9. MOSTBECK, A., PESCHL, L., GISEL, G.: Zur Bedeutung der Leberdurchblutungsmessung mit ^{133}Xenon für klinisch experimentelle Fragestellungen. In: Nuklearmedizin. 9. Jahrestag der Gesellschaft für Nuclearmedizin, Antwerpen 23.–25.9.1971. Stuttgart-New York: F. K. Schattauer Verlag 1973.
10. VETTER, H., FALKNER, R., NEUMAYR, A.: The disappearence rate of colloidal radiogold from the circulation and its application to the estimation of liver blood flow in normal and cirrhotic subjects. J. clin. Invest. **33**, 1594 (1954).
11. YAO, S. T., HOBBS, J. T., IRVINE, W. T.: Ankle pressure measurement in arterial disease of the lower extremities. Br. J. Surg. **55**, 859 (1968).

Discussion Remarks

ANGELINO: A side effect observed by some authors and today also by Dr. YASUI, was edema of the legs. Do you think this could be explained by your observations on peripheral blood flow and venous changes?

PESCHL: In short-term trials we could establish that in the legs capacity previously decreased. Our patients lay in horizontal positions. Whether in long-term experiments under chronic medication, with patients ambulatory and the drug effect lasting, the capacity of the venous system of the lower extremities is perhaps altered, we cannot say.

CHAIRMAN: This means that further investigations will have to be performed to find out exactly what is happening.

The Influence of Adalat on Pulmonary Pressure

D. Vallée

Lungenklinik Heidehaus, Hannover, Fed. Rep. Germany

We studied the question whether and in what ways Adalat might influence the pulmonary pressure. We approached this question with a double-blind cross-over study, the results of which are reported.

Method

Twelve non-coronary patients who had a normal partial pressure of blood gases under resting conditions and under a moderate ergometer stress, took part

Table 1. Initial values of the pulmonary artery pressure on the first and second day of the study

Pat. No.	Medication	Period	$\overline{PA}$(mm Hg)	$\overline{PA}$ difference (mm Hg)
1	Placebo	1st Period	11	6
	Adalat	2nd Period	17	
2	Placebo	1st Period	20	6
	Adalat	2nd Period	14	
3	Adalat	1st Period	11	0
	Placebo	2nd Period	11	
4	Placebo	1st Period	18	2
	Adalat	2nd Period	20	
5	Placebo	1st Period	14	3
	Adalat	2nd Period	17	
6	Adalat	1st Period	07	1
	Placebo	2nd Period	08	
7	Adalat	1st Period	16	2
	Placebo	2nd Period	18	
8	Placebo	1st Period	17	2
	Adalat	2nd Period	15	
9	Placebo	1st Period	17	1
	Adalat	2nd Period	16	
10	Adalat	1st Period	12	2
	Placebo	2nd Period	14	
11	Adalat	1st Period	13	5
	Placebo	2nd Period	18	
12	Adalat	1st Period	13	0
	Placebo	2nd Period	13	

in the study. The subjects were patients of the Dept. of Pulmonary Diseases, Heidehaus, Hannover, with moderate fibroses of lungs and pleura. These patients had not previously received other heart or circulatory medications. All were between 21 and 53 years of age, average age 37. There were 8 males and 4 females. Each patient was given 20 mg Adalat orally, randomly alternating with placebo. The blood pressure was measured with a single volume floating catheter from the Vygon Company. The catheter was floated via the right basilica or cephalica vein. After the exact placement of the tip of the catheter into the pulmonary artery, it was fixed so that the pressure could be measured continuously for 48 h. For single measurements, the catheter was attached with a Statham-element. The pressure was monitored over an amplifier with a four channel recorder, produced by Hellige. Measurements were taken immediately before the administration of the drug, then after 1, 3, 6, and 24 h. The value after 24 h was taken as initial value before the administration of the second medication, which proceeded in the same way as on the first day. All measurements were made under resting conditions and under a continuous ergometer-stress of 50 and 100 watts for a period of 2 min each on a bicycle ergometer with an independent speed of rotation. The

Table 2. Pulmonary artery pressure: values at rest. Differences in mm Hg compared with control (average values)

Medication	day	Time after application				Ø
		1 h	3 h	6 h	24 h	
Adalat	1	1.50	1.67	2.00	1.67	1.71
	2	−0.50	−0.67	−0.67	− 1.17	−0.75
	Ø	0.50	0.50	0.67	0.25	0.48
Placebo	1	−1.00	−0.83	1.17	0.33	−0.08
	2	−0.67	0.67	1.00	− 0.67	0.08
	Ø	−0.83	−0.08	1.08	− 0.17	0.00
	1	0.25	0.42	1.59	1.00	0.81
	2	−0.58	0.00	0.17	− 0.92	−0.33
	Ø	−0.17	0.20	0.87	0.04	0.24

Table 3. Pulmonary artery pressure: load test with 50 watts. Differences in mm Hg compared with control (average values)

Medication	day	Time after administration					Ø
		0 h	1 h	3 h	6 h	24 h	24 h
Adalat	1	5.50	2.83	3.00	4.17	3.67	3.83
	2	4.50	4.17	3.67	5.17	4.67	4.43
	Ø	5.00	3.50	3.33	4.67	4.17	4.13
Placebo	1	5.50	5.00	4.50	6.00	4.50	5.10
	2	3.67	3.33	4.50	4.00	3.17	3.73
	Ø	4.58	4.17	4.50	5.00	3.83	4.42
	1	5.50	3.92	3.75	5.08	4.08	4.47
	2	4.08	3.75	4.08	4.58	3.92	4.08
	Ø	4.79	3.83	3.92	4.83	4.00	4.27

measured values were statistically evaluated with a four-way cross-over analysis of variance. Due to the significant differences of the initial values of the pulmonary artery pressure on both days with individual patients (Table 1), we did not compare the absolute values with each other, but calculated with the difference of the average pressure. In the case of O-stress, this means, that the average pressure was compared with the pre-value under O-stress, and in case of 50 and 100 watt stress, this comparison was performed with the difference of the O-values at the same measurement.

Results

When considering the results, we see that the values measured under resting conditions show no significant differences between the periods after administration of Adalat and after placebo. Likewise, with a stress of 50 watts, there was no significant difference. The results of the analysis of variance are similar to the resting values (Tables 2 and 3). The analysis of variance demonstrated a slight but significant rise in pressure with a stress of 100 watts with Adalat but not with placebo after one and three hours ($p = 0.02$).

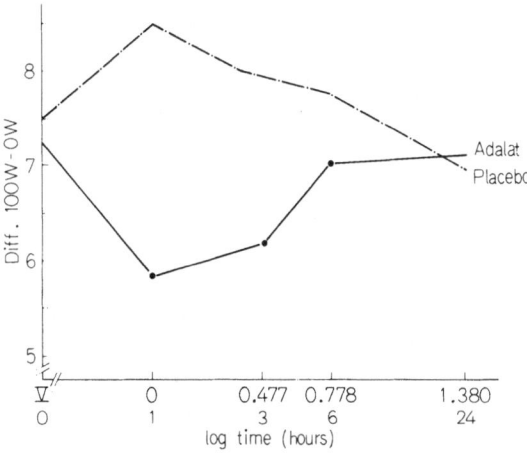

Fig. 1. Pulmonary artery pressure, load test with 100 W

Table 4. Pulmonary artery pressure: load test with 100 watts. Differences in mm Hg compared with control (average values)

Medication	day	Time after administration					Ø
		0 h	1 h	3 h	6 h	24 h	
Adalat	1	7.50	4.83	5.50	6.67	6.67	6.23
	2	7.00	6.83	6.83	7.33	7.50	7.10
	Ø	7.25	5.83	6.17	7.00	7.08	6.67
Placebo	1	8.33	9.33	7.33	7.50	7.00	7.90
	2	6.67	7.67	8.67	8.00	6.83	7.56
	Ø	7.50	8.50	8.00	7.75	6.92	7.73
	1	7.92	7.08	6.42	7.08	6.83	7.06
	2	6.83	7.25	7.75	7.67	7.17	7.33
	Ø	7.37	7.17	7.08	7.37	7.00	7.20

Table 5. Side-effects

Pat. Nr.	Medication	Side-effects
1	Placebo	none
	Adalat	headache
2	Placebo	none
	Adalat	headache
3	Adalat	none
	Placebo	none
4	Placebo	none
	Adalat	none
5	Placebo	none
	Adalat	none
6	Adalat	feeling of heat
	Placebo	none
7	Adalat	feeling of heat, nausea
	Placebo	none
8	Placebo	none
	Adalat	none
9	Placebo	none
	Adalat	none
10	Adalat	none
	Placebo	none
11	Adalat	headache
	Placebo	none
12	Adalat	none
	Placebo	none

After 6 h, this tendency could still be recognized but was no longer statistically significant. There was, on the average, a slight drop of blood pressure of 2–3 mm Hg (Table 4 and Fig. 1). Five patients experienced headaches or sensations of heat in the head about one half to three quarters of an hour after administration of Adalat, one with nausea.

The side-effects lasted 2–3 h and then spontaneously subsided (Table 5). After the administration of placebo, no side-effects were observed. Although they were not extensive, the number of side-effects in this study was relatively high.

Abstract

We demonstrated that in the absence of important alterations in the pulmonary circulation, the rise of blood pressure in the pulmonary artery is on the average 2–3 mm Hg lower 1–3 h after the oral administration of 20 mg Adalat under moderate stress than is the physiological rise in blood pressure. In regard to the mode of action, the question of to what extent Adalat, like the nitrates, influences the capacity vessels with a decreased blood return to the right ventricle, was considered. To clarify this question, further experiments are necessary. In addition, additional investigations should be made to analyse the extent of this effect on persistent pulmonary hypertension.

Comparison of the Effect of Adalat and Propranolol on Exercise Tolerance in Patients with Angina Pectoris

J. D. McArthur, R. G. Murray, A. Tweddel, and T. D. V. Lawrie

University Department of Medical Cardiology, Royal Infirmary, Glasgow, Great Britain

Introduction

Angina pectoris is one of the most distressing manifestations of ischemic heart disease, and its medical management is often difficult. One approach to its treatment has involved the use of vasodilator drugs, of which glyceryl trinitrate is the most commonly used [6]. Unfortunately, while acutely administered glyceryl trinitrate is undoubtedly efficacious, results with so-called "long-acting vasodilators" have been much less impressive [1, 5, 17].

Nifedipine (Adalat) is a new drug which has, among its actions, a vasodilator effect on the coronary arteries [10, 11], and which appears to have a relatively long-lasting effect when administered by the oral route [9]. There is evidence that, when acutely administered (sublingually), the drug improves exercise tolerance [14] and that the number of attacks of angina pectoris are reduced when the drug is taken over a long period of time [3].

If such a drug is to prove a major advance in the treatment of angina pectoris, it should be possible to show that the patient's exercise tolerance is improved when the drug is administered long term by the oral route and that the drug is well tolerated. Beta-adrenergic blocking drugs, which represent a different approach to the treatment of angina pectoris, can be shown to improve exercise tolerance when administered long term [15]. It was planned, therefore, to compare the efficacy of nifedipine with that of propranolol in the improvement of exercise tolerance in patients with angina pectoris. A preliminary study is reported here.

Methods

As a preliminary to a planned double-blind study, a limited study involving five patients (male, aged 40–53 years) with stable angina pectoris (present more than one year) was carried out. All patients had significant ST segment depression on the electrocardiogram on exercise testing and had angiographically proven significant coronary artery disease involving two or more vessels.

While the patients had been treated with beta blocking drugs previously (propranolol, 1 patient; practolol, 4 patients), no one had had any medication other than glyceryl trinitrate as necessary, in the two weeks prior to entering the trial. The patients were familiar with the method of exercise testing, having been tested on the bicycle ergometer at least once before entering the trial.

Each patient was tested at least twice while on no long-term medication and then at weekly intervals while on increasing doses of a) nifedipine and, subsequently, b) propranolol. (In this preliminary study, nifedipine was always given first in view of the prolonged "wash-out" period for propranolol.)

The dose of nifedipine commenced at 10 mg t.i.d. and rose at weekly intervals to 20 mg t.i.d. and 30 mg t.i.d. Administration of the drug was discontinued a) when the 30 mg t.i.d. dose had been taken for one week or b) if intolerable side-effects developed or c) if exercise tolerance appeared to be deteriorating with increasing dose.

Propranolol dosage commenced at 10 mg t.i.d. and rose at weekly intervals to 20 mg q.i.d., 40 mg q.i.d. and 60 mg q.i.d. The drug was discontinued a) when the 60 mg q.i.d. dose had been administered for one week b) if the heart rate fell to less than 60 beats/min c) if intolerable side-effects developed or d) if there was a deterioration in the exercise tolerance with increasing dose.

Each patient was tested in the post-prandial state, which was between $1\frac{1}{2}$ and $2\frac{1}{2}$ h after his last dose of medication. Resting heart rate and blood pressure were recorded and then exercise testing was carried out on the Puch-Tunturi bicycle ergometer. The work load commenced at 300 kilopond-metres/min and was increased by 300 k.p.m. steps at 2 min intervals until a load of 900 k.p.m. for 2 min was sustained or until angina or dyspnoea developed. The total work sustained was obtained by summing the products of the work load by the time sustained.

A careful record of number of attacks of angina pectoris, number of tablets of glyceryl trinitrate consumed and any side-effects volunteered by the patient was kept.

Results

The results are shown in Table 1. There was no significant change in the resting heart rate when nifedipine was taken whereas the heart rate fell by an

Table 1. Pulse, B.P. and exercise tolerance

Patient No.	Pre-treatment			Nifedipine			Propranolol		
	H.R.	B.P.	MAX.E.T. (k.p.m.)	H.R.	B.P.	MAX.E.T. (k.p.m.)	H.R.	B.P.	MAX.E.T. (k.p.m.)
1	90	128/ 88	1350	80	110/70	1250	72	102/70	1600
2	74	138/ 88	1050	80	140/90	1300	58	140/86	1800
3	76	120/ 86	1650	72	126/74	2475	48	142/92	2850
4	80	130/ 90	1400	72	110/70	1500	80	113/72	2100
5	100	150/102	1200	105	130/84	900	60	120/80	1500

H.R.   = Heart rate (beats/min).
B.P.   = Blood pressure (mm Hg).
MAX.E.T. = Maximum exercise tolerance.

Table 2. Side-effects with nifedipine

Gastrointestinal (nausea, epigastric discomfort)	4 Patients
Cardiovascular (flushing, headache, light-headedness)	3
Dyspnoea	2
Pruritus	1

average of 24% when on propranolol. Blood pressure changes were variable and there was no consistent change with either drug.

The maximum exercise tolerance achieved under propranolol medication was clearly increased (average increase 48%) whereas there was no impressive change during nifedipine therapy (average change +12%).

No significant side-effects were reported with propranolol administration but side-effects were reported while on nifedipine therapy. These are shown in Table 2. The gastrointestinal side-effects appeared to be dose related and, in one patient, regressed when he himself reduced the dosage. On the other hand, the cardiovascular side-effects of flushing etc. appeared with the lowest dose but, in two patients, the side-effects regressed even though the nifedipine dose was increased.

Discussion

It should be emphasized that this was a preliminary study, carried out mainly in an attempt to find the optimum effective dose of the two drugs in individual patients, prior to entry into a double-blind trial. Therefore, the study is open to criticism on several points. However, the results are sufficiently striking to justify their reporting here. In our experience, nifedipine does not appear to have a sustained effect on exercise tolerance when administered orally, and its administration is associated with a relatively high incidence of side-effects.

The mechanism whereby vasodilator drugs appear to improve exercise tolerance in patients with angina pectoris is complex but it is generally agreed that at least part of their action is to decrease the peripheral vascular resistance by their action on resistance vessels [13]. Some authors would suggest that they are only useful when this hemodynamic change can be demonstrated [6].

While nifedipine clearly has more actions than simple vasodilation and has, for instance, a Ca^{++} antagonist effect in the excitation-contraction mechanism in muscle [4, 7], its actions, when administered intravenously and sublingually, are very similar to those of glyceryl trinitrate [10, 12] and both produce side-effects (e.g. flushing, headaches) which can be attributed to peripheral vasodilatation. It is not surprising therefore, that improvements in exercise tolerance can be shown after sublingual nifedipine or for a relatively short period after acute oral administration. However, when given as a three-times-a-day regular dosage, it was not possible to demonstrate a beneficial effect on exercise tolerance at a time when there would appear to be an adequate blood level [9]. It may be significant if the action of nifedipine can, in part, be attributed to its peripheral effects, that, at the time of testing, the patients' hemodynamic status, in so far as it could be deduced from resting pulse and B.P. measurements, showed no consistent change from pre-treatment values. It would seem possible that when a vasodilator drug such as nifedipine is administered long term, the body's homeostatic mechanisms tend to counteract the changes brought about by the drug. This could explain why some of our patients found that side-effects which could be attributed to vasodilatation, such as flushing and headaches, regressed, in spite of continued administration of the same or even higher doses of the drug. Workers in nitrite factories likewise become tolerant to the effects of chronic exposure to vasodilator compounds [18].

Methods of assessing the exercise tolerance of individuals and ways of quantitating it vary considerably in different published works [2, 8, 16]. The method used here, which involved the summation of all the work done, may have been relatively less sensitive than some others, as it included quantities of work done at subangina-producing work levels. However, it still clearly demonstrated a beneficial effect on exercise tolerance by propranolol.

As, in this study, no placebo was administered during the period when control exercise tolerance studies were made, it could be argued that the apparent beneficial effects of propranolol were, in fact, a placebo response, but the absence of such a response when nifedipine was administered makes this unlikely.

Other workers have demonstrated a diminution in the number of glyceryl trinitrate tablets consumed by patients under regular nifedipine therapy. Clearly, if the number of attacks of angina pectoris per day is large, benefit from any therapeutic agent would be more easy to demonstrate. Our patients had relatively few attacks of angina per day (2–6 attacks), and no significant effect by nifedipine could be seen.

The incidence of side-effects is, in our experience, disturbingly high [3]. The general level of side-effects reported with nifedipine is around 14%, but other workers have noted a much higher incidence of side-effects (McIlwraith, G., pers. comm.). While the types of side-effect encountered were similar to those reported elsewhere, the relative frequency, with a higher incidence of gastrointestinal side-effects, is different. This may, in part, be due to the use of a rather high dose level in some patients (30 mg three times a day). Naturally, a high incidence of side-effects, as found in this study, would constitute a significant disadvantage.

Abstract

A preliminary study comparing the efficacy of nifedipine with that of propranolol in the improvement of exercise tolerance in patients with angina pectoris is reported. Whereas propranolol improved exercise tolerance significantly and did not cause significant side-effects, nifedipine, under the conditions used in this study, did not significantly improve exercise tolerance and was associated with a significant number of side-effects.

References

1. Battock, D. J., Alvarez, H., Chidsey, C. A.: Effect of propranolol and isosorbide dinitrite on exercise performance and adrenergic activity in patients with angina pectoris. Circulation **39**, 157 (1969).

2. BURKETT, D. A., CHAMBERLAIN, D. A.: Beta-adrenergic blockade in angina pectoris—a method of treadmill assessment. Brit. Med. J. **2**, 500 (1966).
3. EBNER, F.: Summary of results obtained during the world wide clinical investigations on Nifedipine. 2nd International Adalat Symposium. Berlin-Heidelberg-New York: Springer 1975.
4. FLECKENSTEIN, A.: Adalat, a powerful Ca-antagonistic drug. 2nd International Adalat Symposium. Berlin-Heidelberg-New York: Springer 1975.
5. GOLDBARG, A. N., MORAN, J. F., BUTTERFIELD, T. R., NEMICKAS, R., BERMUDEZ, G. A.: Therapy of angina pectoris with propranolol and long-acting nitrates. Circulation **40**, 847 (1969).
6. GOLDSTEIN, R. E., EPSTEIN, S. E.: Mecidal management of patients with angina pectoris. Prog. Cardiovasc. Dis. **15**, 360 (1972).
7. GRÜN, G.: Ca-dependent changes in coronary smooth muscle tone and the action of Ca-antagonistic compounds with special reference to Adalat. 2nd International Adalat Symposium. Berlin-Heidelberg-New York: Springer 1975.
8. HAMER, J., SOWTON, E.: Effects of propranolol on exercise tolerance in angina pectoris. Amer. J. Cardiol. **18**, 354 (1966).
9. HORSTER, F. A.: Pharmacokinetical investigations with labelled Adalat in humans. 2nd International Adalat Symposium. Berlin-Heidelberg-New York: Springer 1975.
10. KIRCHHEIM, H., GROSS, R.: Hemodynamic effects of Adalat in the unanesthetised dog. 2nd Intern. Adalat Symposium. Berlin-Heidelberg-New York: Springer 1975.
11. LICHTLEN, P.: Coronary and left ventricular dynamics under Adalat, in comparison to nitrates, beta blocking agents and dipyridamole. 2nd International Adalat Symposium. Berlin-Heidelberg-New York: Springer 1975.
12. LYDTIN, H., LOHMÖLLER, G., LOHMÖLLER, R., SCHMITZ, H., WALTHER, I.: Hemodynamic studies on Adalat in healthy volunteers and patients. 2nd International Adalat Symposium. Berlin-Heidelberg-New York: Springer 1975.
12. MASON, D. T., BRAUNWALD, E.: The effects of nitroglycerin and amyl nitrite on arteriolar and venous tone in the human forearm. Circulation **32**, 755 (1965).
14. MCILWRAITH, G.: Antianginal efficacy of Adalat under loading conditions. 2nd International Adalat Symposium. Berlin-Heidelberg-New York: Springer 1975.
15. MURRAY, G., TWEDDEL, A., MCARTHUR, J. D., LAWRIE, T. D. V.: Unpublished observations.
16. REDWOOD, D. R., ROSING, D. R., GOLDSTEIN, R. E., BEISER, G. D., EPSTEIN, S. E.: Importance of the design of an exercise protocol in the evaluation of patients with angina pectoris. Circulation **43**, 618 (1971).
17. RUSSEK, H. I.: Therapeutic role of coronary vaso-dilators: glyceryl trinitrate isosorbide dinitrate and pentaerythritol tetranitrate. Amer. J. Med. Sci. **252**, 9 (1966).
18. SCHWARTZ, A. M.: The cause, relief and prevention of headaches arising from contact with dynamite. New Eng. J. Med. **235**, 541 (1946).

Session VII

Clinical Aspects: Proof of Clinical Efficacy

Chairmen: P. Lichtlen (Hannover), L. G. Ekelund (Stockholm)

Nifedipine in Angina Pectoris:
A Multicentric Clinical Trial

F. CAMERINI and S. SCARDI

Divisione di Cardiologia e Centro per la Lotta contro le Malattie Cardiovascolari,
Ospedale Maggiore, Ente Ospedaliero Regionale, Trieste, Italy

The synthesis of nifedipine, the knowledge of its pharmacological action in man and in animals and the first results of its effects in coronary insufficiency induced us to begin a multicentric clinical trial, in order to evaluate the effect of nifedipine, compared to placebo, in patients with angina pectoris.

Materials and Methods

In the six centers[1] taking part in the trial a total of 55 subjects were studied. Of these, 48 (40 males and 8 females aged between 35 and 60, mean age 53) completed the study and have been statistically evaluated. The other 7 cases were dropped from the study because of lack of cooperation or because the data given were unreliable. All patients suffered from typical chronic angina pectoris, after effort and/or at rest, relieved by nitroglycerin.

Patients were taught not to use nitroglycerin prophylactically. All other treatments had been stopped for at least 1 week (in many cases for 2 weeks). No patient presented mental depression. A clinical history of myocardial infarction was not considered as a contraindication, provided at least six months had elapsed after the acute phase. In no case was heart failure or atrioventricular block present. The study was carried out as a double-blind cross-over comparison of nifedipine with placebo. Capsules of the same size, shape and color were used; they were contained in identical bottles, which were differentiated only by a label with the

---

[1] The following centers took part in the project:
Clinica Medica Generale, Cattedra di Malattie Cardiovascolari, Università di Cagliari (M. BINA, A. CHERCHI, R. FONZO).
Divisione di Cardiologia, Ospedale Policlinico S. Matteo, Pavia (P. BOBBA).
Divisione di Cardiologia e Centro per la Lotta contro le Malattie Cardiovascolari, Ospedale Maggiore, Trieste (F. CAMERINI, F. FONDA, S. SCARDI).
Divisione di Cardiologia Ospedale G. B. Guistinian, Venezia (A. BENZONI, G. CATURELLI).
Divisione di Medicina, Ospedale S. Croce, Cuneo (P. F. ANGELINO, R. ALGRANATI, P. TORTORE).
Servizio di Cardiologia, Ospedale Bassini, Milano (G. C. MAGGI).
The data from this project were presented at the First International Nifedipine "Adalat" Symposium, Tokyo, 1973 and are published in *Giornale Italiano di Cardiologia* 4, 575 (1974).

inscription "treatment 1" or "treatment 2". Each bottle contained 50 capsules, enough for 14 days.

The patients were instructed to take 3 capsules a day. Each bottle contained nifedipine (capsules of 10 mg) or placebo, in random order. The patients were clinically examined before the beginning of the experiment and at the end of the first and second cycles of treatment.

Blood pressure and heart rate were measured at the same intervals, an electro-cardiogram was recorded and the following blood tests were carried out: erythro-cyte and leukocyte counts, blood urea nitrogen, glucose, bilirubin, alkaline phos-phatase, SGOT, SGPT, LDH, prothrombine time, serum iron, potassium and calcium, total protein and electrophoresis.

The patients were given two schedules on which they were to mark daily the factors causing angina, the number, duration and severity ("slight", "severe", and "very severe") of attacks, the number of nitroglycerin pills taken daily and any subsequent side effect. The patients were also asked to write down their opinion on the efficacy of the treatment.

The schedules were to be returned after 14 days, and the investigator had to transform the data from the schedules into quantitative values, according to the criteria of evaluation reported in Table 1. For the tabulation of electrocar-diographic data, a particular schedule was used.

The appearance of side effects was analyzed on the basis of carefully collected clinical histories.

The patients were informed that they would use a new drug that had shown promising effects on angina pectoris. For an individual evaluation of the drug, however, a period of investigation was required. The patients were informed

Table 1. Criteria for score (from BIANCHI [1])

	score
1. Factors causing attacks	
a) no cause	0.5
b) slight effort	0.4
c) strong effort	0.3
d) other causes	0.2
2. Number of attacks	1 (for each attack)
3. Duration of pain	
a) transient	1
b) persistent	1
4. Intensity of pain	
a) very severe	3
b) severe	2
c) slight	0.5
5. Consumption of nitroglycerin	1
6. Efficacy of treatment (patients' opinion)	
a) very good	0.1
b) good	0.2
c) no effect	0.5

about the importance of their cooperation, and they were told to take nitroglycerin only in case of pain and not prophylactically. All gave their consent and agreed to follow the criteria suggested.

Statistical Methods

The "clinical-therapeutical total value" (obtained from the addition of the scores derived from the analysis of each symptom during the whole investigation) has been utilized. The analysis of variance for all the data that could be transformed into scores has been used.

In the statistical evaluation of the electrocardiographic data we used for the parameters "heart rate" and "Q-T time" the analysis of variance. For the other electrocardiographic parameters (frequency of ectopic beats, appearance of A-V blocks, changes of repolarization, we preferred, because of the difficulty involved in transforming them into scores, to use qualitative judgements ("improved", "not changed", "worse"). For the statistical analysis of these data the χ^2 calculation (corrected by Yates) was used.

Results

Factors Causing Anginal Attacks

The effect of nifedipine, compared to placebo, on the attacks of angina was studied with the analysis of variance. After nifedipine all types of attacks (analyzed separately) were reduced, although the difference between the results obtained with nifedipine and placebo were not statistically significant. On the other hand, when the total sum of all the factors causing attacks was analyzed, the difference was highly significant ($F = 8.12$; $p < 0.01$). With the use of nifedipine a definite reduction of the attacks of angina was observed (Table 2).

Number of Attacks

The comparison between the number of attacks in the two periods of treatment gave a significant result in favor of nifedipine ($F = 9.52$; $p = 0.01$) (Table 2).

Duration of Pain

The comparison between placebo and nifedipine gave, also for this parameter, a statistically significant result ($F = 5.97$; $p < 0.05$). It must be noted that nifedipine reduces both "transient" and "persistent" attacks of angina, but a statistically significant reduction is obvious only in the "transient" attacks ($p < 0.05$) (Table 2).

Intensity of Pain

The score of the parameter intensity of pain was significantly reduced ($p < 0.05$) after treatment with nifedipine. All types of attacks (pain "very severe", "severe" and "slight") were reduced in number, although the ones characterized by "slight" pain were more evidently reduced ($p < 0.01$) (Table 2).

Table 2. Total clinico-therapeutical value. Mean ± S.E.

	Placebo	Nifedipine	F	p
Factor causing angina	5.61±0.58	3.37±0.53	8.12	<0.01
a) no apparent cause	2.17±0.46	1.09±0.37	3.40	n.s.
b) strong effort	0.57±0.21	0.30±0.11	1.26	n.s.
c) slight effort	2.24±0.37	1.50±0.30	2.40	n.s.
d) other causes	0.63±0.18	0.48±0.14	1	n.s.
Number of attacks	18.5 ±2.4	10.0 ±1.4	9.52	0.01
Duration of pain	22.6 ±3.8	12.1 ±1.9	5.97	<0.05
a) transient	11.6 ±1.35	7.0 ±1.29	5.95	<0.05
b) persistent	10.98±3.4	5.11±1.44	2.53	n.s.
Intensity of pain	16.28±2.71	9.07±1.57	5.30	<0.05
a) very severe	2.2 ±1.0	0.5 ±0.2	2.73	n.s.
b) severe	8.13±1.76	5.57±1.30	1.36	n.s.
c) slight	5.93±0.92	2.99±0.49	7.96	<0.01
Consumption of nitroglycerin	14.42±2.49	5.50±1.08	10.82	<0.01
Efficacy of treatment (patients' opinion)	5.50±0.31	3.23±0.27	30.12	<0.001
a) very good	0.10±0.05	0.40±0.08	9.31	<0.01
b) good	0.82±0.15	1.18±0.16	2.77	n.s.
c) no effect	4.32±0.40	1.65±0.35	25.57	<0.001

Nitroglycerin Consumption

The consumption of nitroglycerin pills was significantly reduced in comparison with placebo, when nifedipine was used ($F = 10.82$; $p < 0.01$) (Table 2).

Patients' Opinions on the Efficacy of Treatment

The opinions given by the patients on the efficacy of the two treatments were clearly in favor of nifedipine ($F = 30.12$; $p < 0.001$).

Influence of Treatment on Blood Tests

The statistical analysis carried out with the results of blood tests (see Materials and Methods) did not show any significant difference between the two periods of treatment. Only the LDH showed a reduction during treatment with nifedipine (mean + 11.6 with placebo and −28.3 with nifedipine; $F = 5.70$; $p < 0.05$).

Blood Pressure

No changes of blood pressure appeared during the two periods of treatment.

Electrocardiogram

The electrocardiogram was studied considering the following data: heart rate, frequency of ectopic beats, appearance of A-V block, changes of the QRS complex, of the repolarization and of the QT interval. No significant changes were noted. Only the heart rate diminished slightly during the period of treatment with nifedipine (placebo: $+1.34$, ± 1.19 beats/min; nifedipine: -3.87, ± 1.21 beats/min).

Side Effects

The following side effects were observed:

Side effects	Placebo	Nifedipine
Headache	2	1
Dyspepsia	3	1
Flush	—	1
Edema of legs	—	2

Discussion

It is well known that the drugs used to treat angina may act via multiple mechanisms. Some drugs, such as the beta blockers, reduce myocardial oxygen consumption while others, such as nitroglycerin, dilate the main coronary arteries and probably also the small collaterals. The action of nitroglycerin is more complex in that it also decreases oxygen consumption by reducing arterial pressure, venous tone, ventricular volume, wall tension, etc.

The studies with nifedipine have shown that this drug acts with a mechanism partially similar to that of nitroglycerin: it causes a dilatation of the coronary vascular bed with consequent increase of flow. Moreover a single oral dose of nifedipine lowers the systemic arterial blood pressure and also the left ventricular external work, with a consequent reduction of oxygen consumption by the heart muscle. These experimental pathophysiological data must, however, be verified clinically, because hemodynamic measurements are insufficient for the assessment of the efficacy of a drug in angina.

This verification has been carried out in our study, which was organized on a multicentric basis; the trial was designed as a double blind cross-over comparison of nifedipine with placebo. This technique is at present considered the most efficient in assessing the effectiveness of a therapeutic agent on a variable and emotionally influenced symptom such as angina.

Nevertheless, a controlled clinical trial, such as the one carried out by us, presents some difficulties and limitations: the patients analyzed must have a history of chronic stable angina, they must be cooperative and have a certain intellectual level. Moreover, if a patient is accustomed to exercise himself up to a certain level of anginal pain, he will increase his exercise tolerance but he may not be able to diminish the nitroglycerin consumption and the daily score.

Notwithstanding these limitations, a controlled multicentric clinical trial is probably the best means to demonstrate the beneficial effect of a drug in angina pectoris. With this technique we were able to demonstrate that nifedipine acts, at least on a short-term basis, be reducing in a statistically significant manner ($p < 0.01$) the occurrence of anginal attacks. In fact the drug diminishes the number of crises determined by all types of factors, thus reducing the absolute number of attacks of angina.

In this study, nifedipine proved significantly more useful than placebo in reducing the duration of attacks (especially transient: $p < 0.05$). A further confirmation of the positive action of the drug is given by the reduction of the intensity of pain ($p < 0.05$) (this reduction is more evident in slight attacks) and by the reduced use of nitroglycerin pills ($p < 0.01$).

Also the patients' opinion on the efficacy of the drug confirms the preceding data ($p < 0.001$).

The literature published thus far, although rich in pharmacological and laboratory data on the drug, is weak in the area of controlled clinical trials.

Our results seem to be in agreement with those of KIMURA et al. [3], who evaluated the efficacy of nifedipine in 16 patients studied with a double-blind cross-over technique and with a sequential analysis. According to these authors, nifedipine was "almost equally effective as isosorbide dinitrate and propranolol".

In a single blind cross-over trial, HAYASE et al. [2] studied a small group of 6 patients: in 5 of the 6, nifedipine given orally in daily doses of 60 mg into 3 divided portions revealed an outstanding preventive effect on the occurrence of anginal attacks.

Tolerance for the drug is good. It has few side effects, and these were never serious enough to cause interruption of the treatment. We did not observe hypotensive reactions, as were observed in one case described by KIMURA et al. [3] and in 4 cases (in a group of 47) studied by KOBAYASHI et al. [4]. Edema of the legs was noticed in only 2 patients, without symptoms or signs of heart failure.

Further we did not observe any significant change in any of the biochemical and hematological parameters studied, except for the LDH, which showed a decrease during treatment. At present we have no explanation for this change.

In conclusion nifedipine, in our double-blind cross-over short term research project, has proved to be an efficient and useful drug, devoid of significant side effects: these results will be confirmed by a long-term clinical experiment. Also the possibility of resistance to nifedipine should be excluded, and the potential utility of its combination with other drugs must be verified.

Abstract

The efficacy of nifedipine has been studied in 55 patients affected by angina pectoris. The experimentation has been carried out in 6 centers as a cross-over double blind study.

The trial demonstrated that nifedipine reduces in a statistically significant way the number and duration of anginal attacks, the intensity of pain and the consumption of nitroglycerin pills.

The efficacy of the drug, which has only a few side effects, has been also confirmed by patients' opinion.

References

1. BIANCHI, C.: La valutazione clinica dei farmaci antistenocardici. In: Atti Simposio sulle metodologie di valutazione dei farmaci nell'uomo. Ed. Ciba, Milano, 1962.
2. HAYASE, S., HIRAKAWA, S., HOSOKAWA, S., MORI, N., KANYAMA, S., IWASA, M.: Hemodynamic and therapeutic effect of BAY a 1040 on the patients with ischemic heart disease. Arzneim.-Forsch. (Drug Res.) **22**, 370 (1972).

3. Kimura, E., Mabuchi, G., Kikuchi, H.: The clinical effect of 4-2'-Nitrophenyl-2,6-di-methyl-3,5-dicarbomethoxy-1,4-dihydropyridine (BAY a 1040) on angina pectoris evaluated by sequential analysis. Arzneim.-Forsch. (Drug Res.) **22**, 365 (1972).
4. Kobayashi, T., Ito, Y., Tawara, I.: Clinical experience with a new coronary-active substance (BAY a 1040). Arzneim.-Forsch. (Drug Res.) **22**, 380 (1972).

Discussion Remarks

Lichtlen: Since the last meeting in Tokyo in November 1973 many more studies have been done on the clinical effects of nifedipine. The clinical efficacy has now become really much clearer and the whole subject been made more interesting for the clinician!

In our discussion, the following topics should be covered: With regard to indications for the drug, special indications should be gone into; also patient selection should be analyzed: Which patients should be given nitrates, which beta-blockers, and which calcium antagonists like nifedipine.

First question: Did you compare Adalat with beta-blocking agents or only with placebos? The second question concerns side effects: How did you explain edema of the legs? My third question: Would you give us your opinion on the indications for use of this drug?

Camerini: To answer your first question: Our study was a double-blind study and we compared nifedipine with placebo; we are now carrying out a new study with multiple comparisons. We noticed in two cases the appearance of edema of the legs; in these cases there were no clinical signs of heart failure and these patients were, from this point of view, in good condition so that we speculated that their edema was of local origin, but we have no explanation for this fact.

As for indications for the drug, we used the drug in the majority of cases in chronic, stable angina and we are now beginning to study the drug in so-called unstable angina.

Lichtlen: Did you use it as a substitute for nitroglycerin or combine it with nitroglycerin; and would you also give it in acute attacks?

Camerini: We have not experience with nifedipine as a substitute for nitroglycerin; we used it as a relatively long-term agent and more for chronic treatment than for acute cases.

An Interim Report on a Cooperative Double-Blind Clinical Trial with Nifedipine

A. SAKUMA and E. KIMURA

Dept. Clin. Pharmacol., Med. Res. Inst., Tokyo Med. and Dent. Univ. 2-3-10 Kanda-Surugadai, Chiyodaku, Tokyo, Japan

Dept. Internal Medicine, Nippon Medical School 1-1-5 Sendagi, Bunkyoku, Tokyo, Japan

A multiclinic, common protocol study was carried out to compare the antianginal utilities of nifedipine (B), molsidomine (S) and propranolol (P). Because the complete analyses including the results of the ECG's are not yet available, this is an interim report of the trial.

Materials and Methods

According to the protocol, anginal patients who fulfilled the following three criteria were selected for the trial: a) ECG showed the ischemic ST depression at rest, during attacks or during exercise tolerance test, b) sublingual glyceryl trinitrate or isosorbide dinitrate (NG) had been effective in relieving the anginal attacks, and c) age from 40–75 years. Furthermore, the number of anginal attacks should be at least 4–5 per week and should be regarded as stable by the attending physician. To eliminate unwanted reactions and interfering factors, patients with glaucoma, cardiac insufficiency, bradycardia, asthma, intermittent claudication and suspected pregnancy were excluded.

All patients were first observed for at least 2 weeks on placebo to determine the frequency and stability of the attacks and to record the control values. Then the patients were randomly allocated to one of three active agents: a) B, 10 mg, b) S, 2 mg, c) P, 20 mg, three times orally per day respectively. Under double-blind conditions, they were observed for a 2-weeks' period of active treatment, and if they were deemed suitable, an optional placebo-follow-up was indicated.

In the case of intolerance, a reduction in dosage or withdrawal of the agent was suggested. Some concomitant treatments were allowed if they constituted medication of continuous background as in the case of hypertension. The prophylactic use of NG was prohibited but its use upon attack was recommended.

The present study covers the period from 1972 to 1974 and is the result of cooperative efforts of 26 hospitals, the full list of which will be given elsewhere.

The patients were instructed to submit weekly a "Patient's Diary" including description of attacks (severity, frequency, time and nature), amount of NG consumption, physical ability in daily life, and impressions of the drug's efficacy during the past week.

A "Doctor's Report Form" consisted of a routine face sheet description, a summary of the patient's report, records of heart rate, blood pressure, exercise tolerance test and ECG at rest and during exercise tolerance test, side-effects, laboratory tests and assessment of drug.

At the end of a 2-week treatment period, each attending physician assessed the degree of comparative overall improvement of his patient's condition and expressed it on a bipolar scale. On the scale, a score of -40 represents the situation in which conditions during the placebo period are definitely better than those during the period of active treatment; 0 means that the two periods are similar; and $+40$ means that the active treatment period is definitely better. Furthermore, the doctor summarized the usefulness of the agent used in the treatment period for each patient on an analog scale where 0 means that the agent should not be given, 40 means that in his opinion the utility of the agent is similar to that of antianginal drugs currently in use, and 80 means that the agent is one of ideal safety and efficacy.

Results

Although more than 100 cases were involved in this trial, 78 patients completed it. Of the latter, the majority exhibited effort (63) and effort-rest (10) angina.

The main reason for rejection involved the stability and frequency of attacks during placebo period.

Upon breaking the key, the patients were cross-classified with respect to some background features, as shown in Table 1. A somewhat biased allocation in terms of the mean number of anginal attacks during placebo period is noted.

The numbers of attacks during the second week of active treatment are (mean excluding dropouts, mean % of placebo): 4.9, 62% for B; 9.5, 79% for S; and 6.9, 66% for P. As compared with the number of attacks during the placebo period, on the average, a reduction in the number of attacks of 3–4 may be expected in 2 weeks of administration of any of these 3 agents.

Examination of the relationship between the number of attacks during the placebo period and the comparative overall judgement or the assessment

Table 1. Some features of the three treatment groups

	Sex		Age			Status		aa(WO)[a]		Dropouts N
	m	f	-49	50–59	60 $-$	out	in	mean	SE	
B	17	8	6	4	15	17	8	7.6	0.83	2	25
S	18	5	6	6	11	19	4	12.8	1.65	2	23
P	20	10	9	10	11	26	4	11.6	1.45	2	30

[a] Average number of anginal attacks during placebo period per week.

Table 2. Summary of the trial

	Comparative overall judgement		Efficacy of the agent		Side-effects cases	N
	mean[a]	SE	mean[b]	SE		
B	16.3	2.92	37.1	4.14	6	25
S	11.1	3.87	35.1	4.67	7	23
P	16.4	3.17	45.1	4.09	4	30

[a] -40: Placebo definitely better; $+40$: Active treatment definitely better.
[b] 0: Better to prohibit use; 80: Ideal safety-efficacy.

of usefulness suggests a slight tendency towards giving a favorable assessment to those experiencing the larger number of attacks during the placebo period. As expected naturally, there is a high correlation between the utility score and the comparative overall judgement. The comparative overall judgement seems to reflect the reduction in the number of anginal attacks, the improvement in physical ability and the patient's impression, while the assessment of usefulness seems to be a summary of the comparative overall judgement and the patient's impression, although the change in ECG was not considered in the present analyses.

The crude results of the two summarizing scores are given in Table 2, with the number of cases in which side-effects occurred. In all 3 groups receiving active treatment, 2 cases in each were recorded as dropout (withdrawal of agent). One case of B and one of P stated that the reason for withdrawal was ineffectiveness; the rest cited disagreeable side-effects, namely, flushing and numbness (B), headache and headache-weakness (S), and gastrointestinal trouble (P).

The utility scores seem to indicate that P is somewhat superior to the other preparations, although a slight correction for the handicapped allocation to B should be considered, as mentioned previously. There are, however, no statistically significant differences at the 5% level among the 3 agents with respect to the comparative overall judgement and the assessment of usefulness.

Abstract

A multiclinic, common protocol study was carried out to compare the antianginal usefulness of nifedipine, molsidomine and propranolol. These active agents were given to a selected group of anginal patients who were observed under double-blind conditions for 2 weeks. On the average, all 3 agents reduced the number of anginal attacks recorded during the preceding placebo-washout period.

Crude results of assessment of usefulness seem to suggest that propranolol is somewhat superior to the other preparations. There are, however, no remarkable differences among these 3 agents in terms of safety-efficacy in anginal patients.

Further analyses of the data are to be completed.

Discussion Remarks

LICHTLEN: Dr. SAKUMA, I think this approach must represent a lot of work. Why is it preferable to the rather ordinary approach for testing antianginal drugs?

SAKUMA: I have been concerned with the design and analysis of this controlled trial. We have tried to define the utility of the drug rather than the efficacy. I think that what the patient wants to have is clinical usefulness, a complex product of efficacy, safety, etc., and not the mechanism of action nor the simple pharmacologic actions. Also, for new drug approval in Japan we have to consider the patient, and his particular condition, in selecting from different types of drugs. As for the analog scale, we decided to use this expression of drug assessment because of its statistical efficiency as compared with those of ordered-categorial ($++$, $+$, $-$, $--$) and dichotomous (yes-or-no) scales.

Results of a Double-Blind Study with Adalat under Short- and Long-Term Treatment

J. MENNA, M. TRAINA, J. C. CASSERA, E. FERREIRÓS, and R. ROHWEDDER

Hospital Italiano, Sociedad Italiana de Beneficencia
Sección Ergometria y Rehabilitación Cardio-Vascular, Buenos Aires, Argentina

The present approach to the treatment of coronary insufficiency requires a therapeutic agent, which relieves the anginal symptomatology, diminishes clearly the incidence and intensity of the attacks and increases the tolerance to physical exercise, without impairment of the cardiac performance. The drug should have a minimum number of adverse reactions.

Based on results of experimental pharmacological and clinical investigations, we undertook a clinical trial with BAY a 1040 (nifedipine, Adalat) in 36 patients suffering from chronic coronary insufficiency. In this presentation, the results concerning the efficacy of the drug are analyzed.

Materials and Methods

The investigations were carried out in 36 out-patients, 29 males and 7 females, aged 38–72 years (average, 53 years) with proved coronary pathology, showing a clinical stable chronic form of angina pectoris, class I or II, according to the criteria accepted by the American Heart Association, without previous infarct or with one or more previous healed infarcts.

The patients were selected after an extensive clinical, radiological and biohumoral examination. For trial selection a graduated ergometric test (Basal-Test) was performed by all patients in order to obtain an acceptable, specific and conclusive result. The universally accepted criterion of positivity was fulfilled with descendent or horizontal changes of the ST segment >0.1 mV, measured within $0.06''$ and $0.08''$ from S. Nadir, at least in 3 complexes, anginal pain $3+/4$, trying to avoid provocation of dangerous arrhythmias.

All the ergometric tests were performed by a stepwise increase of workload during 3-min periods, increasing 25 W in each period, starting from a 1-min warm-up period and a first load of 50 W, on a bicycle ergometer with electromagnetic braking.

A continuous oscilloscopic control was performed, and at the end of every stage, upon immediate recovery and 3 and 5 min thereafter, ECG and blood pressure controls were performed.

Patients with severe hypertension, obesity, diabetes, and emphysema and those under digitalis treatment, with cardiac insufficiency or with signs of disorders of conductibility in the ECG were excluded from this study. The clinical trial was divided into two parts:

a) Short-Term Treatment

During this part, the effects of a single dose of placebo or BAY a 1040 (20 mg) were compared. The study was performed on two consecutive days. The capsules were chewed and their content absorbed sublingually. 30 and 200 min later the ergometric tests were performed, according to the methodology described previously.

b) Long-Term Treatment

In this part, lasting 16 weeks for each patient, the efficacy of placebo and BAY a 1040 was compared, each over an 8-week period. The treatment consisted of the daily administration of 4 capsules. Each capsule of BAY a 1040 contained 10 mg of the active drug. The capsules were taken orally. Every 4 weeks, the patients were asked to come to the consultation without having taken the medication during the previous 12 h.

Two ergometric tests were performed, one without medication, and the other 30 min after the patient had chewed 2 capsules of BAY a 1040 (20 mg) or placebo, respectively.

In addition to the ergometric tests, the number of anginal attacks during weekly periods was also registered.

The investigation was carried out as a double-blind trial. The patients were divided into two groups according to the occurrence of myocardial infarction.

The allocation of the patients to the administration sequence placebo-BAY a 1040 or BAY a 1040-placebo in stages a) and b) was randomized according to aleatory numbers.

Statistical methods: analysis of variability per separated blocks. Each patient was considered as a block. The method was applied to each pathological state and to each sequence of administration [3]. The mean values were compared using the LSD (least significant difference) test [1, 3]. These statistical methods were applied to both the long- and short-term studies.

Results

Five patients were excluded from the results because they did not exhibit a depression of the ST segment >0.1 mV during the ergometric selection test. Two patients did not comply with the long-term treatment.

In order to obtain conclusions regarding the efficacy of the drug, the following parameters were considered: 1. Behaviour of the ST segment; 2. maximum physical exercise performed; 3. number of anginal attacks under treatment with placebo or BAY a 1040.

a) Behaviour of the ST Segment

Changes of the ST segment corresponding to the maximum physical exercise performed by the patients were considered. The experiments were designed so that the exercise performed during the entire course of the study should have been the same.

Tables 1–6 show the results of short- and long-term treatment.

b) Maximum Physical Work Performed

The behaviour of the ST segment under the same exercise performance for each patient was considered in the previous analysis. Tables 7 and 8 show an analysis of the maximum exercise performed by the long-term group of patients,

Table 1. Short-term treatment. ST segment behavior

Sequence of the trial[a]	Group	N	Stand. error	1	2		3		Day
				1 Basal	2 30'	3 200'	4 30'	5 200'	Ergom. Study Ergom. Condit.[b]
With previous infarct	PL→D A	9	0.003	0.163	0.132	0.115	0.112	0.100	
	D→PL B	6	0.005	0.233	0.133	0.118	0.205	0.213	$\bar{X}(-mV)$
Without previous infarct	PL→D C	7	0.004	0.152	0.150	0.124	0.082	0.071	
	D→PL D	9	0.003	0.126	0.117	0.093	0.137	0.140	

[a] Sequence of the trial: PL = placebo, D = Bay a 1040.
[b] Ergometric conditions: 30' = 30 min after 2 capsules adm. subl., 200' = 200 min after 2 capsules adm. subl.

Table 2. Statistical degree of significance of the results from Table 1

Group	1–2	2–3	4–5	2–4	3–5
A	+ +	+ +	+ +	+ +	+ +
B	+ +	−		+ +	+ +
C	−	+ +	+	+ +	+ +
D	−	+ +		+ +	+ +

− : $p > 0.05$ / + : $0.01 < p < 0.05$ / + + : $p < 0.01$.

Table 3. Short-term treatment. ST segment behavior. Percentage reduction of the ST segment depression at 30 and 200 min after sublingual administration of 20 mg BAY a 1040. Reference: Corresponding placebo value ($p < 0.01$)

	Sequence of the trial[a]	30 min	200 min
With previous infarct	PL→D	15.1	13.0
	D→PL	35.1	44.6
Without previous infarct	PL→D	45.3	42.7
	D→PL	14.6	33.6

[a] Sequence of the trial: PL = placebo, D = Bay a 1040.

Table 4. Long-term treatment. ST segment behavior

Sequence of the trial[a]	Group	N	Standard error	Basal	4		8		12		16		Weeks
				1	2	3	4	5	6	7	8	9	Ergom. Study
				B	B	30'	NC	30'	NC	30'	NC	30'	Ergom. Condit.[b] $\bar{X}(-mV)$
With previous infarct													
PL→D	E	5	0.008	0.180	0.142	0.158	0.150	0.148	0.154	0.118	0.122	0.070	
D→PL	F	9	0.013	0.175	0.201	0.130	0.143	0.094	0.147	0.128	0.155	0.134	
Without previous infarct													
PL→D	G	7	0.013	0.134	0.120	0.100	0.121	0.098	0.100	0.074	0.084	0.075	
D→PL	H	7	0.004	0.148	0.130	0.108	0.134	0.114	0.148	0.137	0.148	0.134	

[a] Sequence of the trial: PL = placebo, D = Bay a 1040.
[b] Ergometric conditions: NC = ergometry without capsules, 30' = ergometry 30 min after 2 capsules administered sublingually.

Table 5. Statistical degree of significance of the results from Table 3

Group	1–2	2–4	4–6	6–8	2–3	4–5	6–7	8–9
E	+ +	–	–	+ +	–	–	+ +	+ +
F	–	+ +	–	–	+ +	+	–	–
G	–	–	–	–	–	–	–	–
H	+ +	–	+ +	–	+ +	+ +	+	+ +

$-: p > 0.05$ / $+: 0.01 < p < 0.05$ / $++: p < 0.01$.

Table 6. Long-term treatment. ST segment behavior. Percentage reduction of the ST segment depression 30 min after sublingual administration of BAY a 1040 (20 mg) or placebo. Reference: Ergometry without medication

	Sequence of trial	4	8	12	16
With previous infarct	PL→D	−11.3	1.3	23.4	42.6
	D→PL	35.3	34.3	12.9	13.5
Without previous infarct	PL→D	16.7	20.0	26.0	10.7
	D→PL	16.9	14.9	7.4	9.4

Table 7. Long-term treatment. Behavior of the maximal effort performed by patients without capsules (100%) and 30 min after 2 capsules (placebo or BAY a 1040). Patients with and without previous infarct are considered together

Sequence of the trial	N	4 NC	4 30′	8 NC	8 30′	12 NC	12 30′	16 NC	16 30′	Weeks Ergom. condit.[a]
PL→D	12	100	110.5	100	109.1	100	154.6	100	119.2	Maximal effort[a]
D→PL	16	100	174.4	100	142.7	100	104.9	100	98.3	performed (in?)

[a] Ergometric conditions: NC = ergometry without capsules, 30′ = ergometry 30 min after 2 capsules administered sublingually.

Table 8. Standard errors and statistical significance of the results from Table 7

Sequence of the trial	N	Weeks 4 Std. error	4 Sign.	8 Std. error	8 Sign.	12 Std. error	12 Sign.	16 Std. error	16 Sign.
PL→D	12	9.5	–	8.2	–	31.8	–	11.8	–
D→PL	16	25.2	+	12.2	+ +	4.0	–	3.9	–

$-: p > 0.05$ / $+: 0.01 < p < 0.05$ / $++: p < 0.01$.

Table 9. Long-term treatment. Number of anginal attacks during treatment with placebo or BAY a 1040. Patients with and without previous infarct are considered together

Sequence of the trial	8 weeks		8 weeks	
	N°	%	N°	%
PL→D	740	89.7	85	10.3
D→PL	281	35.3	514	64.7

without medication and after sublingual administration of 2 capsules of placebo or BAY a 1040 (20 mg). A preceding infarct was not taken into consideration.

For a better comparison, the results obtained are expressed in percentages; 100% represents the maximum exercise performed without medication.

c) Number of Anginal Attacks

Table 9 shows the number of anginal attacks reported by the patients during the long-term treatment. As in the previous evaluation, a preceding infarct was not taken into consideration.

Discussion

a) Short-Term Treatment

During the short-term treatment, the pharmacologic effect of a single dose of BAY a 1040 against a single dose of placebo is compared. The parameter considered is the ischemic change of the ST segment in the exercise ECG. This was possible because every patient performed the same workload 30 and 200 min after sublingual administration of the capsules. The differences of ST segment depression observed during administration of BAY a 1040 and placebo indicate the effect of the drug.

Thirty minutes after administration of 20 mg of BAY a 1040 (Tables 1, 2, and 3) a reduction of the ischemic ST segment of between 14.6 and 45.3% was observed, compared with the corresponding values of placebo. This demonstrates that BAY a 1040 prevents to a significant degree the ischemic ECG response to physical effort.

The reduction of the ST segment depression after 200 min was between 13.0 and 44.6%. This indicates a long duration of effect of BAY a 1040.

b) Long-Term Treatment

The regular and prolonged administration of BAY a 1040 leads to the following questions:

1. Does long term treatment with the drug promote improvement of the coronary circulation in ischemic areas?
2. Does the drug induce tachyphylaxis?
3. How is the frequency of anginal attacks affected by the treatment?

ad 1. After long-term administration of BAY a 1040 in dogs, SCHMIER [2] succeeded in inducing the formation of effective collateral circulation in areas of experimental myocardial ischemia. If the same phenomenon occurs in humans, the ergometric tests without medication 12 h before examination should show a substantial reduction of the ischemic ST depression. In our 8-week-treatment study (Tables 4, 5, and 6—ergometry NC), no such influence was observed.

ad 2. The short-term pharmacologic tests (ergometry without medication and ergometry 30 min after sublingual administration of BAY a 1040 or placebo) carried out every 4 weeks during the course of the treatment have proved the persistence of the efficacy of the drug in the course of time, as shown in the observation of the ST segment (Tables 3 and 5) and the effort tolerance (Tables 7 and 8).

ad 3. The difference in the number of anginal attacks during treatment with placebo and with BAY a 1040 is highly significant. In this regard it must be emphasized that a subjective parameter such as the number of anginal attacks is of greater importance in a double-blind investigation, where the sequence of treatment is established on the basis of aleatory numbers.

Conclusions

1. A single dose of 20 mg of BAY a 1040 reduced significantly the cardiac ischemic response to physical effort.

2. This effect still persisted 200 min after administration.

3. BAY a 1040 increased the tolerance to physical effort.

4. Treatment during 8 weeks with a daily dose of 40 mg of BAY a 1040 showed no effect which can be explained by the development of functionally apt collaterals in ischemic areas.

5. No signs of tachyphylaxia were observed during the long-term treatment.

6. The treatment with BAY a 1040 reduced the number of anginal attacks in a highly significant manner.

Abstract

Thirty-six patients with chronic coronary insufficiency in a double-blind study received the new antianginal monosubstance BAY a 1040 (nifedipine, Adalat). The therapeutic sequence placebo/active drug was randomized according to aleatory numbers.

In the first stage of the study (short-term treatment) the efficacy of a single dose of 20 mg BAY a 1040 was compared with that of placebo.

Thirty minutes after sublingual administration of BAY a 1040 (active drug), a significant reduction of ECG ischemic reaction was observed. The therapeutic response persisted for 200 min (long duration of effect).

In the second stage of the study (long-term treatment), the efficacy of BAY a 1040 (a daily dose of 40 mg for 8 weeks) was compared with that of placebo. Two ergometric tests were performed every 4 weeks, one without medication during the previous 12 h and the other 30 min after administration of 2 capsules of either active substance or placebo.

The anginal attacks reported by the patients during weekly periods were also registered.

Analyzing the results of the ergometric tests performed without medication, no evidence further development of functionally apt collaterals in ischemic areas could be observed.

Comparing the results of the ergometric tests performed without medication with those performed under treatment with BAY a 1040, no signs of tachyphylaxia were observed in the course of the 8-week-treatment period.

The reduction of the number of anginal attacks during the treatment with BAY a 1040 was highly significant.

References

1. OWEN, D. B.: Handbook of Statistical Tables, pp. 102–105. London: Addison-Wesley 1962.
2. SCHMIER, J., VAN ACKERN, K., BRÜCKNER, U.: Investigation on Tachyphylaxis and collateral formation after Nifedipine whilst taking into consideration the direction of flow and the mortality-rate due to infarction. 1st International Nifedipine Adalat Symposium, p. 45–52. University of Tokyo Press 1975.
3. SNEDECOR, G. W., COCHRAN, W. G.: Statistical Methods, 6th Ed.. Ames, Iowa: Iowa State Univ. Press 1967.

Discussion Remarks

LICHTLEN: What does the Argentine group think about indications: In which cases do you prefer nifedipine, let us say, against a beta-blocker?

MENNA: We prefer nifedipine in patients who manifest myocardial failure, because in our experience we had a very good response on exercise when the patient had anginal pain and supraventricular extrasystoles under stress. For us such exertional behavior makes us suspect ventricular failure, and we know from hemodynamic studies that the left ventricular end-diastolic pressure is high in these patients.

We had four patients who exhibited this pattern: They developed supraventricular arrhythmia, angina pectoris, and a down-sloping ST segment at 100 watts of work. After administration of nifedipine the supraventricular extrasystoles disappeared. This response with Adalat indicates an improvement of cardiac failure and the hemodynamic condition as opposed to beta-blockers.

LICHTLEN: How about impending infarction and fresh infarction?

MENNA: In Argentine it is very problematic to investigate a new drug in severely ill patients. So I do not use that drug in fresh myocardial infarction.

SAKUMA: Dr. LICHTLEN, I forgot to reply to your general question on indication. Many doctors who have been involved in this trial believe that nifedipine is the drug of choice for patients with a tendency to cardiac failure and for those with Prinzmetal's angina.

LICHTLEN: I was surprised that nobody mentioned Prinzmetal's angina today. In Tokyo there was a lot of talk of nifedipine in the treatment of Prinzmetal's angina.

MENNA: We did an important study on Prinzmetal's angina, how this angina responds to exercise. Comparing this investigation with our knowledge of Adalat, I would think that Adalat would be a good drug for Prinzmetal's angina but I have not used it in such cases.

Long-Term Therapy with Adalat. A Preliminary Report

H. LINKE

Kurklinik für Herz-, Kreislauf- und Gefäßerkrankungen Pitzer KG,
Bad Schwalbach, Fed. Rep. Germany

During the last three years, 40 in- and out-patients with various forms of angina pectoris on effort and/or at rest were treated with Adalat (nifedipine) for a period of one to three months.

The case material, comprising both sexes (26 males, 14 females) between 32 and 78 years of age (average 62 years), includes 22 cases of coronary sclerosis, 8 cases of old myocardial infarction and 10 cases of angina caused by effort under hypertension.

Adalat was administered orally in capsules of 10 mg. The daily dosage was divided into 3 or 4 portions, ranging from 3 to 6 capsules (30–60 mg) given after meals. Most patients received 30 mg daily.

For evaluation of the effect of Adalat in an open clinical study, the following parameters were used, both prior to treatment and during the long-term therapy:

Influence of Adalat on accessory and consecutive symptoms of coronary insufficiency, in particular on consumption of nitroglycerin capsules (0.8 mg) and on number of anginal attacks, moreover on the heart rate, the blood pressure and the ST-segment depression at rest and on exercise ECG under gradually increasing ergometric loading on a bicycle ergometer.

Table 1 shows the influence of Adalat on subjective symptoms of coronary insufficiency, in particular on angina pectoris attacks. Of the patients studied, 27 (67.5%) showed improvement, while in 9 cases (22.5%) no change, and in 4 (10%) a deterioration was observed.

Adalat showed significant antianginal properties (Table 2). It reduced the average nitroglycerin consumption from 8 capsules (0.8 mg) weekly per person to 2.2 capsules, i.e. a 72.5% reduction. Fourteen patients (35%) no longer needed nitroglycerin. The number of anginal attacks was reduced on the average from

Table 1. Influence of Adalat on subjective symptoms (anginal attacks)

Card. diagnosis	No. of cases	Improved	Unchanged	Worse
Coronary sclerosis	22	14	6	2
Old myocardial infarction	8	5	2	1
Angina on effort in hypertension	10	8	1	1
Total	40	27	9	4
Percentage	100	67.5	22.5	10

Table 2. Influence of Adalat on consumption of nitroglycerin capsules (0.8 mg) and on number of anginal attacks before and after 4-week administration of Adalat (average values)

	Before	After administration of Adalat
Nitroglycerin consumption	8.0 caps.	2.2 caps. weekly (-72.5%) No nitroglycerin: 14 patients (35%)
Number of anginal attacks	14.0 attacks	3.5 attacks weekly (-75%) No attacks: 17 patients (42.5%)

Table 3. Influence of Adalat on ECG and subjective symptoms

	No. of cases	Improved	%	Unchanged	Worse
Anginal attacks	40	27	67.5%	9	4
Depression of ST-segments at rest	31	12	39.0%	18	1
Diminution of the depression of ST-segments under ergometric loading	40	22	55.0%	16	2
Influence on work loading, measured by bicycle ergometry	40	28	70.0%	10	2

Table 4. Influence of Adalat on exercise tolerance, measured by bicycle ergometry (average values) 4 weeks post-application

	Before	After application	
Loading time (under maintained work loads)	185 sec	262 sec ($+42\%$)	
Depression of ST-segment			Increase of heart rate:
at rest	0.4 mm	0.25 mm	$+4$/min
after 3 min loading	1.3 mm	0.75 mm	$+7$/min
after 6 min loading	3.0 mm	1.8 mm	$+5$/min
after 1 min rest	1.8 mm	0.85 mm	$+3$/min
after 3 min rest	1.0 mm	0.55 mm	$+4$/min
Work loading	64.2 watts	86.7 watts ($+35\%$)	
Blood pressure at rest			
Systolic decrease		$-$ 12 mm Hg	
Diastolic decrease		$-$ 3.5 mm Hg	

14 attacks per week to 3.5 attacks (i.e. 75% reduction). In 17 patients (42.5%) anginal attacks ceased completely. Intensity and duration of the attacks decreased simultaneously.

In all 40 patients, an ECG at rest and under ergometric loading was recorded before and after application of Adalat for about four weeks (Table 3). Of the 31 cases with depression of ST-segments at rest, 12 (39%) showed an improvement, 18 (58%) no change, and 1 (3.2%) a deterioration. It should be emphasized that the antianginal effect was not always related to an improvement of the ST-segment depression in the resting ECG: While an improvement of anginal attacks in 67.5% of the cases was recorded, a diminution of the ST-segment depression at rest was achieved in only 39%.

Each of the 40 patients was subjected to the exercise test. Compared with results prior to treatment, a reduction of the ST-segment depression under ergometric loading was observed (Table 3 and Fig. 1) during the long-term therapy with Adalat in 22 patients (55%). In 28 persons (70%), the loading time under Adalat was prolonged, and higher work loads were recorded.

Table 4 shows that the average loading time was 185 sec before application and 262 sec after administration (i.e. an increase of 77 sec, or 42%). The depression of ST-segments at rest and under ergometric loading was considerably alleviated, and the heart rate tended toward a very small increase compared with the results prior to administration. The mean work loading after application of Adalat increased from 64.2 to 86.7 watts (i.e. 22.5 watts, or 35%) and the systolic and diastolic blood pressure decreased slightly.

Adalat showed marked efficacy in patients with high blood pressure. Anginal attacks in patients with low blood pressure were less effectively prevented. Furthermore, the response of patients with severe anginal attacks caused by impending or recent myocardial infarction (not included in this report) to Adalat was as weak as that to nitroglycerin. Therefore care should be taken in using it in cases with low blood pressure and in those cases in whom lowering of blood pressure is inadvisable. The onset of the effect of Adalat is apparently slower than that of nitroglycerin, but compared with the effects of other antianginal drugs which were used initially or at intervals between Adalat administration, Adalat acts more frequently, faster and more intensively than isosorbide dinitrate, prenylamine or dipyridamole. On the other hand, Adalat was most effective in combination with propranolol.

Numerous biochemical and hematological parameters (blood sugar, bilirubin, blood urea, alkaline phosphatase, GOT, GPT, LDH, Na, K, total protein, protein electrophoresis, prothrombin time, platelets count, WBC, RBC, Hb and differential leucocyte count) as well as urinalysis did not show any marked pathological changes during the treatment with Adalat. Only minor adverse reactions (short-term headache, flush and nausea) have been observed in individual cases investigation.

We are aware of the limited evidence of the findings obtained so far with Adalat. Nevertheless we think that the existing favorable results justify the use of Adalat in the long-term treatment of ischemic heart disease, in particular in the protection against angina pectoris.

Abstract

Forty in- and out-patients with various forms of angina pectoris and ischemic ST-segment depressions in the ECG were treated with Adalat (Nifedipine) over a period of three months. Adalat was used in capsules of 10 mg orally. The daily

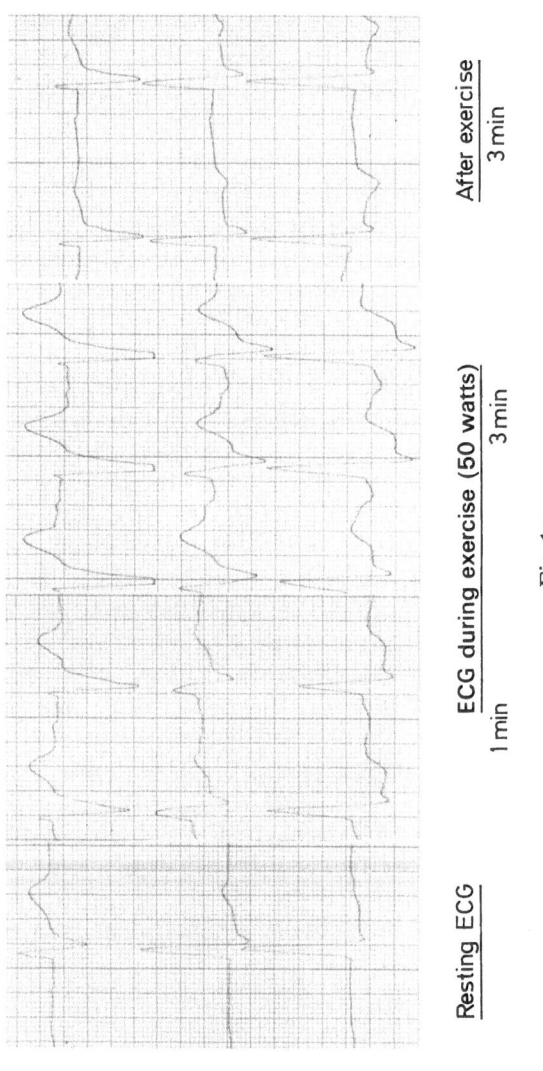

Resting ECG

ECG during exercise (50 watts)
1 min   3 min

After exercise
3 min

a

Fig. 1a

Fig. 1. ECG of a patient with chronic ischemic heart disease and angina pectoris attacks: at rest, during and after exercise (by bicycle ergometry), before and 4 weeks after application of Adalat (30 mg daily). O.R., 53 years, male, August/Sept. 1974

(a) Before Adalat application. The resting ECG showed abnormal ST-T changes in V_5 and in particular in V_6. After one and three min loading (50 watts), the ECG showed a marked fall in ST in V_5 and V_6 and diphasic T-waves in V_6. After three min exercise an anginal attack was elicited. Note also pathologic changes in ST-segment and abnormality of T-waves in V_5 and V_6 in the resting ECG three min after the attack

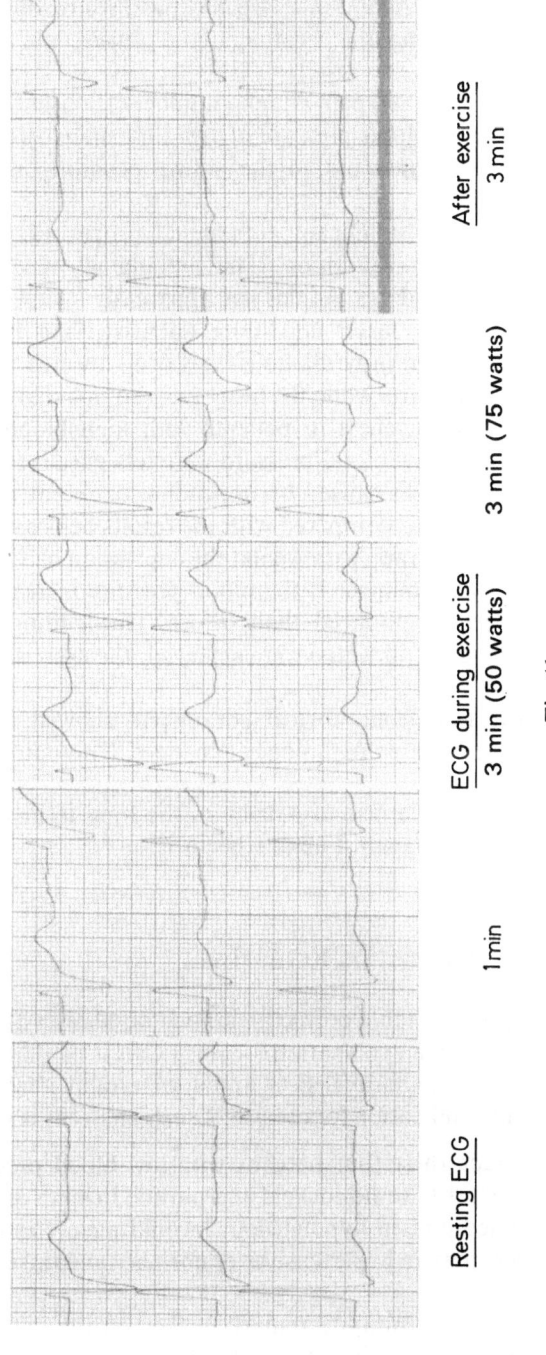

Resting ECG   ECG during exercise

1min   3 min (50 watts)   3 min (75 watts)   After exercise
                                                                    3 min

Fig. 1b

(b) After Adalat administration. A 4-week administration of Adalat (30 mg daily) resulted in a change in the loading ECG. The fall of ST-segment and the changes of T-waves in V_5 and V_6 were reduced, and an attack of angina pectoris was not observed. The loading time was prolonged (from 3 to 6 min), and higher work loads (75 watts instead of 50 watts) could be sustained

dosage ranged from three to six capsules (30–60 mg) after meals, divided in three or four times. The most patients received 30 mg daily.

For evaluation of the effect of Adalat in an open clinical study following parameters were used before starting the treatment and during the long term therapy:

Frequency and intensity of anginal pain attacks, number of consumed capsules of nitroglycerin, heart rate and blood pressure at rest and under gradually increasing ergometric loading, carried out in the sitting position on a bicycle ergometer.

It is shown, that Adalat has significant antianginal properties; it reduced considerably the nitroglycerin consumption. The antianginal effect was not always related to specific ECG findings. Adalat has apparently a slower onset of effect than nitroglycerin, but acts faster and more intensive than PETN, isosorbide dinitrate, prenylamine and dipyridamole. This drug lowered slightly the systolic and diastolic blood pressure, while the heart rate did not change.

Adalat showed marked effectiveness in patients with high blood pressure, anginal attacks in patients with low blood pressure were less effective prevented. Patients with severe anginal attacks caused by impending or recent myocardial infarction respond to Adalat just as compared with the results before starting the treatment during the long term therapy with Adalat the depression of ST-segments under ergometric loading was diminished; the blood pressure increase and the heart rate increase were less pronounced than before. The loading time was prolonged and higher work loads (in watts) were achieved; the exercise tolerance increased.

Numerous biochemical and hematological parameters showed during the treatment with Adalat no remarkable pathological changes. Only minor adverse reactions were observed.

The favorable results justify the use of Adalat in the long term therapy of ischemic heart diseases to protect against angina pectoris.

Discussion Remarks

KAUFMANN: If I interpret the table correctly, in four of 40 cases the anginal attacks worsened. Do you have an explanation for this? Can it be that these patients exhibited a very strong hypotensive effect, and does it follow that with preexisting hypotension, a contraindication for the use of such an agent is indicated?

LINKE: As a matter of fact, these four patients with low blood pressure had already responded unsatisfactorily to β-blockers and nitrate. In spite of this, I see no contraindications for nifedipine in hypotension; I would merely estimate the chances for success to be less than in hypertensives or normals, and this also holds true for β-blockers and nitrates.

I would like to take the opportunity to remark further on the differences in action between the β-blocker propranolol and Adalat. Propranolol is more efficacious when in an episode of angina (e.g., in the climacterium or in strong emotional excitement) a considerable increase in heart frequency in combination with ponounced blood pressure elevation results from a pathologic increase in sympathetic activity to which patients on nifedipine (though not as strong as nitrates) can react with a further increase in heart frequency. In hypertension *without* increased heart frequency we can achieve equally good results with Adalat as with β-blockers.

The combination of β-blockers and Adalat has stood the test repeatedly. Especially in angina pectoris patients with hyperkinetic, hyperdynamic circulatory stoppage, the help of Adalat allowed for a noticeable dose reduction of propranolol and thus decreased the danger—especially in older patients—of an undesirable cardiodepressive action as well as a limitation of the adrenergic regulatory range of the cardiovascular system.

For these reasons our experience with Adalat in coronary patients with hypertensive circulatory stoppage is particularly impressive, whereas we exclude patients with fresh coronary infarction from treatment with Adalat.

LICHTLEN: What are your limitations on the use of nitroglycerin? Would you prefer nitroglycerin, or at least put it on an equal footing? In the event of a difference in method or mode of action, then this point seems to me to be important.

LINKE: Nitroglycerin is, of course, the agent of choice in acute angina pectoris, while the strong point in the application of Adalat lies in its long-term prophylaxis against angina. Here its superiority over PETN and other nitrates is demonstrated; by reason of its action-profile and its hemodynamic effects in patients with chronic coronary insufficiency there is a steady, favorable influence of conclusive determinants of myocardial oxygen supply.

LICHTLEN: I would be very much interested to learn of a double-blind study or at least a comparative study with other nitrates. Many people think long-acting nitroglycerin is of questionable effect. Have you compared nifedipine with long-acting nitrates?

LINKE: Yes. In the framework of short-term angina prevention in patients with coronary blood flow disturbances—especially in situations of physical and mental stress—Adalat is comparable to long-acting nitrates. Over the long term— prolonged therapy of chronic coronary insufficiency—Adalat proves itself superior to nitrates with long-term action, especially in recognition of its ability to retain its efficacy over a period of months. Accordingly, in the work-load tests carried out on the bicycle ergometer at long intervals under Adalat the increase in physical load tolerance of the coronary patients was convincing, as was the improvement in ischemic changes (ST-peak reduction) in the exercise ECG.

LICHTLEN: How long after isosorbide dinitrate did you test?

LINKE: Principally, we undertook the investigations about 9 a.m., namely 1 h after ingestion of long-acting nitrate and 30 min to 1 h after ingestions of nifedipine.

LICHTLEN: Then you were already at the end of the nitrate's effect.

Survey and Summary of Results
Obtained during the World-Wide Clinical Investigations
of Adalat (Nifedipine)

F. EBNER

Pharma-Forschungszentrum/Ressort Medizin, Bayer AG, Wuppertal, Fed. Rep. Germany

Many experimental and clinical findings on Adalat have been reported in detail during this symposium. The different points of view on this new substance, its clinical efficacy, the mechanism of action and the tolerance have been discussed at length.

Not all investigators have been able to take part in this meeting and present their findings—so I should like to summarize the essential clinical trials and the results obtained so far. The aim of all investigations was to gather information on the following questions:

1. What is the effect of Adalat in patients with angina pectoris?
2. Which hemodynamic effects are produced by Adalat in patients with and without coronary disease?
3. What differences occur between intravenous administration and oral (sublingual) administration?
4. Which mechanism of action can be deduced from the results?
5. What is the onset and duration of effect?
6. How well is Adalat tolerated?

Today data from 1233 patients, aged 17–86 years (average age, 54.2 years), are available. Of these patients, nearly two thirds were male.

It is well known that the clinical efficacy of a new antianginal substance can best be demonstrated by standardized exercise tests [21, 37].

Table 1. Antianginal effect of a single sublingual dose. The significant results of 6 controlled studies show the antianginal efficacy of the 10 mg as well as the 20 mg single dose

Invest.	n	mg	Time after administr.	Kind of study	Remark
STEIN [39]	17	10	30'/150'	DBCO/PL	$p<0.024(30')$
EKELUND [7]	10	10	30'	DBCO/PL	$p<0.01$
MCILWRAITH [31]	14	14	15'/100'	DB/PL	$p<0.01$
KALTENBACH [16]	19	19	30'	OKO	$2p<0.01$
STEIN [40]	20	20	30'/150'	DBCO/PL	$p<0.02$
MENNA [32]	32	20	30'/200'	DBCO/PL	$p<0.0005/0.0002$

DBCO/PL = double-blind-cross-over against placebo.
OKO = open-controlled.
DB/PL = double-blind against placebo.

Table 2. Antianginal effect of repeated (subl./oral) doses. Twenty-two long-term studies including 4 double-blind studies show the antianginal efficacy of Adalat during long-term treatment. The average daily dosage was about 30 mg, the longest treatment period was 640 days, the average efficacy, 72%

Author	n	Daily dose mg	Duration of treatment		Route	efficacy %	Remarks
			average	longest			
KIMURA [17]	16	30	14 days	14 days	o	56.2	$p<0.05$
CAMERINI [3]	48	30	14 days	14 days	o	39.9	$p<0.01$
LESSMANN [26]	12	30–60	15 days	21 days	sl	75.0	
KÜHNS [22]	13	20–60	15.7 days	28 days	sl	76.8	
LEMMERZ [25]	16	30	23.7 days	31 days	sl	50.0	
SHIBATA [38]	15	30–40	27.5 days	42 days	o	86.6	
MAGGI [30]	28	30	28 days	28 days	o	80.0	$p<0.003$
CATURELLI [4]	22	30	51 days	120 days	o	95.0	
JINNOUCHI [15]	29	10–30	54 days	126 days	o	73.9	
MENNA [32]	30	60	56 days	56 days	o	31.0	$p<0.01$
BANDO [2]	10	30	58 days	70 days	o	70.0	
NIITANI [35]	30	30–60	65 days	640 days	o	55.1	
HIROSAWA [13]	50	10–40	70 days	213 days	o	80.9	
EBNER [6]	128	30–60	77 days	91 days	o	69.5	
MIZUNO [33]	30	30–60	84 days	525 days	o	83.0	single blind
OGINO [36]	7	30–60	90 days	191 days	o	100.0	
FUKUZAKI [9]	21	20–60	91 days	420 days	o	66.7	
NAKAMOTO [34]	21	30–40	92 days	140 days	o	90.0	single blind
ITOH [14]	62	10–60	99 days	? days	o	56.0	
KOBAYASHI [18]	47	20–60	101 days	456 days	o	80.0	
Germ. coop. [40]	69	30–50	105 days	406 days	o	80.2	
MABUCHI [29]	10	30–40	139 days	360 days	o	90.0	
	714					72.0	

n = number of patients, o = oral, sl = sublingual route

Five investigators in 6 controlled studies under different standardized load conditions showed a significant effect in patients with coronary artery disease (Table 1). These investigations were carried out on 112 patients. In 3 of the studies, the single dose of 10 mg was used, whereas in the other three 20 mg were given. From these results an antianginal effect is evident between 15–200 min after sublingual administration.

Table 2 shows the results of 22 studies on a total of 714 patients. Here one must take into consideration that different reasons, including ethical points of view, limited the number of long-term double-blind studies against placebo. Thus in future we will have to judge the efficacy and tolerance of a new substance in open as well as in controlled trials.

The daily dose ranged from 10–60 mg, mostly given t.i.d., the dose recommended was 30–60 mg. In the different groups the longest average duration of treatment was 139 days; the longest treatment was 640 days. In most cases the capsules were swallowed.

Table 3. Changing of different hemodynamic parameters after sublingual (or oral) administration of nifedipine. The peripheral resistance dropped between 9–34% from control in the different groups. The decreases in the systolic, diastolic and arterial mean pressure are approximately the same as those in left ventricular systolic and enddiastolic pressure

	mg	15 minutes	20 minutes	30 minutes
TPR	10	−29	−32 to −34	−29
	20	−9	−21−14 to −21−27	−27 to −31
Psyst	10	−10		
	20	−10 to −16	−7 to −16	−5 to −8
Pdiast	10	−8		
	20	−6 to −7	−7−10 to −19−28	−6 to −7
Pm	10	−4 to −12	−18 to −20	−17 to −32
	20	−7	−7 to −32	−7 to −19
LVSP	10	−6 to −7		
	20	−5		
LVEDP	10	−19		
	20	−15		
SV	10	−5	+7	0 to +2
	20			+18
CO	10			0
	20		+23	+23 to +25
HR	10	0 to +8	−5	0 to −5
	20	+21	+4(+4) to +16	+7 to +12
Cl	10	+9	+10	+6
	20	+6	0(+4) to +6	
LVWI	10			
	20	+10	−7 to −16	
dp/dt	10	−3		
	20	+12	−4	0 to +25

Twenty-two groups were studied; the average effectiveness of 72% includes the reduced percentage and intensity of attacks as well as the consumption of nitroglycerin. All investigators endeavoured to avoid a competative therapy.

Four double-blind studies showed a significant effect under long-term treatment. Therefore, from the open studies, we can also expect an antianginal effect in the long-term therapy.

BAY a 1040 was investigated in non-coronary as well as in coronary patients. The question was: Are there any significant differences between the 2 groups with respect to hemodynamic reactions caused by nifedipine?

In Table 3 all values are given as a percentage of the initial value; numbers in Roman type represent patients without coronary artery disease and numbers in italics represent patients with coronary artery disease. Measurements were taken 15, 20, and 30 min after sublingual administration. A total of 282 patients were examined by 15 investigators. Therefore variations in the methodology have to be taken into consideration.

The number 10 or 20 indicates the dose given, marked on the left side of the figure. The parameters from top to bottom are: TPR (total peripheral resistance), systolic, diastolic and mean arterial pressure, left ventricular systolic and left ventricular enddiastolic pressure, stroke volume, cardiac output, heart rate, cardiac index, left ventricular work index and dp/dt.

In the individual groups the peripheral resistance dropped to between 9 and 34%. The reductions of systolic, diastolic and arterial mean pressure are approximately the same as those of left ventricular systolic and enddiastolic pressures. Stroke volume and cardiac output as well as the heart rate exhibit a slight or marked tendency to increase. This is certainly dependent on the initial condition of the tonus of the vagal and sympathetic nerves and is also probably dependent on the state of the myocardium.

The directional change in the parameters are the same in both groups of patients. Changes are more distinct 20 and 30 min after administration than after 15 min.

Another question was: Are there any essential differences in the findings after sublingual or i.v. administration?

Table 4 (left side) shows the hemodynamic effects of 6 different groups after sublingual administration of 10 or 20 mg. All patients were tested at a similar time interval. The 3 groups receiving i.v. injections, were on almost the same dosage (right side of the table).

The values for systolic and enddiastolic pressure and the calculation of peripheral resistance show less variation after sublingual and i.v. administration than the heart rate. At the dosage used, the increase in heart rate is greater after i.v. administration. One can therefore assume that the effects measured in the periphery are more constant than the cardiac parameters.

Due to the sensitivity of the solution to light, clinical-pharmacological questions were studied only in a small number of patients after i.v. administration.

LICHTLEN [27] investigated the behavior of the same group of patients under resting and under stress conditions.

Table 5 compares 3 different groups from investigations carried out by HILGER [12] and LYDTIN [28] under resting, and by KURITA [23] under loading conditions.

The doses are similar, but high. As a result, the extent of the changes in blood pressure and heart rate are greater under resting conditions than those obtained after stress conditions. Therefore, the smaller increase in stroke volume, cardiac output, left ventricular work index and tension-time-index under loading conditions—compared with the controls—can be used to explain the antianginal effect under stress. CHERCHI [5] demonstrated the clinical efficacy under loading conditions in patients with coronary artery disease.

Table 6 deals with 2 equally large and similar groups under stress. Although the route of administration is different, we find agreement in the following three important parameters, when compared with controls: drop in the systolic pressure (left ventricular and peripheral), drop in left ventricular enddiastolic pressure and in the tension-time-index.

The heart rate and left ventricular work index are different. According to FLECKENSTEIN [8] and GRÜN [10] the mechanism of action is an influence on the smooth muscle cells of the coronary and peripheral arteries and of the myocardium.

Table 4. Comparison of hemodynamic effects at rest after sublingual or i.v. administration. The values for systolic and enddiastolic pressure and the calculation of peripheral resistance show the same tendency and less variation than the values for heart rate. Ps = systolic, LVED = left ventricular enddiastolic pressure, HR = heart rate, LVWI = left ventricular work index, TPR = total peripheral resistance, CI = cardial index

	LICHTEN [27] n=16	KÖHLER [20] n=5	HAYASE [11] n=6	HAYASE [11] n=8	KOCHSIEK [19] n=4	KALTENBACH [16] n=16	HILGER [12] n=9	LYDTIN [28] n=10	ANGELINO [1] n=20
Dosis	20 mg 15' p.A.	20 mg 20' p.A.	20 mg 20' p.A.	20 mg 20' p.A.	10 mg 20' p.A.	10 mg 15' p.A.	0.03 mg/kg/3'	0.015 mg/kg/1.5'	0.015 mg/kg/3'
Ps	− 4.9 (LV)	−6.5 (A)	−16.0 (P)	− 9.0 (P)	− 9.1 (A)	− 6.2 (LV) − 9.9 (A) −18.7	−20.7 (P)	− 4.0 (P)	− 2.7 (P)
LVED	−15.0								
HR	+ 21.5	−1.8	+ 4.3	+ 4.2	− 5.0		+ 25.0	+27.3	+ 2.6
LVWI	+ 10.1		−16.5	− 7.0				+32.5	
TPR	− 8.9		−20.7	−13.8	−33.6			−33.7	
CI	+ 6.2		+ 3.7	+ 5.9	+ 9.0			+44.0	+20.2

Table 5. Hemodynamic effects after i.v. administration at rest and during stress. The changes in blood pressure and heart rate are greater under resting conditions than those obtained under stress conditions

	Hilger [12] n=9	Lydtin [28] n=10	Kurita [23] n=9	i.v.
Dose	0.03 mg/kg − 3′	0.015 mg/kg − 1.5′	0.02–0.03 inf.	
	valve def. at rest	healthy vol. at rest	C.A.D. after stress: K	
O$_2$-Sat.	+90.3%			Oxygen saturation
Ps	−20.7%	− 4.0	− 3.5	systolic pressure
Pd	−23.7	− 7.9		diastolic pressure
Pm		− 6.3		mean art. pressure
LVSP			+ 2.6	left ventr. syst. pr.
LVEDP			− 10.7	left ventr. endd. pr.
SV		+ 12.6	− 8.6	stroke volume
HR	+25.0	+ 27.3	− 11.1%	heart rate
CO		+ 44.2	− 5.4	cardiac output
LVET		− 2.2		left ventr. ej. time
LVWI		+ 32.5	− 6.9	left ventr. work index
TTI		+ 16.3	− 14%	tension time index
CI		+ 44.0		cardiac index
dp/dt			− 7.1	contr. index
TPR		− 33.7		tot. periph. res.
PBF		+179.2		periph. blood flow

Table 6. Comparison of two groups suffering from coronary artery disease under stress conditions (all data are expressed as percent of control value). Under loading conditions we find agreement in the following 3 important parameters, when compared with controls: drop in systolic pressure (Ps), left ventricular enddiastolic pressure (LVEDP) and in the tension time index (TTI)

	Lichtlen [27] n=9 20 mg s.l. 15′ p. appl.	Kurita [23] n=9 0.03 mg/kg i.v./inf.
Ps	− 4.2 (LV)	− 3.5 (P)
LVEDP	−14.3	−10.7
HR	+ 7.2	−11.1
SV		− 8.6
SVI	+ 1.4	
LVWI	+ 7.1	− 6.9
TTI	− 2.3	−14.0
dp/dt	+11.1	− 7.1

As a result a change in different hemodynamic parameters is caused in the intact organism. The findings of Vater [41] indicate a twofold mechanism resulting in decrease the myocardial oxygen consumption: one is peripheral and the other, myocardial.

Table 7. Onset and duration of effects. The increases of oxygen saturation and of pO$_2$ are in close agreement with the experimental findings. Black arrow patients without CAD, light arrow patients with CAD

Coronar	10 mg												20 mg												
	1	2	3	4	5	10	15	20	30	40	50	60 min	1	2	3	4	5	10	15	20	30	40	50	60	180 min
Ox. sat.	–	↗																⇐		⇐	⇐	⇐			
pO$_2$		↑	↑			↑	↑	↑	↑	↑	↑	↑						↑		↑	↑	↑			
flow (AVDO$_2$)					↑	↗	↑	↑	↑	↑	↑	↑						↑	⇐	↑	↑	↑			
coron. res.																			⇒						

Table 8. Onset and duration of effects. If measured, the change of the hemodynamic parameters begins in the second minute after administration and lasts longer than 180 min

Several (hemodynamic) parameters at rest

Cardial	10 mg												20 mg												
	1	2	3	4	5	10	15	20	30	40	50	60 min	1	2	3	4	5	10	15	20	30	40	50	60	180 min
Ps			↗	↗	⇒	⇒	⇒	→	⇑↓	→	→							⇒	⇑↓	⇑↓	→	→			
Pd				=	⇗	→	⇒	→	⇑↓	→	→								⇑↓	⇑↓	⇑↓	→			
Pm				–	↗	⇒	→	→	⇑↓	→	→								⇑↓	⇑↓	→				
LVSP				↗	⇒	→	↑	↗										⇒							
LVEDP				–	↗	→	↑	↑	↑									⇒	→						
HR	↗				↗↘	↑=	↑↗	↑										↑	↑↗	↑	↑			↗	
CO					↗	↗↘	↑	↑											↑						
SV																									
CI																									
LVWI																	⇐	↑↑	↑↑					
dp/dt	⇒		⇒	↗	↗	↗	↑	↑	↑↑									⇐	↑↓	↑↗	↗				
TTI																		⇐							
TPR				↗	→	→	→	→	→									⇒	⇑↓	⇑↓	→				
PBF										↗								↑			↑	↑			↑

Table 9. Different kinds of laboratory results. In 1430 different analyses from a total of 400 patients, no significant deviation compared with normal values is visible

	No of investig.	No of analyses	Normal value bef. and after N.	Remarks
SGOT	10	182	170	10 path. val. improved 1 path. val. slight increase (18–28) 1 real increase (9–21)
SGPT	10	200	191	5 × decrease of pathol. value 2 × increase of pathol. value 2 × normal v. increased: 12–30, 14–22
AP	7	105	104	1 × path. val. decreased
LDH	5	50	50	
Bili	3	60	60	
Serum protein	4	69	69	
Electrophoresis	3	24	24	
				1 × increase
Cholesterol	8	141	138	2 × decrease
Triglyceride	3	65	63	2 × slight increase
Blood sugar	15	133	133	until 8 months
p.p. blood sug.	2	58	55	1 path. val. changed to normal 2 path. val. unchanged
Creatinine	5	89	89	
Urea	6	49	49	
Uric acid	14	65	65	
Sodium (Na)	2	30	30	
Potassium	2	31	31	
Calcium	1	9	9	
Urine status	1	70	67	3 × trace of protein

Not only are the mechanism of action and the time-dependent change in the hemodynamics of interest, but also the onset and duration of effects to establish the duration of the antianginal effect.

Table 7 shows the findings on pO_2 in the coronary sinus and the coronary circulation of a total of 52 patients in 4 different studies. After 10 mg, the first measurements are made earlier than after 20 mg. These results are in close agreement with the experimental findings.

The survey of a total of 282 patients from 15 different groups clearly shows the rapid onset and the long duration of the effects (Table 8). I would like to compare these results with those of the loaded tests, which have demonstrated an antianginal effect for up to 200 min.

Investigations on biological tolerance have been carried out by numerous investigators. Table 9 summarizes the findings from about 400 patients who received Adalat for more than 14 days. The first column shows the number of investigators, the second, the number of analyses and the third, the results.

Table 10. Side-effects. Side-effects such as headache, facial flush, dizziness and vomiting may be caused by the substance. But it must be taken into consideration that concomitant therapy also causes side-effects that are hidden in this summary

n = 1233 patients
without side-effects: 1051
        side-effects: 182 (14.7%)

Cardiovascular		
Headache	63 ×	5.1%
Facial flush	61 ×	4.9%
Dizziness	35 ×	2.8%
Nausea	30 ×	2.4%
Heat sens.	28 ×	2.2%
Tiredness	26 ×	2.1%
Retching	15 ×	1.2%
Hypotension	11 ×	0.8%
Sweating	7 ×	0.5%
Reddening	5 ×	0.4%
Itching	6 ×	0.4%
Palpitation	5 ×	0.4%
Tinnitus	4 ×	0.3%
Paresthesia	4 ×	0.3%
Collapse	3 ×	0.2%
Gastrointestinal tract		
Diarrhoea	8 ×	0.6%
Anorexia	6 ×	0.4%
Heartburn	7 ×	0.5%
Skin		
Exanthem	4 ×	0.3%

There is no evidence of intolerance. The most important parameters such as liver enzymes, blood sugar and serum-creatinine are within the normal range. Only one slight increase in SGOT and 2 in SGPT are reported, but these are not definitely pathologic values.

In 182 patients out of 1233 (14.7%), side-effects that probably could be attributed to the administration of nifedipine were observed. Here one must take into consideration the fact that the assessment is made difficult because many patients needed concomitant therapy (Table 10).

There is only a small group without additional therapy. One third of the patients had glycoside therapy and a high percentage had additional medication.

In my opinion, side-effects such as headache, facial flush, dizziness, vomiting and sensation of heat are caused by the peripheral vasodilatory effect of the drug. Moreover, some sensitive patients may show a decrease in blood pressure which may be undesirable. However, the 3 collapses were observed only during the initial stage of the investigations. Within the last month, however, a 4th has been reported: a patient who had taken a higher dose of propranolol + nifedipine + nitroglycerin. It seems that in this case, the major fall in blood pressure was the cause. On the other hand, there are some patients receiving the combination of beta blocking agents + BAY a 1040 without any adverse effects.

Table 11. Treatment discontinued due to side-effects (1233 patients). The most frequently occurring side-effect leading to discontinuance of treatment is facial flush. But compared with the total number of patients, the percentage is very low

Facial flush	5 (0.4%)
Heat sens.	4 (0.3%)
Nausea	4
Headache	3 (0.2%)
Hypotension	5 (0.4%)
Palpitation	1
Exanthema	4 (0.3%)
Total	26 (2.1%)

The rare occurrence of premature termination of therapy is proof of the good tolerance of nifedipine: in only 2.1% of cases was therapy discontinued because of side-effects (Table 11).

Discussion

Most striking in the hemodynamics is the fact that while the behavior of some parameters shows the same tendency, that of other parameters exhibits greater variations.

In this regard, I would comment that patients who react with small changes in pressure and frequency save more oxygen via a negative inotropic component than other patients, who react more via a peripheral component to reduce oxygen consumption.

I would, however, consider the following components to be important for all patients: The local vascular effect of the substance causes an increase in blood flow in the different regions of the body, such as myocardium, muscles, skin, kidneys and liver. This, depending on the intensity of local effect, produces a higher arterial blood uptake and redistribution of the blood.

The decrease in coronary and peripheral resistance—in other words, a prolongation and enlargement of the Windkessel[1]—and hence the shifting from pressure work into volume output, certainly are essential factors. This, in connection with the decrease in the enddiastolic filling pressure, leads to a decrease in pre- and afterload and to a better circulation in the inner myocardial layers during diastole.

Finally the influence on oxygen consumption is the decrease due to the slightly reduced contractility of the myocardium.

The balance of all these effects must override the increased oxygen consumption of the baroreceptor mechanism.

After sublingual absorption, the first sites of effect are the muscles of the coronary vascular system and the myocardium. Increased circulation and a slightly negative inotropism and in part also, a slightly dromotropism result. In

---

[1] The term "Windkessel" describes the action whereby during systole the elastic aortic wall is distended and during diastole the natural contraction to the resting state facilitates a continued smooth blood flow initiated by the heart muscle.

addition a number of intracellular processes occur in the myocardium. If, during the first few minutes after administration, an antianginal effect can be demonstrated, then it can only occur via the myocardial component.

A reduction in the coronary resistance can be correlated with a reduction in the work done by the heart. Due to the pronounced peripheral effect a delayed reduction of the peripheral resistance occurs, which, like the nitrites, leads to reduced myocardial oxygen consumption in the final stage. However, the tissue concentration required for these effects is still unknown.

The drop in peripheral resistance also causes a drop in arterial and enddiastolic pressure. As a result the stroke volume increases more than the heart rate, depending on the condition of the body and the increases in peripheral flow.

Because the drop in blood pressure and the increase in flow cannot be counterregulated, the left ventricular enddiastolic as well as the intracoronary and intramyocardial pressures fall.

Therefore pressure relief and distribution of blood appear to be the main effects of nifedipine. In conclusion: Adalat is a single chemical entity with rapid and complete sublingual and enteric absorption, and long-lasting, antianginal effect that is demonstrable clinically.

Abstract

A great variety of clinical investigations were conducted with Adalat comprising many volunteers and patients. The tests aimed at solving the following questions:

1. What is the effect of BAY a 1040 in patients with angina pectoris?
2. Which hemodynamic effects are produced by BAY a 1040 in healthy persons and in patients with coronary diseases?
3. What differences occur between intravenous application and oral (sublingual) application?
4. Which mechanism of action is indicated by the results?
5. How does the action profile develop with time?
6. What is the tolerance of Adalat?

The report, based on 1400 thoroughly examined persons to date, tries to answer these questions.

References

1. ANGELINO, P. F., ALGRANATI, R., TORTORE, P.: Hemodynamic studies. New Therapy of Ischemic Heart Diseases, Adalat-Symp. Tokyo University press, **221**, 1975.
2. BANDO, I.: pers. comm.
3. CAMERINI, F.: New Therapy of Ischemic Heart Diseases, Adalat-Symp. Tokyo University press, **260**, 1975.
4. CATURELLI, G.: New Therapy of Ischemic Heart Diseases, Adalat-Symp. Tokyo University press, **214**, 1975.
5. CHERCHI, A.: New Therapy of Ischemic Heart Disease, Adalat-Symp. Tokyo University press, **85**, 1975.
6. EBNER, F., BRAASCH, W., TROLL, V.: in press.

7. EKELUND, L. G.: New Therapy of Ischemic Heart Diseases, Adalat-Symp. Tokyo University press, **144**, 1975.
8. FLECKENSTEIN, A., TRITTHART, H., DÖRING, H.-J., BYON, K. Y.: Arzneim.-Forsch. (Drug Res.) **22**, Nr. 1, 22–32 (1972).
9. FUKOZAKI, H., OKAMOTO, R., YOKOYAMA, M., TOMOMATSU, T.: New Therapy of Ischemic Heart Diseases, Adalat-Symp. Tokyo University press, **205**, 1975.
10. GRÜN, G., FLECKENSTEIN, A.: Arzneim.-Forsch. (Drug Res.) **22**, Nr. 2, 334–343 (1972).
11. HAYASE, S., HIRAKAWA, S., HOSOKAWA, S., MORI, N., KANYAMA, S., IWASA, M.: Arzneim.-Forsch. (Drug Res.) **22**, Nr. 2, 370–373 (1972).
12. HILGER, H. H.: pers. comm.
13. HIROSAWA, K., HOSADA, S.: pers. comm.
14. ITOH, Y., TAWARA, I., ITOH, T.: New Therapy of Ischemic Heart Diseases, Adalat-Symp. Tokyo University press, **251**, 1975.
15. JINNOUCHI, F., MIMURA, G., KODERA, M.: New Therapy of Ischemic Heart Diseases, Adalat-Symp. Tokyo University press, **216**, 1975.
16. KALTENBACH, M.: New Therapy of Ischemic Heart Diseases, Adalat-Symp. Tokyo University press, **126**, 1975.
17. KIMURA, E., MABUCHI, G., KIKUCHI, H.: Arzneim.-Forsch. (Drug Res.) **22**, Nr. 2, 365–367 (1972).
18. KOBAYASHI, T., ITO, Y., HAWARA, I.: Arzneim.-Forsch. (Drug Res.) **22**, Nr. 1, 380–389 (1972).
19. KOCHSIEK, K., NEUBAUR, J.: Arzneim.-Forsch. (Drug Res.) **22**, Nr. 2, 353–358 (1972).
20. KÖHLER, F. J.: II. Internat. Adalat-Symposion Amsterdam 1974, Springer Verlag, in press.
21. KUBICEK, F.: Herz/Kreislauf **5**, 9, 363–368 (1973).
22. KÜHNS, K.: pers. comm.
23. KURITA, A., KANAZAWA, M., HAMAMOTO, H.: New Therapy of Ischemic Heart Diseases, Adalat-Symp. Tokyo University press, **121**, 1975.
24. LANG, E., SCHOEDEL, J., WOIKE, N.: pers. comm.
25. LEMMERZ, A. H.: pers. comm.
26. LESSMANN, N., SCHIRMEISTER, J.: pers. comm.
27. LICHTLEN, P.: New Therapy of Ischemic Heart Diseases, Adalat-Symp. Tokyo University press, **114**, 1975.
28. LYDTIN, H., LOHMÖLLER, R., WALTER, I.: New Therapy of Ischemic Heart Diseases, Adalat-Symp. Tokyo University press, **97**, 1975.
29. MABUCHI, G., KISHIDA, H., SUZUKI, K.: New Therapy of Ischemic Heart Diseases, Adalat-Symp. Tokyo University press, **177**, 1975.
30. MAGGI, G. C.: New Therapy of Ischemic Heart Diseases, Adalat-Symp. Tokyo University press, **160**, 1975.
31. MCILWRAITH, G.: II. Internat. Adalat-Symposion Amsterdam, 1974, Springer Verlag, in press.
32. MENNA, J., TRAINA, M., CASSERA, J. C., FERREIROS, E., ROHWEDDER, R.: II. Internat. Adalat-Symposion Amsterdam, 1974, Springer Verlag, in press.
33. MIZUNO, Y.: New Therapy of Ischemic Heart Diseases, Adalat-Symp. Tokyo University press, **163**, 1975.
34. NAKAMOTO, K.: New Therapy of Ischemic Heart Diseases, Adalat-Symp. Tokyo University press, **279**, 1975.
35. NIITANI, H., FUJIMAKI, T.: New Therapy of Ischemic Heart Diseases, Adalat-Symp. Tokyo University press, **268**, 1975.
36. OGINO, K.: pers. comm.
37. REDWOOD, D. R., ROSING, D. R., GOLDSTEIN, R. E., BEISER, G. D., EPSTEIN, ST. E.: Circul. Vol. XLIII, 618–628 (1971).
38. SHIBATA, N.: New Therapy of Ischemic Heart Diseases, Adalat-Symp. Tokyo University press, **235**, 1975.
39. STEIN, G.: New Therapy of Ischemic Heart Diseases, Adalat-Symp. Tokyo University press, **192**, 1975.
40. STEIN, G.: II. Internat. Adalat-Symposion Amsterdam, 1974, Springer Verlag, in press.
41. VATER, W.: II. Internat. Adalat-Symposion Amsterdam, 1974, Springer Verlag, in press.

Discussion Remarks

MCILWRAITH: Mr. President, Dr. EBNER in his summary referred to his incidence of side effects on a world-wide basis. I think he said that of the total number of patients, in the order of 1400 patients, about 14.6% of them had side effects and only 2.1% of these patients actually needed to discontinue nifedipine. I am wondering if, in fact, he might have any more recent information indicating that the incidence of side effects could be different from this?

EBNER: I am aware of the problem. Until now, unlike your results, the world-wide studies concur with what I have shown in my paper. Your last data are not included in my results. I cannot say why this difference has come up. Perhaps it is a difference in the use of drugs, in treatment, or in the population. This is my observation, but I am unable to answer your question at the moment.

MCILWRAITH: Do you know if there are other studies being conducted, with final results yet to come, where they are getting side effects similar to the incidence in my study?

EBNER: No. But when you are talking about side effects you should also bear in mind that there are many other influences. For instance, concomitant therapy: Do you have a concomitant therapy and, if so, which one? I know from a long-term study of about 140 patients, that the 20 patients without concomitant therapy had no side effects. We must study large groups because small groups could give us a false impression. I think it might well be that some side effects will come up because individuals differ in their reaction.

LINKE: A number of our patients with coronary diseases treated with Adalat suffered at the same time from peripheral arterial occlusive disease. It is noteworthy that some of them reacted to Adalat with sensations of heat, flushing, and headaches of vascular origin, the same vasomotor symptoms seen with nitroglycerin and the nicotinic-acid derivatives (Complamin, Ronicol retard). I believe that in that patient group, a special vasomotor lability, an individually increased reaction to vascular expanding agents is displayed. In my opinion, this uniform reaction to different vasoactive agents is harmless in individual vasolabile patients under observation, and is in no case grounds for stopping treatment.

LICHTLEN: I think all vasodilators have some of these side effects and this has to be taken into account.

I think we have to stop here. In summary, we can say, that there is no doubt as to the clinical efficacy of nifedipine. Many new investigations were carried out during the last year; the question of indications has surely to be looked into further, also selection of patients, and the clinical differences vs. treatment with beta-blocking agents and nitrates. Long-term studies have also to be performed in order to analyze further the question of side effects.

Closing Remarks

W. Lochner

We have arrived at the end of our Symposium: two full, very interesting and fruitful days lie behind us. There remains now only the task of giving a short resume—a quick backward glance—and the opportunity to outline again various lines of discussion and several crucial points. I do not propose to review all of the material—there was too much for that. I shall discuss various papers, chosen more or less randomly, so my choice should not be taken as an evaluation in comparison to those not chosen. I should like to note that all of the papers have contributed toward giving us a picture of Adalat, which is the reason why we have come here together.

Most of the papers were devoted to *clinical studies*. In my introduction, I advocated the viewpoint that clinical results constitute the conclusive factor in judging a new substance such as Adalat, because no matter how carefully the mechanism of action and the therapeutic principles are formulated, it is not possible to make beforehand a definite statement concerning the clinical efficacy of such a substance in the sense of an antianginal therapeutic agent. Therefore it was certainly right that a large number of clinical studies were presented to us.

I am very thankful to the Chairman of the last session this afternoon, Dr. Lichtlen. In a very pithy statement, he summarized his opinion and said that from the data reported to us, *there can be no doubt about the clinical efficacy of Adalat*. I also made a note to say—just as he did—that the problem of the differential application of an antianginal substance certainly has not yet been sufficiently discussed; it can be predicted that all those who in the near future will be working with Adalat also will have to study this problem more exactly. I am not a clinician, but it appears doubtful that all cases should be treated according to one method.

Although there is no doubt that *Adalat is an efficacious substance* and although we have been presented with excellent studies, which certainly stand up under critical analysis, one is nevertheless once again reminded of the importance and necessity of such a critical analysis. I am very thankful to Dr. Blümchen for demonstrating that the investigation of ST segments, with their cyclic oscillations, presents difficulties and problems. Finally, it should be emphasized that, behind the impressive diagrams and tables we have seen, stands again and again the very complex physician-patient relationship, which also should be included in a critical analysis of the situation.

Dr. Ebner gave such a comprehensive survey of all the clinical results that I believe no further commentary is necessary. It is interesting to note that nitroglycerin, as a comparative substance, played a large role in the assessment of Adalat, obviously because no other substance is so convincing in its clinical efficacy. It is, therefore certainly justifiable to inquire about the mode of action of nitroglycerin in analyzing the effect of the new substance Adalat. Although many facets of the mechanism of action of nitroglycerin are known, no one wishes to offer a final, conclusive statement. This probably cannot be otherwise. I would say that this point was also made by several speakers.

All investigations are in agreement on one point, regardless of whether they were carried out with complex or simple methods: Adalat, administered in sufficient doses, leads to an increase in coronary blood flow, to a certain lowering of blood pressure with a more or less clear heart rate acceleration. Studies with both anesthetized and unanesthetized animals show this, as well as studies with healthy human subjects. There can be no doubt that the decrease of peripheral resistance and the decrease of venous tone, which I will soon speak about, are the critical mechanisms. Findings in dogs of an increase in heart rate are difficult to carry over to humans, which was also clearly pointed out. Moreover, differences in the circumstances of the point of departure must not be neglected. I would agree unequivocally with Dr. KRONEBERG's analysis that the increase in heart rate, when it occurs, must have a reflex origin. One must determine further whether one is dealing with an effect via the vagus nerve or via the sympathetic system. A reflex increase of the heart rate can certainly be mediated over either system. All investigators agreed that Adalat increases the coronary blood flow. This was evident in healthy human subjects and in experimental animals. Adalat produces a primary coronary dilatation, since experiments were also reported in which it was shown that there is a sharp increase of O_2 saturation in coronary venous blood.

In my introduction, I referred to the *question of collaterals*. Along these lines, Dr. SCHMIER communicated findings about the development of collaterals after long-term application of Adalat in dogs. It should be pointed out that it is not a question of a specific effect of Adalat that results in the formation of collaterals, but rather it is the general effect of an increase of coronary blood flow that is decisive. The formation of collaterals therefore is caused by the latter phenomenon, just as through anoxia or muscle training.

The *baroreceptor reflex mechanism*, caused by the fall in blood pressure, does not operate only on the heart rate, rather it also prevents the negative inotropic effect of Adalat on the heart, which can be observed in the isolated heart. In any case, whether completely or less completely rigorous methods were used, all investigators agreed that a negative inotropic effect in intact hearts *in situ* was not observed. In this connection, the investigations of HOLLMAN are interesting; he investigated maximal work capacity in healthy subjects and analyzed the behavior of the heart rate and cardiac output. It is interesting that insofar as the general sympathetic activation through work leads to that end, the primary existing effects of Adalat were abolished. This finding can be interpreted as showing that the sympathetic nervous system predominates and that the Ca-antagonistic effect does not become as predominant, as in the resting condition. However, this finding requires further study, because, as we heard, the antianginal effect can be observed particularly clearly upon loading of the body.

The question of an effect of Adalat on the *venous return* emerges repeatedly in the discussions. I should like to attempt to organize somewhat the problems involved. It depends on how one defines venous return. There is no single, short definition. Secondly, the venous return flow must always be equal to the cardiac output, because only that which is pumped through the heart can flow back to the heart. According to this definition, Adalat has a promoting effect on the venous return. In all studies, the cardiac output increased with effective doses. There is dispute over the degree, but it definitely increases. This increase must be attributed to a decrease of peripheral circulatory resistance, since the blood pressure remains the same or falls. If, in such a circulatory machine, nothing more were to happen than a decrease of peripheral circulatory resistance, the cardiac output would have to increase, if we can be sure, that the pump transports all that is offered to it, and because of a decrease of peripheral resistance, it is offered more. In addition, there is a moderate reflex increase in heart rate. In several studies the stroke volume of the heart was also somewhat increased, while in some it remained the same or decreased. It may very well have been somewhat decreased, because of the heart rate effect.

The venous return will be influenced not only through the resistance but also through the venous tone, i.e. the tone of the capacitance vessels. We heard two papers on this theme: one of them was from a colleague of mine in Düsseldorf. There can be no doubt that Adalat not only decreases the tone of the smooth muscles of the arterioles, but also that of the postcapillary capacitance vessels and that this mechanism of action is not insignificant in the general picture of action. What is its role? If a substance widens only arterioles, we get an increase of venous return with a moderate increase of enddiastolic pressure and an increase of stroke volume. If we had a substance that widened only the capacitance system selectively—there is no such substance—then the result would be a decrease of cardiac output with a decrease of enddiastolic filling pressure. The entire circulatory work would sink to a low level. It would happen somewhat like a venesection.

Also the enddiastolic pressure, the filling pressure of the heart, is related to the venous return. In the case of Adalat, it appears to me that for most of the studies to hold true, the enddiastolic filling pressure should decrease rather than increase. A decrease would mean that a relieving—a diminution—of the heart occurred, similar to what we assume as the mechanism of action of nitroglycerin. Dr. HAGEMANN could present a result from our laboratory whereby Adalat—like other substances—also has an effect on the capacitance system. It turned out that of all the substances tested, nitroglycerin has the greatest effect on the venous system. When nitroglycerin is infused in an adequate dose, a fall of arterial pressure occurs, but barely an increase of cardiac output. The latter remains the same because dilatation of the arterioles is compensated through the dilatation of the capacitance vessels. In the foregoing description, I have paraphrased the peripheral spectrum of effect of Adalat and believe that my analysis is in agreement with most of the findings presented here.

Perhaps in this regard I should mention something about the indirect effect of Adalat on the heart. If it is true that the enddiastolic filling pressure falls, that could be the reason for a redistribution of the blood flow of the heart muscle, which Dr. LICHTLEN also accepts, and which is, by all means, possible. I believe that this argument is more probable than the assumption of a selective effect on the collaterals or arterioles. Such an indirect effect is also likely for nitroglycerin: a redistribution based on an alteration of extravascular factors, i.e. of extravascular components of circulatory resistance.

I would like to make still another point—concerning the mechanism of action at the cellular level. The data on calcium antagonism were presented to us by FLECKENSTEIN and GRÜN in a very interesting manner. I would like to raise once again in this regard the question of the vascular-specific effect. An organ-specific material—which influenced primarily only the blood flow of the brain, the heart or the skeletal muscles—would certainly be welcome. Criteria for such a phenomenon are certainly not easy to find. What is the situation in regard to the specificity of coronary dilatators? A definite specificity must be assumed from observing the pattern of the effect of the coronary dilatators.

The effect of Adalat appears to depend upon the calcium-mediated tonus of the coronary vessels. I agree with DR. KRONEBERG, that α-receptors in the coronary vessels play hardly any role. One could, however, assume yet another type of specificity, which could be designated as secondary specificity, in the sense that reflexively, through the baroreceptors, other vessels come under a definite constrictive influence, while the coronary vessels, because they have no α-receptors, are not influenced. Here, after a careful differential analysis, the effect of Adalat on the various vascular regions and the change in effect with the circulatory reflexes could be evaluated more precisely. In this connection, and I believe this was not said, the inhibition of the circulatory effect of Adalat through methylxanthine is not possible, as it is with other dilatators, some of which have been classified in the group which works by means of the "adenosine-mechanism".

As I come to the end of my remarks, I hope that I have succeeded in pulling together several important lines of thought from the extensive material presented to us. In my introduction I expressed the wish that the material would be presented in a comprehensive and critical manner. I believe that has happened. We were particularly well informed by the discussion this afternoon about clinical questions. I had, in my introduction, also expressed the wish that Adalat would serve to stimulate further research and would provide us broader knowledge about the character of ischemic heart disease and thereby also its therapy. I believe that this has indeed happened, although with the current status of the situation, such steps in knowledge can only be small. We have in Adalat a new tool which can certainly be of help in our efforts towards new knowledge.

In summary, therefore, I think that it was good and necessary that we took the time—particularly since not all of us are so amply blessed with time—to listen and to discuss, not in the least for the well being of the patients, for whom all of our efforts are of value. In this sense, I would like to thank all participants very much.

I do not wish to close without thanking profusely the organizing staff, headed by Dr. BRANDAU and Mr. KERSCHER. Both made this meeting not only possible but also pleasurable.

Subject Index

H. SELYE
Experimental Cardiovascular Diseases
In two parts, not sold separately
1970. 73 figures, some in color
XVIII, VIII, 1155 pages
ISBN 3-540-05010-8 Cloth DM 238,–
ISBN 0-387-05010-8 (North America) Cloth $68.00

A critical survey of over 6300 publications and
40 years of personal research on the experimental
cardiovascular diseases, their mechanisms and clinical
implications.

Atherosclerosis 3
Proceedings of the 3rd International Symposium,
24-28 October 1973. Editors: G. Schettler, A. Weizel
1974. 349 figures, 22 tables. XXXV, 1034 pages
ISBN 3-540-06909-7 Cloth DM 78,–
ISBN 0-387-06909-7 (North America) Cloth $32.00
Distribution rights for Japan:
Maruzen Co. Ltd., Tokyo

These symposium proceedings embody the views
of a number of internationally known experts
on the causes, initiation, course, prevention, and
treatment of atherosclerosis. The principal themes
are the metabolic disorders that lead to the deposition
of lipids in the artery walls, the role of enzymes,
reactions in the collective tissue, and immunological
questions. There is a detailed discussion of prevention
by correct diet and drug treatment of atherosclerosis.

**New Aspects of Storage and Release
Mechanisms of Catecholamines**
Bayer-Symposium II
Editors: H.J. Schümann, G. Kroneberg
1970. 116 figures. X, 301 pages
ISBN 3-540-05051-5 Cloth DM 60,–
ISBN 0-387-05051-5 (North America) Cloth $15.90

International experts – among them two Nobel Price
Winners 1970 – attending an International Symposium,
report latest results of this research field on sympathetic
transmitting substances.

**Springer-Verlag
Berlin
Heidelberg
New York**

Prices are subject to change without notice

A.J. CLARK

General Pharmacology

2nd reprint of the 1st edition Berlin 1937
1973. 79 figs. (2) VI, 228 pages (Handbook of Experimental
Pharmacology, Supplement, Vol. 4)
ISBN 3-540-04845-6 Cloth DM 86,–
ISBN 0-387-04845-6 (North America) Cloth $37.00

The book contains the fundamentals of general pharmacology
which are still valid.

A. LABHART

Clinical Endocrinology

Theory and Practice. With a foreword by G.W. Thorn
In collaboration with numerous experts. Translators: A. Trachsler,
J. Dodsworth-Phillips
1974. 400 figs. XXXII, 1092 pages
ISBN 3-540-06307-2 Cloth DM 125,–
ISBN 0-387-06307-2 (North America) Cloth $48.00
Distribution rights for Japan: Igaku Shoin Ltd., Tokyo

This textbook covers the whole field of clinical endocrinology,
including gynecological and pediatric endocrinology and the
different aspects of diabetes. The pharmacological application
of hormones is also touched upon. The authors have combined
morphological and clinical viewpoints with description of the
biochemistry and pathogenesis of the various illnesses discussed,
but the main emphasis is on clinical aspects. Every chapter is
followed by a listing of relevant literature; these bibliographies
are mainly concerned with the most recent review articles up to
the end of 1972. This book is thus a reference work with the
status of an encyclopedia.

European Journal of Clinical Pharmacology

Pharmacologia Clinica
Managing Editors: H.J. Dengler, F. Gross

The **European Journal of Clinical Pharmacology** accepts for
publication original papers on all aspects of pharmacology and
drug therapeutics in man. This heading comprises studies on
pharmacokinetics, drug metabolism, and drug interactions as
well as therapeutics trials, reports on adverse reactions, and
general problems in therapeutics. Methodological papers on
the topics mentioned are welcome. Trends in the development
and safe use of drugs, and structural aspects of clinical pharmacology, especially those common to various European
countries, are covered by editorials and invited papers. Review
articles on special problems related to clinical pharmacology
or other fields of therapeutics are regularly issued. The journal
is intended primarily to provide a means of communication
in the rapidly developing field of clinical pharmacology and
therapeutics.

Sample copies as well as subscription and back-volume
information available upon request.

Please address:
Springer-Verlag, Werbeabteilung 4021
D 1000 Berlin 33, Heidelberger Platz 3
or
Springer-Verlag, New York Inc., Promotion Department
175 Fifth Avenue, New York, N Y 10010

Prices are subject to
change without notice

Springer-Verlag
Berlin
Heidelberg
New York